Textbook of Iatrogenic Pathology

Edited by:

Simona Gurzu

Department of Pathology, University of Medicine and Pharmacy, Tirgu-Mures, Romania

&

Ioan Jung

Department of Pathology, University of Medicine and Pharmacy, Tirgu-Mures, Romania

Textbook of Iatrogenic Pathology

Editors: Simona Gurzu and Ioan Jung

eISBN (Online): 978-1-68108-514-2

ISBN (Print): 978-1-68108-515-9

First published in 2017.

BENTHAM SCIENCE PUBLISHERS LTD.

End User License Agreement (for non-institutional, personal use)

This is an agreement between you and Bentham Science Publishers Ltd. Please read this License Agreement carefully before using the ebook/echapter/ejournal (**"Work"**). Your use of the Work constitutes your agreement to the terms and conditions set forth in this License Agreement. If you do not agree to these terms and conditions then you should not use the Work.

Bentham Science Publishers agrees to grant you a non-exclusive, non-transferable limited license to use the Work subject to and in accordance with the following terms and conditions. This License Agreement is for non-library, personal use only. For a library / institutional / multi user license in respect of the Work, please contact: permission@benthamscience.org.

Usage Rules:

1. All rights reserved: The Work is the subject of copyright and Bentham Science Publishers either owns the Work (and the copyright in it) or is licensed to distribute the Work. You shall not copy, reproduce, modify, remove, delete, augment, add to, publish, transmit, sell, resell, create derivative works from, or in any way exploit the Work or make the Work available for others to do any of the same, in any form or by any means, in whole or in part, in each case without the prior written permission of Bentham Science Publishers, unless stated otherwise in this License Agreement.
2. You may download a copy of the Work on one occasion to one personal computer (including tablet, laptop, desktop, or other such devices). You may make one back-up copy of the Work to avoid losing it. The following DRM (Digital Rights Management) policy may also be applicable to the Work at Bentham Science Publishers' election, acting in its sole discretion:

- 25 'copy' commands can be executed every 7 days in respect of the Work. The text selected for copying cannot extend to more than a single page. Each time a text 'copy' command is executed, irrespective of whether the text selection is made from within one page or from separate pages, it will be considered as a separate / individual 'copy' command.
- 25 pages only from the Work can be printed every 7 days.

3. The unauthorised use or distribution of copyrighted or other proprietary content is illegal and could subject you to liability for substantial money damages. You will be liable for any damage resulting from your misuse of the Work or any violation of this License Agreement, including any infringement by you of copyrights or proprietary rights.

Disclaimer:

Bentham Science Publishers does not guarantee that the information in the Work is error-free, or warrant that it will meet your requirements or that access to the Work will be uninterrupted or error-free. The Work is provided "as is" without warranty of any kind, either express or implied or statutory, including, without limitation, implied warranties of merchantability and fitness for a particular purpose. The entire risk as to the results and performance of the Work is assumed by you. No responsibility is assumed by Bentham Science Publishers, its staff, editors and/or authors for any injury and/or damage to persons or property as a matter of products liability, negligence or otherwise, or from any use or operation of any methods, products instruction, advertisements or ideas contained in the Work.

Limitation of Liability:

In no event will Bentham Science Publishers, its staff, editors and/or authors, be liable for any damages, including, without limitation, special, incidental and/or consequential damages and/or damages for lost data and/or profits arising out of (whether directly or indirectly) the use or inability to use the Work. The entire liability of Bentham Science Publishers shall be limited to the amount actually paid by you for the Work.

Bentham Science Publishers Ltd.
Executive Suite Y - 2
PO Box 7917, Saif Zone
Sharjah, U.A.E.
Email: subscriptions@benthamscience.org

BENTHAM SCIENCE

CONTENTS

FOREWORD

The Textbook of Iatrogenic Pathology represents a transdisciplinary collection of the main effects of drugs and medical interventions encountered in daily practice. It is edited by two pathologists with significant experience in autopsy who are also teaching the under- and postgraduate students in field of iatrogenic pathology.

The book is split in two parts. The first part that comprises 13 chapters was mainly synthesized by pathologists based on the literature data and practical aspects observed during daily autopsies. In the 6 chapters of the second part, the doctors involved in the clinical practice have presented the specific aspects of their surgical or medical specialties.

This book is a necessity for all persons involved in the patient's care, from student to professor and represents at the moment the largest collection of aspects related to iatrogenic pathology. It is an original and complex book that include the newest aspect of iatrogenesis. It is always important to learn all our life not only from direct/positive evidences, but also from missing facts or/and medical errors.

I strongly recommend publication of the Textbook of Iatrogenic Pathology as a necessity for awareness of medical staff in the field of consequences of the medical facts.

Prof. Marius Raica
Rector of the University of Medicine and Pharmacy,
Timisoara,
Romania

PREFACE

The Textbook of Iatrogenic Pathology concerns doctors and medications. Iatrogenic is a word that derives from the Greek "iatros", which means "doctor" or "medicine", and "genic", which means "induced by". Thus, the book comprises a basic synthesis of the consequences of medical diagnostic or therapeutic procedures, as well as the main side effects of medications in daily use.

In the present book, the authors aimed to present the interdisciplinary features of iatrogenic lesions. The book is based on the opinions of doctors from several disciplines, including pathology, surgery, intensive care, neurology, metabolic diseases, *etc*. In reviewing the existing literature, we did not find complex studies or large syntheses in this field, and therefore consider this book to be very useful to clinicians of all medical specialties. Moreover, the co-editor of the book founded the Department of Iatrogenic Pathology in our university and we offer, every year, lectures in this field for medical students (MD students, dental medicine students and nurses). Our practical experience (editor and co-editor) based on the lectures and everyday autopsies (we perform more than 200 autopsies per year), along with collaboration with clinicians, guarantees the complexity and originality of the present book.

The book is organized into two main parts. The first (13 chapters) is written by pathologists and describes iatrogenic lesions (adverse drug reactions, lesions occurring during diagnosis and as consequences of therapeutic interventions) of the organs and systems. These chapters include practical examples from our daily practice in the Department of Pathology. The second part (six chapters) is written by clinicians and describes specific lesions induced by surgery, neurology, *etc.*

The following main chapters will be included: adverse drug reactions; radiation-induced lesions (through radiotherapy); iatrogenic immunopathology (including pathology regarding organ and tissue transplantation); iatrogenic lesions of the cardiovascular system; iatrogenic lesions of the lung and airways; iatrogenic lesions of the digestive tract (mouth, pharynx, esophagus, stomach, small and large bowel); iatrogenic lesions of the peritoneum and abdominal cavity; iatrogenic lesions of the liver, bile ducts and pancreas; iatrogenic lesions of the kidney and urinary tract; iatrogenic lesions of the female genital organs and breast; iatrogenic lesions of the male genital organs; iatrogenic lesions of the bone marrow and lymphoid tissue; iatrogenic lesions of cutaneous tissue; iatrogenic lesions in endocrinology; iatrogenic lesions in neurology; iatrogenic lesions in anesthesiology and intensive care; iatrogenic lesions in general and thoracic surgery; iatrogenic lesions in gynecology and obstetrics; and iatrogenic lesions in neurosurgery.

This book is for those who already have a basic understanding of the mysteries of the human body and have decided that they are ready to treat it. It is for young residents who believe that they already know all about medicine and its pitfalls. If you decide to read it, try to perform a self-assessment of your medical aptitudes. If you feel that the medical mistakes outlined here can easily occur, try to discover how they can be prevented. If you feel that they cannot happen to you, try to read more on the subject.

Finally, do not forget that honesty is a doctor's best policy and that the real physician is one who chooses to learn, to study, to be informed and to collaborate with his/her colleagues.

To treat and help others, to be a doctor, can be a pleasure and can be a challenge, but it is also a daily choice. From time to time, a doctor cannot treat or help a given patient, and may make mistakes. This is a reality. To judge, to know, to think, to ask – these are the grounding secrets of a physician, and are mandatory to prevent mistakes becoming habits.

Prof. Simona Gurzu
Head of Department of Pathology,
University of Medicine and Pharmacy,
Tirgu-Mures,
Romania

&

Prof. Ioan Jung
Department of Pathology,
University of Medicine and Pharmacy,
Tirgu-Mures,
Romania

List of Contributors

Leonard Azamfirei	Department of Anestesiology and Intensive Care, Rector of University of Medicine and Pharmacy, Tirgu-Mures, Romania
Iudita Badea	Department of Anestesiology and Intensive Care, University of Medicine and Pharmacy, Tirgu-Mures, Romania
Rodica Balasa	Head of Department of Neurology, University of Medicine and Pharmacy, Tirgu-Mures, Romania
Tivadar Bara	Department of Surgery, University of Medicine and Pharmacy, Tirgu-Mures, Romania
Tivadar Jr. Bara	Department of Surgery, University of Medicine and Pharmacy, Tirgu-Mures, Romania
Vlad Butiurca	Department of Surgery, University of Medicine and Pharmacy, Tirgu-Mures, Romania
Nicolae Dorin Gherasim	Department of Neurosurgery, Clinical County Emergency Hospital, Tirgu-Mures, Romania
Simona Gurzu	Head of Department of Pathology, University of Medicine and Pharmacy, Tirgu-Mures, Romania
Ioan Jung	Department of Pathology, University of Medicine and Pharmacy, Tirgu-Mures, Romania
Imre Kun	Department of Endocrinology, University of Medicine and Pharmacy, Tirgu-Mures, Romania
Alexandru Madaras	Department of Neurosurgery, Clinical County Emergency Hospital, Tirgu-Mures, Romania
Bogdan Andrei Suciu	Department of Surgery, University of Medicine and Pharmacy, Tirgu-Mures, Romania
Bela Szabo	Head of Department of Obstetrics and Gynecology, University of Medicine and Pharmacy, Tirgu-Mures, Romania
Sabin Gligore Turdean	Department of Pathology, University of Medicine and Pharmacy, Tirgu-Mures, Romania

ABBREVIATIONS

5-FU = 5-fluorouracil
ACE = angiotensin-converting enzyme
ADR = adverse drug reaction
AGEP = acute generalized exanthematous pustulosis
AIH = amiodarone-induced hypothyroidism
AIT = amiodarone-induced thyrotoxicosis
ALI = acute lung injury
AMP = cyclic adenosine monophosphate
AMPK = adenosine monophosphate-activated protein kinase
ARDS = acute respiratory distress syndrome
ASCUS = atypical squamous cells of undetermined significance
ATLS = advanced trauma life support
ATP = adenosine triphosphate
BBB = blood-brain barrier
BCG = Bacillus Calmette–Guerin
BMI = body mass index
BMS = bare metal stent
BPH = benign prostatic hyperplasia
BVS = bioresorbable vascular scaffold
CBD = common bile duct
CBG = corticosteroid-binding globulin
CIN = cervical intraepithelial neoplasia
CK = creatine kinase
CMV = cytomegalovirus
CN = Consciousness
CNS = central nervous system
COPD = chronic obstructive pulmonary disease
CSF = cerebrospinal fluid
CT = computed tomography
CTP = corticotroph tumor progression
CU-ADR = cutaneous adverse drug reaction
CYP3A4 = cytochrome-oxidase 3A4

D_2 receptor = dopaminergic receptor 2
DCO = damage control orthopedics
DES = drug eluting stent
DETA = Diethylenetriamine
DHEA = dehydroepiandrosterone
DIC = disseminated intravascular coagulation
DIND = drug-induced neurological disorders
DM = diabetes mellitus
DRBA = dopamine receptor-blocking agent
DRESS = drug reaction with eosinophilia and systemic symptoms
EBV = Epstein-Barr virus
ECG = electrocardiogram
EEG = electroencephalography
EGF = epidermal growth factor
EGFR = epidermal growth factor receptor
EMA = European Medicines Agency
EORTC = European Organization for Research and Treatment of Cancer
EP = encephalopathy
ePTFE = polytetrafluoroethylene
EPPER = eosinophilic, polymorphic and pruritic eruption associated with radiotherapy
EQ-5D = EuroQol five dimensions questionnaire
ERC = European Resuscitation Council
ERCP = endoscopic retrograde cholangiopancreatography
ESR = erythrocytes sedimentation rate
EUS = endoscopic ultrasonography
FAP = Familial Adenomatous Polyposis
FDA = Food and Drug Administration
FEF = forced expiratory flow
FEV = forced expiratory volume
FGF = fibroblast growth factor
FGS = female genital system
FNA = fine needle aspiration
FRC = functional residual capacity
FSH = follicle stimulating hormone

GAPPS = gastric proximal polyposis of the stomach
GAVE = gastric antral vascular ectasia
GERD = gastro esophageal reflux disease
GH = growth hormone
GI = gastrointestinal
GnRH = gonadotropin-releasing hormone
HBV = hepatitis B virus
HCC = hepatocellular carcinoma
HCV = hepatitis C virus
HE = Hematoxylin-Eosine
HHV = human herpes virus
HIV = human immunodeficiency virus
HLA = human leukocyte antigen
HPV = human papilloma virus
H-SIL = high-grade squamous intraepithelial lesion
HTLV = human T-cell lymphotropic virus
HV = herpes virus
IBD = inflammatory bowel disease
ICU = Intensive Care Unit
Ig = immunoglobulin
IL = interleukins
IR = insulin-resistance
ITP = idiopathic thrombocytopenic purpura
IUD = intrauterine device
JCV = John Cunningham polyomavirus
JGCA = Japanese Gastric Cancer Association
LG = lethargy
LKB1 = liver kinase B1
LSD = Lysergic acid diethylamide
L-SIL = Low-grade squamous intraepithelial lesion
MDMA = 3,4-Methylenedioxymethamphetamine
MET = mesenchymal-epithelial transition
MRCP = magnetic resonance cholangiopancreatography
MRI = magnetic resonance imaging
MS = muscular system

MSOF = multisystem organ failure
mTOR = mammalian target of rapamycin
mTORC1 = mammalian TOR-complex 1
NAION = non-arteritic ischemic optic neuropathy
Nd:YAG = neodymium-doped YAG
NGAL = neutrophil gelatinase-associated lipocalin
NHLBI = National Heart, Lung and Blood Institute
NMJ = neuromuscular junction
NO = nitrogen monoxide
NS = non-specific
NSAIDs = non-steroidal anti-inflammatory drugs
PCI = Percutaneous Coronary Intervention
PDE = phosphodiesterase
PDGF = platelet-derived growth factor
PEEP = positive-end expiratory pressure
PML = Progressive multifocal leukoencephalopathy
PNS = peripheral nervous system
PONV = postoperative nausea and vomiting
PPAR = peroxisome proliferator-activated receptor
PPI = proton pump inhibitor
PRL = prolactin
PTCA = Percutaneous Coronary Angioplasty
RET = rearranged during transfection
rhGH = recombinant human-type growth hormone
RTOG = Radiation Therapy Oncology Group
SIADH = syndrome of inappropriate antidiuretic hormone secretion
SIL = squamous intraepithelial lesion
SIRS = systemic inflammatory response syndrome
SIRT = selective internal radiation therapy
SJS = Stevens-Johnson syndrome
SM = somnolence
SN = syncope
ST = stupor
STK11 = Serine/Threonine Kinase 11
T3 = triiodothyronine

T4 = thyroxine
TAPP = transabdominal pre-peritoneal
TEN = toxic epidermal necrolysis
TGF = transforming growth factor
TNF = tumor necrosis factor
TRAIL = tumor necrosis factor-related apoptosis-inducing ligand
TRALI = transfusion-related acute lung injury
TRH = thyrotropin-releasing hormone
TSH = thyroid stimulating hormone
TTP = Thrombotic thrombocytopenic purpura
TUR = transurethral resection
TUR-P = transurethral resection of the prostate
UK = United Kingdom
UPA = ulipristal acetate
VAS = Visual Analog Scale
VEGF = vascular endothelial growth factor
WHO = World Health Organization
Wnt = Wnt-β-catenin signaling
Y = yttrium
YAG = yttrium aluminum garnet

CHAPTER 1

Adverse Drug Reactions

Ioan Jung and **Simona Gurzu***

Department of Pathology, University of Medicine and Pharmacy, Tirgu-Mures, Romania

Abstract: This chapter includes general aspects regarding the definitions and mechanisms of occurrences of adverse drug reactions (ADRs). They can be realized through non-immunological (type A reaction) or immunological (type B reaction) pathways and can be dose-dependent or independent. A new type of ADR is encountered in oncology departments in patients taking monoclonal antibodies. It is known as drug-induced apoptosis and is presented in this chapter. The mechanisms and classification of the severity of these reactions, as well as the particularities of acute, chronic and chronic-delayed ADRs, are also explored. The severity can be patient- or drug-related. In the chapters that follow, specific system- and organ-related ADRs are presented.

Keywords: Acute, Adverse drug reaction, Allergy, Apoptosis, Ahronic, Hypersensitivity, Iatrogenic, Idiosyncrasy, Monoclonal antibodies, Recurrent.

INTRODUCTION

Adverse drug reactions (ADRs) are defined as unwanted reactions associated with drug intake [1]. According to the World Health Organization (WHO), an ADR is defined as "a response to a drug which is noxious and unintended, and which occurs at doses normally used in man for the prophylaxis, diagnosis, or treatment of disease, or for the modification of physiological function" [1]. It has been estimated that ADRs are associated with 10-20% of all drugs, yet the real incidence is unknown and the importance of these side effects is often underestimated [2, 3].

Based on their severity, ADRs are classified as low, moderate or severe, and can have a lethal evolution. The Food and Drug Administration (FDA) considers a serious adverse event to be one that impacts the patient's outcome in one the following ways: leads to a threat to the patient's life or induces the patient's death; leads to prolonged hospitalization; gives rise to a congenital anomaly (in pregnant females); or induces disability or requires supplementary interventions

* **Corresponding author Simona Gurzu:** Department of Pathology, University of Medicine and Pharmacy, Tirgu-Mures, Romania; Tel: 0040-745-673550; Fax: 0040-372-653250; E-mail: simonagurzu@yahoo.com

to avoid permanent disability [4]. The main ADRs that can induce the patient's death are the following: fulminant bleeding from an iatrogenic peptic ulcer or occurring as a side effect of anticoagulant or chemotherapeutic drugs, severe aplastic anemia, hepatorenal failure, septic shock, anaphylactic shock, *etc.* [5].

In the United States, it has been estimated that approximately 3-7% of all hospital admissions are due to an ADR [6], 10-20% of which are severe [7]. The incidence of ADR-induced mortality is about 0.5-0.9%, but this is known to be an underestimate [8].

An ADR is a multifactorial process that can affect the skin, liver, kidneys, bone marrow, blood vessels, gastrointestinal (GI) tract, lungs and other organs and tissues. In this chapter, basic features regarding ADRs are presented, while system- or organ-related reactions are included in the following chapters of this book.

Types and Mechanisms of ADRs

Based on the ***time of appearance***, ADRs are classified as acute, chronic or chronic-delayed reactions. They occur during a single dose or a single cycle of therapy (*acute ADRs*), or can be dose- and time-related. A drug-induced reaction that occurs after 10-12 months of treatment is considered a *chronic ADR,* whereas *chronic-delayed* effects are realized years after treatment. *Recurrent ADRs* can also be identified in clinical practice [9].

Regarding the ***mechanism of occurrence***, in 1977 it was observed that ADRs could be *pharmacologically-induced (type A)* or the result of *idiosyncratic lesions (type B)* [10]. The most common ADRs (80%) are type A reactions that are dose-dependent and can be reversible after drug cessation [7, 11]. About 75-80% of type A reactions are predictable [11]. Type B reactions are immune-mediated, cannot be predicted, are dose-independent and occur only in susceptible individuals [1, 7].

Based on their mechanisms, ADRs are also classified as specific (immune mechanisms and nonallergic hypersensitivity) and non-specific. *Non-specific or non-immunological reactions (type A)* can be induced by overdose, direct side effects or drug interactions [1, 12]. The toxic effect can be dose-dependent or a result of metabolic disorders (slow hepatic detoxification) or renal failure (delayed elimination). Non-medical drug overdose, whether accidental or intentional, is not considered an ADR. Pharmacological side effects refer to drug-induced disorders at therapeutic doses [12].

In hospitalized patients, sedatives and hypnotics, respectively opiates and narcotics, are considered the leading sources of ADRs, followed by steroids, antibiotics and anticoagulants. As a result of drug interaction, a specific effect of a medical agent can be diminished or amplified. For example, barbiturates such as phenobarbital can diminish other drug effects as a result of hepatic enzymes activation. The antibiotic drug rifampin accelerates the renal elimination of drugs used in cardiology, such as verapamil. The histamine receptor antagonist cimetidine affects the metabolism and inhibits the excretion of several drugs, such as the antimalarial hydroxychloroquine, psychoactive medications and nifedipine, and doubles the half-life of zolmitriptan (used for migraine attacks) [5].

A distinct mechanism of non-immunological ADRs is *drug-induced apoptosis*. This is specific to the latest monoclonal antibodies used in medical oncology for individualized treatment (*e.g.*, bevacizumab, rituximab, adalimumab, cetuximab, trastuzumab, *etc.*) and other drugs such as the anti-acne isotretinoin (13-ci--retinoic acid). Apoptosis is a consequence of drug-induced formation of apoptotic protein tumor necrosis factor-related apoptosis-inducing ligand (TRAIL) and neutrophil gelatinase-associated lipocalin (NGAL). Due to the risk of teratogenicity, oligohydramnios and poor neonatal outcomes, these drugs are not recommended for use during pregnancy. In animals, drug-induced apoptosis has been proven to decrease hypothalamic cell numbers and to induce depression [13, 14].

Specific or immunological reactions (type B) are dose-independent, difficult to predict and occur at doses tolerated by normal subjects. They include immune-mediated lesions and nonallergic hypersensitivity [1, 11].

Nonallergic or pseudoallergic hypersensitivity which is also known as idiosyncrasy or intolerance, is defined as the unusual or unpredictable effect that might be induced in a particular patient at usual doses as a result of enzymatic deficiency or through a genetic mechanism [1]. It can be a life-threatening disorder.

Immune mechanisms or allergic (IgE-mediated and non IgE-mediated) hypersensitivity reactions are the result of activation of one of the four hypersensitivity reactions: type I (IgE-mediated), type II (cytotoxic), type III (immune complex) or type IV (cell-mediated) [1, 5, 11]. Anaphylactic reactions (type I hypersensitivity) can be mild, moderate or severe (anaphylactic shock) and are not dose-dependent. They are realized as cutaneous eruptions, fever, eosinophilic pneumonia and, infrequently, thrombocytopenia and anemia. Other rare manifestations of allergies are vasculitis (*e.g.*, penicillin, sulfonamides, iodine, *etc.*), interstitial nephritis (methicillin) and hepatic injury [5]. Cytotoxic reactions (type II hypersensitivity) are involved in the pathomechanism of drug-induced hematological disorders (quinidine-induced thrombocytopenia, penicillin or methyldopa-induced hemolytic anemia). Immune complex-mediated reactions (type III hypersensitivity) occur as a result of the antigenic role of medications [5]. Serum sickness is a specific self-limiting disease characterized by vasculitis, hematological disorders and cutaneous lesions that occur approximately 10 days after passive immunization as a result of a type III hypersensitivity reaction to proteins from a non-human animal antiserum (*e.g.*, antitetanic, anti-lymphocyte, anti-diphtheritic anti-botulinic serum) or drugs. Chronic-delayed ADRs are mediated by T lymphocytes through cell-mediated (type IV) hypersensitivity. The specific lesions induced through the four hypersensitivity reactions are presented in Chapter 3.

Adverse reactions induced by non-steroidal anti-inflammatory drugs (NSAIDs) are considered a new specific group of ADRs that involve both non-immunological (type A) and immunological (type B) mechanisms. They are also known as *NSAID-induced hypersensitivity reactions*, are dose-related and occur as a result of the direct pharmacological action of the drug (anti-prostanoid, anti-cyclooxygenase) [1]. The criteria of classification were proposed in 2001 by Stevenson et al. and were later modified by the European Academy of Allergy and Clinical Immunology's Task Force on NSAIDs Hypersensitivity [1, 15]. The type A effects of NSAIDs are dose-related and mainly relate to the GI disorders that are presented in Chapter 6. The type B effects of NSAIDs are grouped according to allergic and nonallergic effects. The allergic (selective) effects of NSAIDs are rare and include urticaria, angioedema, anaphylaxis and NSAIDs-induced delayed hypersensitivity. The nonallergic/non-immunological effects (the old idiosyncrasy) are cross-reactive and can be responsible for the occurrence of urticaria, angioedema or exacerbation of a cutaneous or respiratory disorder [1].

Severity of ADRs

The patient-related factors of severity of non-immune ADRs are the following: female gender, older age, associated severe comorbidities (renal failure, hepatic disorders, systemic lupus erythematosus), polypragmasia, associated viral infections (*e.g.*, human immunodeficiency virus [HIV], herpes virus, cytomegalovirus), alcohol consumption, etc. Females, asthmatic patients, users of beta blockers and patients with HIV and other autoimmune disorders, such as systemic lupus erythematosus, have a higher risk of developing hypersensitivity-related ADRs [11, 16].

The Drug-Related Factors of Severity refer to the *chemical properties and molecular weight* of the drug. For example, it is known that heterologous sera (non-human proteins) are highly immunogenic, but other drugs may also have immunogenic properties by coupling with proteins to form haptens (antigen-antibody immunogenic complexes) [11]. The risk of developing hypersensitivity-related ADRs also depends on *the route of drug administration*. The most common allergic phenomena occur after intramuscular or intravenous drug administration [11].

In Chapters 4 to 13, the specific system- and organ-related ADRs (drug-induced lesions) will be presented in detail. Drug-induced neurological disorders are presented in Chapter 14 and endocrine disorders are included in Chapter 15. The specific disorders occurring in intensive care units are presented in Chapter 16, those related to gynecology and obstetrics are covered in Chapter 18 and drug-induced ototoxicity is extensively examined in Chapter 21.

CONFLICT OF INTEREST

The authors confirm that this chapter content has no conflict of interest.

ACKNOWLEDGEMENTS

Declared none.

REFERENCES

[1] Kowalski ML, Makowska JS. Seven steps to the diagnosis of NSAIDs hypersensitivity: how to apply a new classification in real practice? Allergy Asthma Immunol Res 2015; 7(4): 312-20. [http://dx.doi.org/10.4168/aair.2015.7.4.312] [PMID: 25749768]

[2] Nebeker JR, Barach P, Samore MH. Clarifying adverse drug events: a clinicians guide to terminology, documentation, and reporting. Ann Intern Med 2004; 140(10): 795-801. [http://dx.doi.org/10.7326/0003-4819-140-10-200405180-00017] [PMID: 15148066]

[3] Pirmohamed M, Breckenridge AM, Kitteringham NR, Park BK. Adverse drug reactions. BMJ 1998; 316(7140): 1295-8. [http://dx.doi.org/10.1136/bmj.316.7140.1295] [PMID: 9554902]

[4] Phillips KA, Veenstra DL, Oren E, Lee JK, Sadee W. Potential role of pharmacogenomics in reducing adverse drug reactions: a systematic review. JAMA 2001; 286(18): 2270-9. [http://dx.doi.org/10.1001/jama.286.18.2270] [PMID: 11710893]

[5] Jung J, Ed. Patologie iatrogenă. Tîrgu-Mureş, Romania: University Press 2006.

[6] Tarloff JB. Merck Manual: Adverse drug reactions. 2012. Available at: www. msdmanuals.com.

[7] Einarson TR. Drug-related hospital admissions. Ann Pharmacother 1993; 27(7-8): 832-40. [http://dx.doi.org/10.1177/106002809302700702] [PMID: 8364259]

[8] Tarloff JB. Adverse Drug Reactions Clinical Pharmacology 2007. Available at: www.merckmanuals.com.

[9] Reynoso-von Drateln C, Gómez-Hernández N, Rodríguez-Martínez N, Torres-Lozano C. Recurrent toxic epidermal necrolysis syndrome: a report of two cases. Drug Saf Case Rep 2016; 3(1): 9. [http://dx.doi.org/10.1007/s40800-016-0032-x] [PMID: 27747689]

[10] Rawlins MD, Thompson JW. Mechanisms of adverse drug reactions. In: Davies DM, Ed. Textbook of Adverse Drug Reactions. Oxford: Oxford University Press 1991; pp. 18-45.

[11] Riedl MA, Casillas AM. Adverse drug reactions: types and treatment options. Am Fam Physician 2003; 68(9): 1781-90.
[PMID: 14620598]

[12] Rang HP. Pharmacology. Edinburgh: Churchill Livingstone 2003; p. 146.

[13] Sarno MA, Mancari R, Azim HA Jr, Colombo N, Peccatori FA. Are monoclonal antibodies a safe treatment for cancer during pregnancy? Immunotherapy 2013; 5(7): 733-41.
[http://dx.doi.org/10.2217/imt.13.64] [PMID: 23829624]

[14] Melnik BC. Apoptosis may explain the pharmacological mode of action and adverse effects of isotretinoin, including teratogenicity. Acta Derm Venerol 2017; 97(2): 173-81.
[http://dx.doi.org/10.2340/00015555-2535] [PMID: 27671426]

[15] Stevenson DD, Sanchez-Borges M, Szczeklik A. Classification of allergic and pseudoallergic reactions to drugs that inhibit cyclooxygenase enzymes. Ann Allergy Asthma Immunol 2001; 87(3): 177-80.
[http://dx.doi.org/10.1016/S1081-1206(10)62221-1] [PMID: 11570612]

[16] Barranco P, López-Serrano MC. General and epidemiological aspects of allergic drug reactions. Clin Exp Allergy 1998; 28 (Suppl. 4): 61-2.
[PMID: 9761035]

CHAPTER 2

Radiation-Induced Lesions

Simona Gurzu* and **Ioan Jung**

Department of Pathology, University of Medicine and Pharmacy, Tirgu-Mures, Romania

Abstract: This chapter includes general aspects regarding the mechanisms of radiation-induced lesions and specific organ-related effects of radiotherapy, from the cardiovascular system to bone marrow. For oncologists, understanding the mechanisms of radiation-induced carcinogenesis and knowing the estimated time taken for post-radiotherapy occurrence of metachronous tumors is mandatory for proper patient follow-up. We here analyze all lesions of the skin and internal organs, leaving aside tumors for this chapter. The acute and chronic effects of radiotherapy are presented in detail, and the grading system of oral mucositis is also outlined.

Keywords: Actinic enterocolitis, Bone marrow, Bronchiolitis obliterans, Dermatitis, Endarteritis obliterans, EPPER-syndrome, Iatrogenic, Malignancy, Mucositis, Pneumonitis, Radiation enteropathy, Radiodermatitis, Radiotherapy, Reticuloid syndrome, Sweet's syndrome, Vasculitis.

INTRODUCTION

In medical practice, radiation is used for diagnosis (0.1-10 mSv per procedure) or therapeutic purposes (20-60 Gy per targeted tissue). Two types of ionizing radiation are used for radiotherapy: photon radiation (X- or gamma-rays) and particle radiation (electrons, protons, neutrons, carbon ions, alpha and beta particles). Photon radiation is used for deep tumors, while electron beams are produced by a linear accelerator and are useful for treatment of cutaneous tumors and cancers that are close to the surface of the body. Proton beam radiation therapy requires highly advanced equipment and is not performed in all oncology departments. Neutron beams are useful for head, neck and prostate carcinomas, as well as for inoperable tumors. Their use severely affects the surrounding normal tissue. For radio resistant tumors, carbon ion radiation (heavy ion radiation) can be helpful. Alpha and beta particles are contained in radioactive particles that can be injected, swallowed or inserted into the body [1].

* **Corresponding author Simona Gurzu:** Department of Pathology, University of Medicine and Pharmacy, Tirgu-Mures, Romania; Tel: 0040-745-673550; Fax: 0040-372-653250; E-mail: simonagurzu@yahoo.com

Radiotherapy using photon radiation can involve the whole human body (*e.g.*, bone marrow transplant) but, in most cases, is used for localized therapy. Based on the radiation source, radiotherapy is classified into two main groups: external beam radiotherapy (wherein the X-ray tube is placed outside the patient's body) and brachytherapy (wherein irradiation is performed using an isotope, such as cadmium-226, cesium-137, iridium-192, iodine-125 or carbon ion, that is inserted into a tumor or within a cavity). Several medical procedures that involve radiation, such as stereotactic surgery, intensity-modulated radiation therapy, accelerated/hypo- or hyper-fractioned whole- or partial-breast irradiation, brachytherapy, intraoperative radiation therapy and fluoroscopic-guided procedures are responsible for iatrogenic lesions that range from minimal damage to chronic injuries, carcinogenic effects and radiation-induced death [2 - 7].

EFFECTS OF RADIATION – GENERAL DATA

Ionizing radiation causes DNA damage *via* direct toxicity with DNA breakage and subsequent cellular death. The indirect mechanism is based on the radiation-induced formation of free radicals with further fragmentation of the DNA or ionization of water or other molecules within the cell. The damaged tissues and vessels are then replaced by fibrocytes that are unable to synthesize collagen [8, 9].

Mucosal injuries consist of inflammatory reactions. In first steps, they are characterized by the death of mucosal cells, the breakdown of the mucosal homeostasis and the activation of pro-inflammatory cytokines, chemokines and growth factors [10]. Later, fibrosis occurs as a result of the activation of interleukins (IL-6, IL-8) and growth factors (transforming growth factor [TGF], tumor necrosis factor [TNF], *etc.*) [11, 12].

The effects of radiation depend on several factors, including the following [2, 9, 13, 14]:

- *Size of irradiation field, dose fractionation and total dose*: in the whole body, irradiation of 100-300 rad can induce acute radiation sickness, while higher doses can lead to death within approximately one month (350-500 rad) or a couple of days (>1000 rad). The main causes of death are heart/renal failure, bone marrow suppression and septicemia.
- *Exposure time and time interval between fractions:* the first effects are decreasing serum levels of erythrocytes and leukocytes (bone marrow injury), followed by mucosal damage (gastrointestinal [GI] tract injuries) and central nervous system disorders. Radiation-induced malignancy usually occurs years after radiotherapy.

- *Type and technique of irradiation*: the most aggressive form of radiation is alpha particle radiation, followed by beta radiation. X-rays have a highly penetrative effect with minimal tissular damage, but can destroy the weak bonds between nucleic acids and induce chromosomal alterations.
- *Radiation sensitivity of tissue:* hair follicles, mucosa of the GI tract, bone marrow, lymphatic tissue, ovarian follicles and testes present high sensitivity, while medium sensitivity is noted for connective tissue, blood vessels and urothelium. Cartilaginous tissue, muscles, corpus luteum and ovarian stroma are relatively radio resistant, as are the liver, kidneys, pancreas and brain.
- *Individual susceptibility*: the consequences of radiotherapy are more severe in patients who have previously received radiotherapy, and also depend on the patient's age at exposure, gender, associated comorbidities and genetic factors.

POST-RADIATION MALIGNANCY

Ionizing radiation can induce carcinogenesis. Approximately 0.5-2.2% of patients develop a histopathologically independent second tumor within 5-7 years of radiotherapy, in a dose-dependent manner. The first known instance of radiation-induced cancer was reported in 1902, on ulcerated skin, and leukemia in radiation workers was reported in 1911. Moreover, in recent history, the leukemia risk of radiologists has been found to be nine times higher than in other medical specialties, proving that whole-body radiation is a high-risk factor for bone marrow disorders [2, 13, 15, 16].

Secondary tumors are primarily located in or near the first irradiated tumor site. The most common malignant tumors are cutaneous carcinomas, carcinomas of the GI tract (30%), head and neck tumors (10%), lymphomas (10%), breast cancer (9%), sarcomas (9%) and lung cancer (8%). Radiation-induced benign tumors can also develop [2, 15, 16].

Radiotherapy performed for head, neck and mediastinal tumors can be followed by occurrence of thyroid papillary carcinoma and/or laryngeal carcinoma at 8-20 years respectively 20-40 years after radiotherapy. In 22% of the cases, the second cancer is developed in extra-laryngeal places such as lung and prostate [16, 17].

In patients with GI tract carcinomas, radiotherapy can be followed by a secondary tumor of the GI tract but extra-GI tumors such as prostate carcinoma were also reported [18]. In cases with radiation-induced damages of the pancreatic parenchyma and chronic pancreatitis, secondary neuroendocrine tumors seem to derive from the intralobular ducts lining epithelium that presents a radiation-induced endocrine differentiation [2, 19].

In patients with breast cancer, radiotherapy alone is primarily associated with a risk of lung cancer, followed by contralateral breast cancer. Malignant tumors of the GI tract and genital system can also occur [20].

Pelvic radiotherapy can give rise to the development of malignancies of the genital organs and intestines. Colorectal carcinomas (median dose = 50 Gy) and carcinosarcomas of the uterine body were reported between months and five years following treatment [16, 21, 22].

Squamous cell carcinoma can occur at 8-50 years after skin radiotherapy. It can develop on relatively normal skin or in the context of chronic radio dermatitis. Other tumors, such as Merkel cell carcinoma, can also occur [23].

Post-radiation sarcomas are rare and are mainly realized as fibrosarcoma (90%), osteosarcoma, synovial sarcoma and malignant fibrous histiocytoma [24]. Approximately 1.5-6.9% of primary bone tumors are radiation-induced sarcomas occurring 4-20 years after radiotherapy [25, 26]. Chondroid differentiation can be seen in about 89% of radiation-induced osteosarcomas [27]. Chondrosarcoma of the bladder has been reported at 19 years after radiotherapy [28]. Maxillofacial chondrosarcoma can develop at about six months following radiotherapy for basal cell carcinoma [29]. Brain irradiation can induce genesis of radiogenic primary sarcoma of the brain [30]. Breast irradiation is a risk factor for breast angiosarcoma, which is developed years after radiotherapy [30]. Osteosarcomas, undifferentiated spindle cell or pleomorphic sarcomas and fibrosarcomas can occur in patients with desmoid tumors at 5-21 years after radiotherapy, originating from CTNNB1 wild- or mutated-type desmoid fibromatosis cells [31].

In children, radiation-induced benign tumors have been reported. Single or multiple osteochondromas develop in more than 10% of patient receiving radiotherapy [32, 33]. Dose-dependent radiation-induced peripheral nerve tumors, such as neurofibromas, have been reported at 5-31 years following radiotherapy [15].

RADIATION-INDUCED NON-TUMOR LESIONS

Cutaneous Lesions

Acute Radiodermatitis

Cutaneous lesions can occur within a few days or weeks of radiotherapy. The effects present as erythematous rash, plaques, ulcerations or necrosis and are less severe after the use of high- and medium-energy accelerators. The hair follicles and nails can also be affected. There are four grades of acute dermatitis, based on severity. Grades 1 and 2 are the most common (90%), while grades 3 and 4 are relatively rare [34 - 36]:

- *Grade 1* is characterized by erythema, a burning sensation, edema, dry desquamation and reversible hair loss in the affected area.
- *Grade 2* is similar to grade 1 but is associated with exudative plaques (moist desquamation of the skin folds and creases).
- *Grade 3* is characterized by exudative dermatitis, with skin shedding (moist desquamation other than skin folds and creases), ulceration and bleeding induced by minor trauma or abrasion. This grade occurs in cases where the dose exceeds 40 Gy. After re-epithelization, dyschromia or alopecia is often permanent.
- *Grade 4* involves dose-dependent radio necrosis that usually develops within a few days of treatment. It is a painful plaque comprising necrosis, ulceration and hemorrhage of the full thickness of dermis, which can extend to muscles, tendons and bones.

Simultaneous use of radio chemotherapy and targeted drugs, such as epidermal growth factor receptor (EGFR) inhibitors (*e.g.,* cetuximab), advanced age and severe immunodeficiency are risk factors for grade 3 and 4 radio dermatitis. The risk is lower in patients receiving cisplatin-based chemotherapy as compared to those receiving anti-EGFR agents. Moreover, radio dermatitis presents earlier in patients receiving radiotherapy alone as compared to those receiving radiotherapy and anti-EGFR drugs (1-2 weeks *versus* 3-5 weeks after radiotherapy). In the latter group, immune-mediated dermatitis is characterized by xerosis, crust formation, well-defined subepidermal inflammatory infiltrate and high risk of super infection [36].

Chronic Radiodermatitis or Actinic Reticuloid Syndrome

Radiation-induced chronic cutaneous lesions encompass a wide spectrum that is dominated by chronic dermatitis. Such lesions are characterized by ulceration, superficial prominent telangiectasia, dermal fibrosis (Fig. **2-1**) and epidermal atrophy. Hyperkeratosis and the pseudolymphomatous (reticuloid) aspect are also characteristic. Chronic radio dermatitis occurs months to years after radiotherapy and can be an indicator of premalignancy. Excessive fibrosis is induced by abnormally high levels of cytokines (IL-4, IL-5, TGF-β) that stimulate the secretion of extracellular matrix and activation of fibroblasts. Fibrosis of the hair follicles leads to alopecia, while nail irradiation can be followed by nail loss. The sebaceous and sweat glands can also be damaged. The severity of chronic dermatitis depends on the radiation dose. A dose of over 50 Gy induces severe lesions [2, 4, 23, 37, 38].

Other Skin Lesions

Sweet's Syndrome(Acute Febrile Neutrophilic Dermatosis) is characterized by post-radiotherapy inflamed or blistered skin and mucosal lesions associated with fever [39].

Eosinophilic, Polymorphic and Pruritic Eruption Associated with Radiotherapy (EPPER) Syndrome is a rare radiation-induced lesion that primarily affects the lower limbs of females and is characterized by pruriginous papules and vesicles. Under the microscope, deep perivascular lymphohistiocytic infiltrate rich in eosinophils is characteristic. It can be an acute or late complication of radiotherapy [40].

Other Late Radiation-Induced Cutaneous Lesions are hyperpigmentation, parakeratosis, cellulitis, recall dermatitis, pemphigoid, erythema multiforme, lichen sclerosis, lupus-like lesions, inflammatory acne, pruriginous rashes, late wound healing, morphea (a localized scleroderma characterized by pain and disfiguration of the affected area) and subcutaneous calcinosis [2, 4, 23, 37].

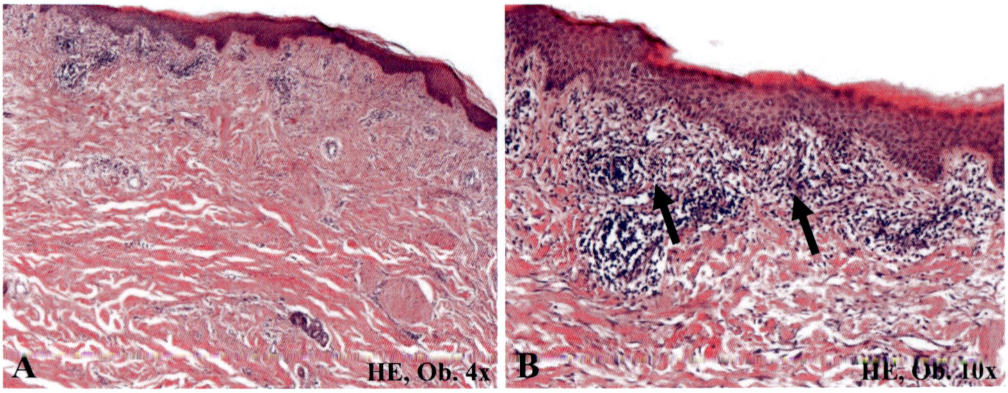

Fig. (2-1). Radio dermatitis with dermal fibrosis (**A**) and well-defined sub epidermal lymphoid infiltrate (**B**).

CARDIOVASCULAR LESIONS

Vascular Injuries

Large blood vessels present medium sensitivity when subject to radiotherapy. Common effects are endarteritis, thrombosis and necrosis. These can involve acute lesions followed by endarteritis obliterans (Fig. **2-2**), atherosclerosis, perivascular fibrosis and compression of the surrounding tissues [41, 42]. Local radiation for the treatment of head and neck cancer can induce carotid atherosclerosis, especially in patients at elevated risk for atherosclerosis (diabetes mellitus [DM], hypertension, hypercholesterolemia, smoking) [43].

In such cases, the capillaries, arterioles and venules are more sensitive to radiation, showing endothelial swelling and endarteritis, possibly due to the release of free oxygen radicals. In late stages, endothelial hyperplasia, usually without clinical impact, and vascular fibrosis can be seen in medium-sized vessels [41]. Vascular changes are induced by a dose of about 50 Gy [44].

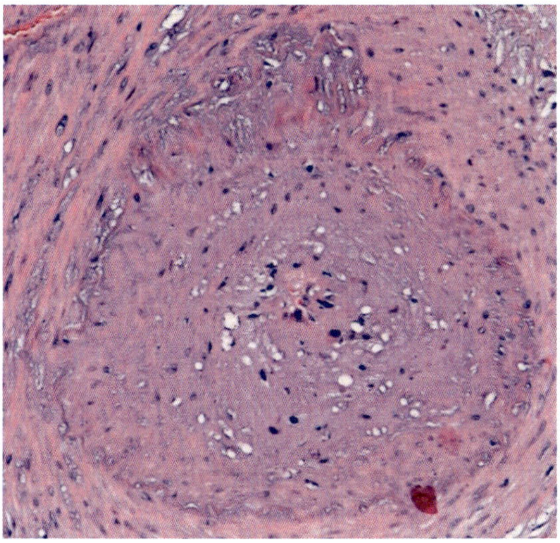

Fig. (2-2). Radiation-induced endarteritis obliterans in a patient with rectal cancer. Luminal obstruction, thickening of the media and perivascular fibrosis are characteristic. HE, 10x.

Lesions of the Heart

Radiation-induced heart disease primarily means coronary vessel injury, but lesions of the pericardium, myocardium, heart valves and conduction system may also occur. This is a dose-dependent effect associated with an immune component. The consequences of this effect are more severe at younger ages and in patients with coexisting heart diseases. Relatively safe doses are 60 Gy for 25% of heart volume and 45 Gy for 65% of heart volume, both at 2 Gy/24 hours [41, 45, 46].

Radiation-Induced Coronary Artery Injuries involve an accelerated atherosclerosis with fibrous thickening of the intima and luminal narrowing. By comparison with non-radiation-induced coronary sclerosis, the media are more affected, with loss of smooth muscle cells, and the adventitia is markedly fibrotic and thick. Coronary disease occurs at 10-15 years after radiotherapy [45, 47, 48].

Pericardial Lesions occur at months to years after radiotherapy and include pericarditis (acute, delayed or constrictive), pericardial effusion and pericardial-myocardial fibrosis [45, 49, 50].

Myocardial Injuries (Radiation-Induced Cardiomyopathy) are rare and occur most commonly in patients receiving radiotherapy for mediastinal tumors. The pathomechanism is based on radiation-induced microvascular damage with further decrease of myocardial perfusion. The main consequences are myocardial fibrosis, diastolic dysfunctions, occurrence of congestive cardiomyopathy and heart failure [45, 51]. The main risk factors for myocardial lesions are coexisting heart diseases (heart malformations, valvulopathies, preexisting myocarditis, hypertension, *etc*.). High serum levels of troponin can be an indicator of radiation-induced cardiotoxicity, but this finding is controversial [2, 52].

Valvular Damage primarily involves the aortic and mitral valves, and is seen at 3-5 years following radiotherapy [53, 54].

Conduction Disorders are revealed by changes in electrocardiogram (ECG) readings that include ST-T abnormalities, low voltage, bundle branch blocks and/or complete atrioventricular block [55, 56].

LESIONS OF THE LUNGS AND AIRWAYS

Lung and airway injuries are frequently seen in patients receiving radiotherapy for esophageal carcinomas or mediastinal lymphomas (especially Hodgkin's lymphoma) and are seen rarely in females with breast cancer [3, 57].

Lung Lesions

Radiation-induced dose-dependent damage to lung parenchyma is relatively common after stereotactic body radiotherapy. The cartilaginous tissue is a relatively radio resistant structure [58].

Post-Radiotherapy Bronchiolitis Obliterans Organizing Pneumonia also known as ***secondary organizing pneumonia,*** is the most common variant of radiation pneumonitis and is characterized by the presence of granulation tissue in the distal airways extending into the alveolar ducts. Bilateral patchy infiltrates are seen on the chest radiographs, with ground-glass opacities on computed tomography (CT). This is a rare but serious complication (5% mortality rate) of breast cancer radiotherapy. The symptoms occur for between a number of weeks and one year after treatment completion. They are similar to those of classic pneumonia (fever, cough, shortness of breath, fatigue) but do not improve with antibiotic therapy – steroids are instead required [3].

Acute Radiation Pneumonitis is a type of diffuse alveolar damage with an associated severe vascular component (fibrinoid necrosis and thrombosis of the arterioles and congested venules), edematous widening of the septa, presence of intra-alveolar fluid and hyaline membranes (acute respiratory distress syndrome; ARDS) [3].

Chronic Radiation Pneumonitis with Fibrosis can occur after acute pneumonitis or if its appearance is insidious, without an acute phase. The arterioles are obliterated by intimal fibrosis and recanalized thrombi. Fibrotic enlargement of the alveolar septa is characteristic, as is peribronchial and perivascular fibrosis [59].

Late Pulmonary Damage is seen following stereotactic therapy for pulmonary cancer and includes – besides tumor remnants – consolidation, volume loss and ground-glass changes corresponding to interstitial damage. Radiographic evaluation, by comparison with the pre-radiotherapy evaluation, is reported as increased, stable, decreased, obscure or not present [58].

Radiation Recall Pneumonitis refers to chemotherapy-induced inflammation in healthy pulmonary areas previously exposed to irradiation. It can be related to erlotinib exposure [60].

Lesions of the Upper Airways

Laryngeal Edema can develop in patients receiving radiotherapy for head, neck or mediastinal tumors. In patients with laryngeal cancer, carbon ion therapy can induce laryngeal edema, necrosis and stenosis [5].

Nasopharyngeal Granuloma has been reported in patients receiving radiotherapy for nasopharyngeal carcinoma. The clinical symptoms are nasal obstruction, purulent discharge, headaches, epistaxis, foreign body sensation and/or hearing impairment. This granuloma can mimic a tumor recurrence [61].

Lesions of the Digestive System

The mucosa of the GI tract presents high sensitivity to radiation, being frequently affected during systemic radiotherapy. The lesions are acute (mainly inflammatory lesions) or chronic (fibrosis of the GI wall) and can involve one or multiple GI tract segments.

Radiotherapy-Related Nausea and Vomiting

These are usually associated with pain flare and are the most common side effects in patients receiving palliative radiotherapy for symptomatic bone metastases [62].

Oral Complications

Acute complications in this regard are mucositis, xerostomia, dysphagia, dysgeusia and opportunistic infections (Gram-negative bacteria and fungi). Chronic lesions refer to trismus, fibrous sialadenitis, radiation caries, osteoradionecrosis and changes of the periodontal attachment. The periodontium is radio resistant [9, 63]. All patients receiving head and neck radiation (60-70 Gy) present oral mucositis, but in mild forms in most cases. Proper oral hygiene decreases the risk of periodontitis and tooth loss [9, 36, 63]. The rate of Candida colonization ranges from 56.7% during radiation to 63.3% post-radiation. Candida albicans is the most common type, followed by Candida parapsilosis, tropicalis and glabrata [64].

Oral mucositis is classified by the World Health Organization (WHO) according to the following grades, based on severity [36, 63]:

- *Grade 1 (mild mucositis)* = oral erythema and soreness
- *Grade 2 (moderate mucositis)* = ulcers and difficulties eating solids
- *Grade 3 (severe mucositis)* = ulcers and difficulties taking liquids
- *Grade 4 (life-threatening lesion)* = oral alimentation is not possible

The National Cancer Institute's Common Terminology Criteria for Adverse Events include the presence or absence of pain and classify mucositis severity as follows [36, 63]:

- *Grade 1* = asymptomatic or mild symptoms
- *Grade 2* = moderate pain not interfering with oral intake
- *Grade 3* = severe pain interfering with oral intake
- *Grade 4* = life-threatening mucositis
- *Grade 5* = death

Radiation Esophagitis

Radiation esophagitis is characterized by desquamative and/or fungal inflammation, with late fibrosis, stenosis and functional esophageal disorders [63].

Radiation Gastritis, Duodenitis and Peptic Ulcerations

The antrum, pylorus and duodenum are commonly affected as a result of selective internal radiation therapy (SIRT), whereby microspheres emitting yttrium-90 (Y-90) are intra-arterially infused in patients with primary or metastatic tumors of the liver, to produce radioembolization. During biopsy, the Y-90 microspheres can be identified as small round-shaped black foreign bodies [65]. After external beam radiation of the right hypochondrium and epigastrium, performed to treat hepatic carcinomas (more than 55 Gy) or for gastric lymphomas, life-threatening diffuse hemorrhagic gastritis was reported, in one study, three months after radiotherapy. This involved acute vasculopathy characterized by edema, obliterative endarteritis, vasculitis, endothelial proliferation, mucosal ischemia, telangiectasias and gastric ulcerations [18].

Radiation Recall Gastritis refers to chemotherapy-induced inflammation in healthy gastric areas previously exposed to irradiation. It can be related to anthracyclines, taxanes, gemcitabine, capecitabine and erlotinib exposure [60].

Bowel Lesions

Radiation-Induced Diarrhea is graded by the National Cancer Institute's Common Terminology Criteria for Adverse Events according to five grades:

- *Grade 1* = fewer than four stools per day over the baseline
- *Grade 2* = between four and six stools per day over the baseline
- *Grade 3* = up to seven stools per day over the baseline; associated with incontinence and limited self-care activities of daily living
- *Grade 4* = life-threatening diarrhea
- *Grade 5* = death

Changes in bowel habits occur in 90% of patients receiving pelvic radiotherapy, with half of these reporting an impact on their quality of life [63, 66].

Radiation Enteropathy or Actinic Enterocolitis concerns the majority of patients treated for pelvic cancers (gynecological cancer, prostate, rectal cancer, *etc.*). For severe painful pelvic bowel damage and dysfunction, the term of *"pelvic radiation disease"* is usually accepted. Radiation enteropathy is an ulcerative enterocolitis (Fig. **2-3**) characterized by epithelial desquamation, atrophy, perivascular fibrosis with intramural necrosis and progressive fibrosis of the submucosa and underlying layers. Diarrhea or constipation occurs in early phases (stage I), followed by the presence of stools with desquamated membranes (stage II), mucinous/hemorrhagic stools (stage III) and intestinal strictures with changes in bowel habits (stage IV). Fistulae, perforation, malabsorption syndrome, ileus and peritoneal adherences can be associated [2, 8, 67, 68].

Radiation Proctitis or Proctopathy occurs following pelvic radiotherapy performed to treat tumors of the cervix, prostate, bladder or rectum. It is a dose-dependent lesion that is usually associated with cystitis. The incidence ranges from 2% for patients receiving up to 5000 cGy to 18-29% for patients receiving 8001 cGy or more to the rectum. It is more common in patients with preexistent inflammatory bowel diseases and more severe when co-occurring with vitamin D deficiency. Acute proctitis occurs within the first three months of initiation of treatment, while chronic radiation proctitis occurs between eight and 12 months following treatment completion. The clinical symptoms are rectal bleeding, rectal pain, tenesmic, diarrhea, bloating, fecal incontinence, *etc*. Besides mucosal injuries and intramural fibrosis, mesorectal disorders include fibrosis (95%), vasculitis with perivascular fibrosis (51%), and sclero-hyalinosis of the lymph nodes with pericapsular and perineural fibrosis (23% and 13%, respectively). The remedy for acute proctitis comprises treatment cessation, hydration and supportive treatment with anti-inflammatory, antidiarrheal and steroid drugs. For chronic proctitis, non-invasive treatment comprises administration of non-steroidal anti-inflammatory drugs (NSAIDs), antioxidants, sucralfate, short chain fatty acids and hyperbaric oxygen. Invasive treatment includes formalin injection, endoscopic yttrium aluminum garnet (YAG) laser or argon plasma coagulation, radio frequency tumor ablation, cryoablation or surgery [6, 22, 44, 66, 69 - 71].

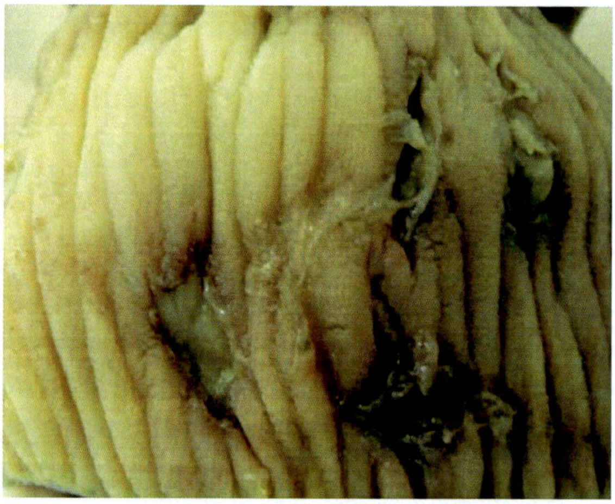

Fig. (2-3). Stage I radiation enteropathy with multiple fibrin-covered ulcerations.

Anastomosis-Related Complications can occur in patients with rectal cancer who have undergone long-course radiotherapy (45.0-50.4 Gy) with concurrent 5-fluorouracil (5-FU)-based chemotherapy [72].

Radiation-Induced Retroperitoneal Fibrosis

A very rare consequence of radiotherapy, radiation-induced retroperitoneal fibrosis is characterized by an extensive fibrosis of the periaortic retroperitoneum.

It can entrap the ureters causing obstructive uropathy. Spontaneous regression can be observed [73, 74].

Hepatic and Pancreatic Injuries

Hepatic and Biliary Injuries are rarely encountered, these structures being relatively radio resistant. The radiation hepatopathy comprises hyperemia, centrilobular necrosis, veno occlusive disease, Budd-Chiari-like syndrome and infrequent cholecystitis and/or biliary damage. Radio frequency tumor ablation can be followed by bleeding, while hematoma is visible as low attenuation on unenhanced CT scans [2]. Radiation-induced hepatitis B virus reactivation is a life-threatening complication (60% mortality rate) that has been reported during radiotherapy for hepatocellular carcinoma (HCC) with portal vein tumor thrombosis. The risk of reactivation is related to baseline HBV-DNA levels and HBeAg positivity [75].

Pancreatic Injuries are rare, this organ being relatively radio resistant. They refer to acute or chronic pancreatitis, the latter being a premalignant lesion [19].

LESIONS OF THE KIDNEY AND URINARY TRACT

Radiation Nephropathy

This is a rare lesion, the kidney parenchyma being relatively radio resistant. This dose-dependent lesion (the safety dose is 10 Gy) emerges from six months to years after radiotherapy and is more commonly reported after total body irradiation for bone marrow transplantation. It is characterized by hypertension, proteinuria, impairment of urine concentration, anemia and progressive renal failure. Microscopically, stepwise nephropathy includes lesions of the glomeruli (endothelial and mesangial cell damage, thickening of the basement membrane, hyalinization, thrombotic microangiopathy and nephrosclerosis) followed by renal tubes injury (epithelial denudation, necrosis and atrophy), lesions of the interstitium (edema, inflammation and gradual tubulointerstitial scarring) and vascular injuries (fibrinoid necrosis and vascular wall fibrosis). Ataxia telangiectasia syndrome can co-occur [2, 14].

Urinary Tract Injuries

These injuries involve mucosal ulcerations and epithelial damage in early phases, followed by proliferation of poorly vascularized fibrotic tissue and strictures. Urothelium presents a medium radio sensitivity [2].

Ureteral Obstruction (Obstructive Uropathy) emerges as a result of the direct effect of radiotherapy or as a consequence of external compression exerted by radiotherapy-induced retroperitoneal fibrosis [73, 74].

Urethral Strictures occur in about 11% of patients receiving radiotherapy for prostate cancer or pelvic radiotherapy. It emerges at a median time of 26 months after brachytherapy. The associated risk factors are transurethral resection of the prostate (TUR-P) prior to radiation, age, non-white race and associated comorbidities [8].

Recto-Urethral Fistulae occur in 0.2% of patients with prostate cancer receiving brachytherapy. The risk is higher if biopsies are taken from the rectum following radiation, as well as in patients with preexisting microvascular disorders and smokers [42].

Radiation Cystitis

This is a common dose-dependent complication of external beam radiotherapy or MRI-guided brachytherapy to the pelvic area [8, 76].

Conventional Radiation Cystitis is a stepwise lesion that is firstly characterized by epithelial degenerative changes, ulcerations, necrosis and vascular disorders (endothelial proliferation, perivascular fibrosis). Then, a severe intramural fibrosis of the urinary bladder occurs at about three years after radiotherapy (*"radiation bladder"*). The main consequences are micturition disorders, recurrent and ascending infections, septicemia, *etc.* [2].

Radiation-Induced Hemorrhagic Cystitis Also Known As ***Radiation Recall Syndrome,*** occurs in 3% of patients receiving up to 5000 cGy and about 12% of patients receiving a dose greater than or equal to 8001 cGy to the bladder. It is a sterile cystitis that can occur from days or months (acute cystitis) to 15 years (delayed cystitis) after radiation. The symptoms of acute onset are hematuria, dysuria and anemia. Depending on the severity of hematuria, it is graded by the Radiation Therapy Oncology Group (RTOG) and the European Organization for Research and Treatment of Cancer (EORTC) according to the following groups:

- *Grade I* = microscopic hematuria
- *Grade II* = macroscopic hematuria
- *Grade III* = macroscopic hematuria with clots
- *Grade IV* = urinary tract obstruction with clots

In late onset, the acute-onset symptoms are associated with sphincter dysfunction, reduced bladder capacity, ulceration, perforation and infrequent fistulization. The treatment comprises treatment cessation, hyperhydration and continuous bladder irrigation with saline, aluminum potassium sulfate (alum), silver nitrate, mesna (sodium 2-mercaptoethane sulfonate), sodium hyaluronate, formalin or phenol. Hyperbaric oxygen therapy, endoscopic laser coagulation with neodymium-doped YAG (Nd:YAG) and intravesical administration of tacrolimus, cranberry juice, prostaglandin or chondroitin sulfate are also suggested [69, 70, 76, 77].

LESIONS OF THE GENITAL SYSTEM

Ovaries and testes are highly sensitive to radiotherapy, 5-15 Gy being enough to affect their functioning. The ovary follicles are more sensitive than the testis, while the corpus luteum and ovarian stromal cells are radio resistant structures [2].

Lesions of the Female Genitalia

Vesico-Vaginal Fistulae occur following pelvic radiotherapy performed to treat tumors of the cervix, bladder or rectum, especially in elderly patients. It is difficult to differentiate these from tumor fistulae. Following surgical repair, a vesico-vaginal fistula can be complicated by urinary incontinence [78].

Radiation-Induced Sterility can be a consequence of irradiation of the uterus and is the most common complication with long-term effects in females. Recent studies have shown that, in young patients receiving sterilizing pelvic radiotherapy, cryopreserved ovarian cortical tissue can be re-transplanted after treatment. This method has been successfully used in some patients for fertility preservation [79]. Acute radiation sickness is followed by late effects that comprise amenorrhea and fibrosis of the uterus and ovaries in the second year following exposure. The patient's estradiol levels can also decrease, while follicle-stimulating hormone and luteinizing hormone levels increase in the first year [80].

Endometrial And Myometrial Changes include fibrosis/hyalinization and uterine shrinkage at about three months following completion of treatment [81].

Vaginal Injuries can arise from pelvic radiotherapy or brachytherapy performed to treat an endometrial, cervical or vulvar cancer. The incidence of vaginal atrophy is 36% after brachytherapy and 18% after external beam therapy. However, modern radiotherapy techniques aim to decrease the rate of vaginal damage. The acute vaginal lesions that occur in first two to three months after radiotherapy are edema, erythema, mucosal desquamation, mucositis and submucosal hyperemia. The chronic lesions are vascular injuries (endarteritis obliterans, telangiectasia and bleeding), mucosal ulceration and necrosis, fistulae, fibrosis, atrophy, decreased vaginal elasticity and vaginal stenosis. Injuries to the vulva and occurrence of pain during sexual intercourse are common in the first month after radiotherapy [6].

Radiation-Induced Female Sexual Dysfunctions are primarily the consequence of vaginal/vulvar/perineal injuries and include hypoactive sexual desire, arousal and orgasm, as well as sexual pain disorders. Dyspareunia and decreased sexual satisfaction are also reported consequences. Postradiotherapy sexual dysfunction was reported in 50-81% of the females studied [6].

Radiation-Induced Embryo-/Fetopathies

The incidence of such embryo-/fetopathies depends on the age of the embryo/fetus, the dosage and time span of radiotherapy and the localization of the mother's tumor. Depending on the time of implantation, the following complications can occur: embryonic death, external/internal malformations (in the case of radiotherapy during embryo-/organogenesis), growth disorders (low height and weight), neurological maldevelopment, mental retardation, hydrocephalus (in the case of radiotherapy during fetal period), *etc*. In utero, fetal irradiation with diagnostic X-rays increases the risk of childhood cancer at an organ dose of 10 mGy [7, 13, 82].

Breast Lesions

Intraoperative Radiotherapy for early breast cancer induces complications in one third of patients. Such complications include infections, wound dehiscence, skin necrosis, bleeding and formation of hematoma or seroma [83].

Breast Fibrosis is a common complication occurring as a result of radiation-induced CD8 T-lymphocytes apoptosis. The risk of fibrosis is higher in smokers and females receiving adjuvant hormonal therapy and is not increased by concomitant chemotherapy [35].

Atypical Vascular Lesions can be complications of the radiotherapy of the breast and should be differentiated from radiation-induced vascular tumors. It was recently reported that *MYC* and *FLT* gene amplification is detected in more than 75% of radiation-induced angiosarcomas, but not in atypical vascular lesions, thus being proposed as a differentiator between the two lesion types [30].

Lesions of the Male Genitalia

Sterility is the main consequence of radiotherapy, followed by the tumorigenic risk. In patients with acute radiation sickness, late effects include a decreased sperm count and abnormal sperm morphology, but exclude testosterone level disorders [80].

Sexual Dysfunctions occur in 51% of patients receiving pelvic radiotherapy. They include dose-dependent erectile difficulties (17%) and changes to the seminal fluid. Change in potency is induced by a dose to the penile bulb greater than 50 Gy [66, 84, 85]. In patients receiving brain radiation, sexual disturbances can be the result of damage to the hypothalamic-pituitary axis [86].

Prostatic Necrosis can be a result of pelvic radiation, as a primary lesion or a secondary rectoprostatic fistula in patients with radiation proctitis [8, 87].

Penile Necrosis is very rare, occurring between one and two years after prostate brachytherapy. It is a complication of a radiation-induced recto-urethral fistula with further spread of infection in the corpus spongiosum, corpora cavernosa, surrounding soft tissues and scrotum. Radiation-induced chronic hyalinization of vessels within the corpora cavernosa and corpus spongiosum is a conducive factor for infection spread. Its clinical symptoms are urinary incontinence, dysuria and pelvic and perineal pain. In some cases, penectomy is necessary [42].

LESIONS OF THE BONE MARROW AND HEMATOLOGICAL DISORDERS

Bone marrow is one of the most radiosensitive tissues in terms of dose-volum--time dependency. It is especially affected by whole-body radiation but pelvic, ribs or brain radiation can also influence recruitment of peripheral myeloid cells. The most common adverse effect is decrease of the hematopoietic function of the red marrow, reducing the number of hematopoietic cells and sharply increasing the bone marrow adipose tissue. This results in an increase of the proportion of yellow marrow, hypoplasia/aplasia/gelatinous atrophy and myelofibrosis. Bone marrow suppression induces a high risk of infection, septicemia and hemorrhage. Blood serum analysis shows lymphopenia (first hours), neutropenia (first days/weeks) and thrombocytopenia (weeks/months). The erythrocytes present the highest radioresistance and anemia occurs in later phases. Several months are necessary for bone marrow regeneration [2, 88 - 90].

LESIONS OF THE LYMPHATIC TISSUE

The direct effects of ionizing radiation on the *lymph nodes* are dose- and time-dependent. The stepwise disorders firstly comprise a diffuse hyperplasia of lymphocytes attempting to compensate for lymphopenia. Follicular hyperplasia of the lymph nodes is also characteristic, without clinical impact (Fig. **2-4**). Then, macrophages take in the cellular detritus and old degenerated lymphocytes and the injured area is replaced by fibrous tissue. The final effect is the sclero-hyalinosis of the lymph nodes with pericapsular fibrosis [2, 44].

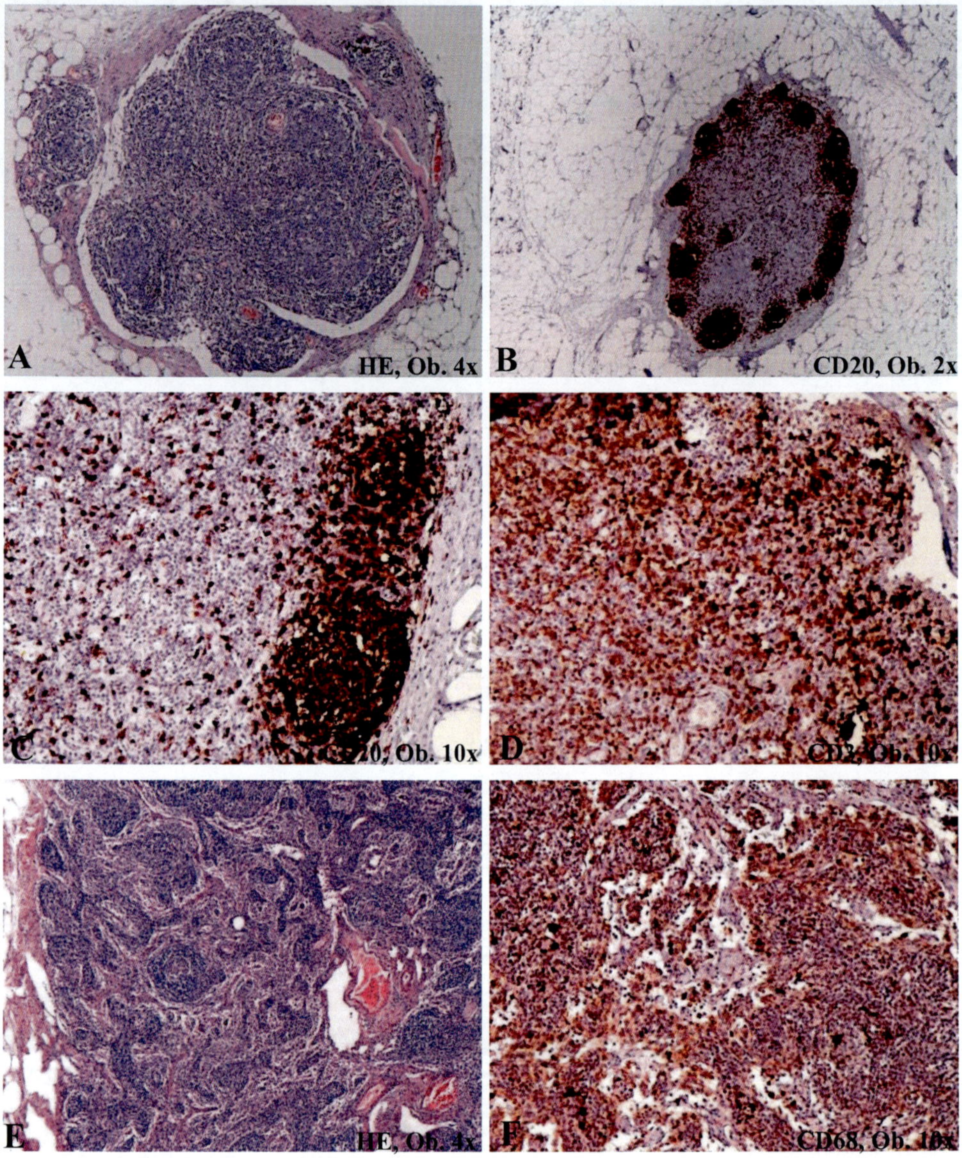

Fig. (2-4). Radiation-induced morphological disorders of the lymph nodes. A-D: Diffuse lymphoid hyperplasia (A) with few CD20 positive B-cells (B, C) and predominance of proliferated CD3 positive T-cells (D). E-F: Sinusal hyperplasia with rich CD68 positive macrophagic infiltrate (F).

In the *spleen*, chemoradiotherapy can induce erythrophagia that is associated with hemosiderosis and fibrosis of the red pulp, with further decrease of spleen volume to 37% at four years after radiotherapy, usually without clinical impact. Sepsis can be a fatal complication [2, 91].

BONE AND JOINTS LESIONS

Bone Injuries

Abscopal Effect of Irradiation is a term used to indicate local radiotherapy used to treat metastatic cancers that has not only local but also systemic effects, inducing shrinkage of distant metastases, including bone metastases. Any tumor radiation therapy for prostate, pancreatic, cervical, rectal or endometrial cancers involves skeleton exposure. The severity of bone lesions depends on the radiation dose and field, the age of the patient and dose fractionation. The bonc absorbs up to half of the radiation dose used for pelvic malignancies. Moreover, single bone irradiation can induce time-dependent disorders of the skeleton outside the radiation field, mediated by bone marrow changes (*e.g.,* femoral injuries in patients receiving local radiotherapy for breast cancer) [89, 92].

Bone Lesions in Adults mainly involve a rapid increase in osteoclastogenesis (one week after radiotherapy) and decrease of the number of osteoblasts. This can result in a decrease of trabecular bone volume, regional or systemic osteopenia, decrease of bone mineral density (osteoporosis), osteoradionecrosis and pathological fractures [2, 26, 89]. Osteoradionecrosis, which occurs between six and 17 months after radiotherapy, is the result of decreased matrix production given diminished osteoblast function and is a contributory factor for pathological fractures [89, 93, 94]. Bone necrosis and atrophy are caused by radiation-induced obliterative endarteritis [9]. Radiation-induced bone marrow suppression of the hematopoiesis also contributes to bone mineral loss and increases fracture risk [88].

Bone Lesions in Children primarily refer to altered bone growth that can be caused by a targeting dose of 12 Gy. Epiphysis is the most sensitive bone area to irradiation, followed by metaphysis. The diaphysis is relatively radio resistant. The effects comprise irregular ossification and slipped femoral epiphysis. The radiotherapy-induced micro vascular lesions and dircct cellular damage are followed by degeneration of chondrocytes and osteocytes, and by fibrogenesis. Diaphyseal irradiation leads to periosteal new bone formation, metaphyseal fraying and sclerosis. Other clinical effects are bone fracture, platyspondyly (flattened vertebral bodies), spinal deformity and genu valgum [2, 26, 33, 95].

Joint Damage

Dose-dependent radiation effects upon synovial tissues are poorly understood. Radiation-induced arthropathy includes degenerative changes and decreased mobility. In children, painful valgus knee joints after irradiation have been reported [33].

OTHER NON-TUMOR LESIONS

Optical Disorders

The neuro-optic structures (optic nerves, chiasm and retina) can be injured during brain radiation therapy. The main dose-dependent effects are dry eye (7%), cataract (11%) and chronic retinopathy. The lacrymal glands are affected at a median dose of 1.47 Gy, the lenses at 1.05 Gy, and cataract can be induced by a dose of 2-10 Gy [80, 96]. In patients with acute radiation sickness, the later effects on the eye lenses include opacity (six months after exposure) and gradual deterioration in visual acuity [80]. Another complication of radiation to the head and neck area (especially to the sella or skull base) is ocular neuromyotonia. This is characterized by periodic involuntary extraocular muscle contraction as a result of injury to the sixth cranial nerve [97].

Cerebral and Neurological Lesions

Damage to the Brain Parenchyma and Nervous Fibers are rare. These structures are relatively radio resistant and are only affected at high doses. Radiation can induce acute and persistent increases in the numbers of CD3+ and CD11c+ cells in the central nervous system, and can lead to a process of inflammatory. Myelin tract injuries (demyelination) and white substance necrosis can occur at median doses of 20-30 Gy. Multifocal necrotizing leukoencephalopathy (focal necrosis of the white matter of the pons) and myelitis is realized in more than one third of adult patients. Sensorineural hearing loss can also occur. Endothelial cells, oligodendrocytes and astrocytes have high radiation sensitivity. Perivascular fibrosis can be a consequence of radiation. In children, neurodevelopmental disorders are the most common effects of radiation. Long-term complications of craniospinal irradiation with 18-36 Gy include uni- or bilateral ototoxicity, with hearing loss in 12% of cases and alteration of processing speed and verbal comprehension, without modifications of the working memory [2, 90, 98, 99].

Peripheral Neuropathy/Paresis/Paralysis are very rare lesions that can occur months or years after radiotherapy (*e.g.*, neuropathy of the brachial nerves after radiotherapy performed for breast cancer). Neurological involvement has been reported as an extracutaneous manifestation of Sweet's syndrome (neuro-Sweet disease) in patients receiving radiotherapy for oral squamous cell carcinoma [39]. In patients with head and neck cancers, *trismus* has been reported in 47.1% of patients, with depression associated with 8.7% of such cases [100].

Endocrine Disturbances

The most common radiotherapy-related endocrine sequelae are the disorders of the hypothalamic-pituitary axis. Pituitary injuries occur in 80% of patients receiving craniocerebral radiotherapy. The main clinical effect is progressive and irreversible hypopituitarism. This can be followed by a compensatory increase in hypothalamic release activity. In adults, growth disorders, body image, skeletal health, fertility, sexual function and physical and psychological health are impacted. In children with neuroblastomas, craniospinal irradiation induces neuroendocrine deficits in 55% of patients, most of whom present growth hormone (GH) deficits. Other effects of childhood radiotherapy are puberty disorders, thyroid and parathyroid dysfunctions, obesity and metabolic syndrome, alterations in glucose metabolism and decreased bone mineral density [86, 98].

CONFLICT OF INTEREST

The authors confirm that this chapter content has no conflict of interest.

ACKNOWLEDGEMENTS

Declared none.

REFERENCES

[1] http://www.cancer.org/treatment/treatmentsandsideeffects/treatmenttypes/radiation/radiationtherapyprinciples/radiation-therapy-principles-types-of-radiation. Accessed at 30 of August 2016.

[2] Jung J, Ed. Patologie iatrogenă. Tîrgu-Mureş, Romania: University Press 2006.

[3] Epler GR, Kelly EM. Systematic review of postradiotherapy bronchiolitis obliterans organizing pneumonia in women with breast cancer. Oncologist 2014; 19(12): 1216-26. [http://dx.doi.org/10.1634/theoncologist.2014-0041] [PMID: 25361622]

[4] Herz-Ruelas ME, Gomez-Flores M, Moxica-Del Angel J, *et al.* Ulcerated radiodermatitis induced after fluoroscopically guided stent implantation angioplasty Case Rep Dermatol Med 2014; 2014: 768624. [http://dx.doi.org/10.1155/2014/768624] [PMID: 25276441]

[5] Demizu Y, Fujii O, Nagano F, *et al.* Unexpected radiation laryngeal necrosis after carbon ion therapy using conventional dose fractionation for laryngeal cancer. Jpn J Clin Oncol 2015; 45(11): 1076-81. [http://dx.doi.org/10.1093/jjco/hyv121] [PMID: 26355161]

[6] Jensen PT, Froeding LP. Pelvic radiotherapy and sexual function in women. Transl Androl Urol 2015; 4(2): 186-205. [PMID: 26816824]

[7] Kanter DJ, OBrien MB, Shi XH, *et al.* The impact of ionizing radiation on placental trophoblasts. Placenta 2014; 35(2): 85-91. [http://dx.doi.org/10.1016/j.placenta.2013.12.011] [PMID: 24418702]

[8] Hofer MD, Gonzalez CM. Management of radiation-induced urethral strictures. Transl Androl Urol 2015; 4(1): 66-71. [PMID: 26816812]

[9] Kassim N, Sirajuddin S, Biswas S, Rafiuddin S, Apine A. Iatrogenic damage to the periodontium caused by radiation and radiotherapy. Open Dent J 2015; 9: 182-6. [http://dx.doi.org/10.2174/1874210601509010182] [PMID: 26312083]

[10] Ong ZY, Gibson RJ, Bowen JM, *et al.* Pro-inflammatory cytokines play a key role in the development

of radiotherapy-induced gastrointestinal mucositis. Radiat Oncol 2010; 5: 22. [http://dx.doi.org/10.1186/1748-717X-5-22] [PMID: 20233440]

[11] Langberg CW, Hauer-Jensen M, Sung CC, Kane CJ. Expression of fibrogenic cytokines in rat small intestine after fractionated irradiation. Radiother Oncol 1994; 32(1): 29-36. [http://dx.doi.org/10.1016/0167-8140(94)90446-4] [PMID: 7938676]

[12] Wang J, Boerma M, Fu Q, Hauer-Jensen M. Significance of endothelial dysfunction in the pathogenesis of early and delayed radiation enteropathy. World J Gastroenterol 2007; 13(22): 3047-55. [PMID: 17589919]

[13] Shah DJ, Sachs RK, Wilson DJ. Radiation-induced cancer: a modern view. Br J Radiol 2012; 85(1020): e1166-73. [http://dx.doi.org/10.1259/bjr/25026140] [PMID: 23175483]

[14] Baradaran-Ghahfarokhi M. Radiation-induced kidney injury. J Renal Inj Prev 2012; 1(2): 49-50. [PMID: 25340106]

[15] Lai V, Wong YC, Poon WL, Fu YP, Lam TC, Yuen SC. Radiation-induced peripheral nerve neurofibromata in a patient receiving hypofractionated radiation therapy. Am J Neuroradiol 2008; 29(10): 1995-7. [http://dx.doi.org/10.3174/ajnr.A1219] [PMID: 18653682]

[16] Welte B, Suhr P, Bottke D, *et al.* Second malignancies in high-dose areas of previous tumor radiotherapy. Strahlenther Onkol 2010; 186(3): 174-9. [http://dx.doi.org/10.1007/s00066-010-2050-4] [PMID: 20339826]

[17] Khan MK, Koyfman SA, Hunter GK, Reddy CA, Saxton JP. Definitive radiotherapy for early (T1-T2) glottic squamous cell carcinoma: a 20 year Cleveland Clinic experience. Radiat Oncol 2012; 7: 193. [http://dx.doi.org/10.1186/1748-717X-7-193] [PMID: 23164282]

[18] Tatsis V, Peponi E, Papadopoulos G, Tsekeris P, Fatouros M, Glantzounis G. Subtotal gastrectomy for diffused hemorrhagic gastritis induced by radiation, following liver resection for hilar cholangiocarcinoma. A case report. Int J Surg Case Rep 2016; 18: 30-2. [http://dx.doi.org/10.1016/j.ijscr.2015.11.014] [PMID: 26686486]

[19] Landreau P, Facy O, Ravoire A, *et al.* Radiation-induced pancreatitis: search for the neoplasm. Clin Res Hepatol Gastroenterol 2012; 36(3): e48-9. [http://dx.doi.org/10.1016/j.clinre.2011.11.012] [PMID: 22285641]

[20] Marcheselli R, Marcheselli L, Cortesi L, *et al.* Risk of second primary malignancy in breast cancer survivors: a nested population-based case-control study. J Breast Cancer 2015; 18(4): 378-85. [http://dx.doi.org/10.4048/jbc.2015.18.4.378] [PMID: 26770245]

[21] Zwierzchowska A, Panek G, Gajewska M. Postradiation carcinosarcoma of the corpus uteri a case report. Eur J Gynaecol Oncol 2015; 36(6): 746-9. [PMID: 26775366]

[22] Min M, Chua B, Guttner Y, *et al.* Is pelvic radiation disease always the cause of bowel symptoms following prostate cancer intensity-modulated radiotherapy? Radiother Oncol 2014; 110(2): 278-83. [http://dx.doi.org/10.1016/j.radonc.2013.11.012] [PMID: 24412017]

[23] Ansai S, Noro S, Ogita A, Fukumoto H, Katano H, Kawana S. Case of Merkel cell carcinoma with squamous cell carcinoma possibly arising in chronic radiodermatitis of the hand. J Dermatol 2015; 42(2): 207-9. [http://dx.doi.org/10.1111/1346-8138.12737] [PMID: 25510284]

[24] Smith J. Postradiation sarcoma of bone in Hodgkin disease. Skeletal Radiol 1987; 16(7): 524-32. [http://dx.doi.org/10.1007/BF00351266] [PMID: 2827314]

[25] Weatherby RP, Dahlin DC, Ivins JC. Postradiation sarcoma of bone: review of 78 Mayo Clinic cases. Mayo Clin Proc 1981; 56(5): 294-306. [PMID: 6939953]

[26] Mitchell MJ, Logan PM. Radiation-induced changes in bone. Radiographics 1998; 18(5): 1125-36. [http://dx.doi.org/10.1148/radiographics.18.5.9747611] [PMID: 9747611]

[27] Barker JP, Monument MJ, Jones KB, Putnam AR, Randall RL. Secondary osteosarcoma: is there a predilection for the chondroblastic subtype? Orthopedics 2015; 38(5): e359-66. [http://dx.doi.org/10.3928/01477447-20150504-51] [PMID: 25970361]

[28] Sule N, Xu BO, El Zein D, *et al.* Radiation-induced chondrosarcoma of the bladder. Case report and review of literature. Anticancer Res 2015; 35(5): 2857-60. [PMID: 25964567]

[29] Yang S, Tang W, Tang XF, *et al.* Case report: postradiation chondrosarcoma with a short latency period of 6 months. Int J Biol Markers 2014; 29(4): e440-4. [http://dx.doi.org/10.5301/jbm.5000109] [PMID: 25385242]

[30] Cornejo KM, Deng A, Wu H, *et al.* The utility of MYC and FLT4 in the diagnosis and treatment of postradiation atypical vascular lesion and angiosarcoma of the breast. Hum Pathol 2015; 46(6): 868-75. [http://dx.doi.org/10.1016/j.humpath.2015.02.014] [PMID: 25864386]

[31] Verschoor AJ, Cleton-Jansen AM, Wijers-Koster P, *et al.* Radiation-induced sarcomas occurring in desmoid-type fibromatosis are not always derived from the primary tumor. Am J Surg Pathol 2015; 39(12): 1701-7. [http://dx.doi.org/10.1097/PAS.0000000000000510] [PMID: 26414222]

[32] el-Mahdi AM, Marks R Jr, Thornton WN, Constable WC. Sequelae of pelvic irradiation in infancy. 25-year followup. Radiology 1974; 110(3): 665-6. [http://dx.doi.org/10.1148/110.3.665] [PMID: 4811688]

[33] Hutchinson ID, Olson J, Lindburg CA, *et al.* Total-body irradiation produces late degenerative joint damage in rats. Int J Radiat Biol 2014; 90(9): 821-30. [http://dx.doi.org/10.3109/09553002.2014.927935] [PMID: 24885745]

[34] Mateus C, Thomas M. Radiation dermatitis. In: Therapeutics in dermatology A reference book on the management of skin diseases www.therapeutique-dermatologique.org. Accessed at 14th of January 2016.

[35] Azria D, Riou O, Castan F, *et al.* Radiation-induced CD8 T-lymphocyte apoptosis as a predictor of breast fibrosis after radiotherapy: results of the prospective multicenter French trial. EBioMedicine 2015; 2(12): 1965-73. [http://dx.doi.org/10.1016/j.ebiom.2015.10.024] [PMID: 26844275]

[36] Zhu G, Lin JC, Kim SB, *et al.* Asian expert recommendation on management of skin and mucosal effects of radiation, with or without the addition of cetuximab or chemotherapy, in treatment of head and neck squamous cell carcinoma. BMC Cancer 2016; 16: 42. [http://dx.doi.org/10.1186/s12885-016-2073-z] [PMID: 26817597]

[37] Spalek M, Jonska-Gmyrek J, Gałecki J. Radiation-induced morphea - a literature review. J Eur Acad Dermatol Venereol 2015; 29(2): 197-202. [http://dx.doi.org/10.1111/jdv.12704] [PMID: 25174551]

[38] Dawe RS, Ferguson J. Diagnosis and treatment of chronic actinic dermatitis. Dermatol Ther (Heidelb) 2003; 16(1): 45-51. [http://dx.doi.org/10.1046/j.1529-8019.2003.01607.x] [PMID: 12919126]

[39] Wallett A, Newland K, Foster-Smith E. Radiation therapy-induced neuro-Sweet disease in a patient with oral squamous cell carcinoma. Australas J Dermatol 2017; 58(2): e51-3. [http://dx.doi.org/10.1111/ajd.12442] [PMID: 26821310]

[40] Lam Cham Kee HX, Charra-Brunaud C, Cuny JF, Reigneau M, Vogin G, Peiffert D. [Case report of EPPER Syndrome (eosinophilic polymorphic pruritic eruption associated with radiotherapy) in a patient treated against endometrial cancer]. Cancer Radiother 2013; 17(1): 54-7.

[http://dx.doi.org/10.1016/j.canrad.2012.10.012] [PMID: 23291008]

[41] Yusuf SW, Sami S, Daher I. Radiation-induced heart disease: A clinical update. Cardiol Res Pract 2011; 2011: 317659.
[http://dx.doi.org/10.4061/2011/317659] [PMID: 21403872]

[42] Kinahan J, Pai H, Martens M, *et al.* Penile necrosis requiring penectomy complicating recto-urethral fistula post prostate cancer external beam radiation and brachytherapy. Can Urol Assoc J 2014; 8(1-2): E57-9.
[http://dx.doi.org/10.5489/cuaj.1112] [PMID: 24454604]

[43] Pereira EB, Gemignani T, Sposito AC, Matos-Souza JR, Nadruz W Jr. Low-density lipoprotein cholesterol and radiotherapy-induced carotid atherosclerosis in subjects with head and neck cancer. Radiat Oncol 2014; 9: 134.
[http://dx.doi.org/10.1186/1748-717X-9-134] [PMID: 24919963]

[44] Reggiani Bonetti L, Domati F, Farinetti A, Migaldi M, Manenti A. Radiotherapy-induced mesorectum alterations: histological evaluation of 90 consecutive cases. Scand J Gastroenterol 2015; 50(2): 197-203.
[http://dx.doi.org/10.3109/00365521.2014.983153] [PMID: 25515346]

[45] Kucharska W, Negrusz-Kawecka M, Gromkowska M. Cardiotoxicity of oncological treatment in children. Adv Clin Exp Med 2012; 21(3): 281-8.
[PMID: 23214190]

[46] Martinou M, Gaya A. Cardiac complications after radical radiotherapy. Semin Oncol 2013; 40(2): 178-85.
[http://dx.doi.org/10.1053/j.seminoncol.2013.01.007] [PMID: 23540743]

[47] Brosius FC III, Waller BF, Roberts WC. Radiation heart disease. Analysis of 16 young (aged 15 to 33 years) necropsy patients who received over 3,500 rads to the heart. Am J Med 1981; 70(3): 519-30.
[http://dx.doi.org/10.1016/0002-9343(81)90574-X] [PMID: 6782873]

[48] Virmani R, Farb A, Carter AJ, Jones RM. Pathology of radiation-induced coronary artery disease in human and pig. Cardiovasc Radiat Med 1999; 1(1): 98-101.
[http://dx.doi.org/10.1016/S1522-1865(98)00010-9] [PMID: 11272363]

[49] Veinot JP, Edwards WD. Pathology of radiation-induced heart disease: a surgical and autopsy study of 27 cases. Hum Pathol 1996; 27(8): 766-73.
[http://dx.doi.org/10.1016/S0046-8177(96)90447-5] [PMID: 8760008]

[50] Ling LH, Oh JK, Schaff HV, *et al.* Constrictive pericarditis in the modern era: evolving clinical spectrum and impact on outcome after pericardiectomy. Circulation 1999; 100(13): 1380-6.
[http://dx.doi.org/10.1161/01.CIR.100.13.1380] [PMID: 10500037]

[51] Adams MJ, Hardenbergh PH, Constine LS, Lipshultz SE. Radiation-associated cardiovascular disease. Crit Rev Oncol Hematol 2003; 45(1): 55-75.
[http://dx.doi.org/10.1016/S1040-8428(01)00227-X] [PMID: 12482572]

[52] Kozak KR, Hong TS, Sluss PM, *et al.* Cardiac blood biomarkers in patients receiving thoracic (chemo)radiation. Lung Cancer 2008; 62(3): 351-5.
[http://dx.doi.org/10.1016/j.lungcan.2008.03.024] [PMID: 18462828]

[53] Carlson RG, Mayfield WR, Normann S, Alexander JA. Radiation-associated valvular disease. Chest 1991; 99(3): 538-45.
[http://dx.doi.org/10.1378/chest.99.3.538] [PMID: 1995208]

[54] Tamura A, Takahara Y, Mogi K, Katsumata M. Radiation-induced valvular disease is the logical consequence of irradiation. Gen Thorac Cardiovasc Surg 2007; 55(2): 53-6.
[http://dx.doi.org/10.1007/s11748-006-0070-x] [PMID: 17444176]

[55] Slama MS, Le Guludec D, Sebag C, *et al.* Complete atrioventricular block following mediastinal irradiation. a report of six cases. Pacing Clin Electrophysiol 1991; 14(7): 1112-8.

[http://dx.doi.org/10.1111/j.1540-8159.1991.tb02842.x] [PMID: 1715548]

[56] La Vecchia L. Physiologic dual chamber pacing in radiation-induced atrioventricular block. Chest 1996; 110(2): 580-1.
[http://dx.doi.org/10.1378/chest.110.2.580-a] [PMID: 8697881]

[57] Gross NJ. Pulmonary effects of radiation therapy. Ann Intern Med 1977; 86(1): 81-92.
[http://dx.doi.org/10.7326/0003-4819-86-1-81] [PMID: 319723]

[58] Raziee H, Hope A, Faruqi S, *et al.* Classification and reporting of late radiographic changes after lung stereotactic body radiotherapy: proposing a new system. Clin Lung Cancer 2015; 16(6): e245-51.
[http://dx.doi.org/10.1016/j.cllc.2015.05.008] [PMID: 26077096]

[59] Castellino RA, Glatstein E, Turbow MM, Roesnberg S, Kaplan HS. Latent radiation injury of the lung and heart activated by steroid withdrawal. Ann Intern 1974; 80: 595-9.
[http://dx.doi.org/10.7326/0003-4819-80-5-593]

[60] Graziani C, Hegde S, Saif MW. Radiation recall gastritis secondary to erlotinib in a patient with pancreatic cancer. Anticancer Res 2014; 34(12): 7339-43.
[PMID: 25503169]

[61] Yang L, Li H, Wang H, *et al.* Nasopharyngeal granulomatous mass after radiotherapy for nasopharyngeal carcinoma. Auris Nasus Larynx 2016; 43(3): 330-5.
[http://dx.doi.org/10.1016/j.anl.2015.10.005] [PMID: 26791589]

[62] Chiu N, Chiu L, Popovic M, *et al.* Latest advances in the management of radiation-induced pain flare, nausea and vomiting. Ann Palliat Med 2016; 5(1): 50-7.
[PMID: 26841815]

[63] Peterson DE, Boers-Doets CB, Bensadoun RJ, Herrstedt J. Management of oral and gastrointestinal mucosal injury: ESMO Clinical Practice Guidelines for diagnosis, treatment, and follow-up. Ann Oncol 2015; 26 (Suppl. 5): v139-51.
[http://dx.doi.org/10.1093/annonc/mdv202] [PMID: 26142468]

[64] Zhang YY, Li AQ, Wang NN, Liu LN, Cui JL. [Oral candida species distribution in patients receiving radiotherapy for head and neck cancer]. Shanghai Kou Qiang Yi Xue 2014; 23(5): 605-8.
[PMID: 25543608]

[65] Baumann J, Lin M, Patel C. An unusual case of gastritis and duodenitis after yttrium 90-microsphere selective internal radiation. Clin Gastroenterol Hepatol 2015; 13(5): xxiii-v.
[http://dx.doi.org/10.1016/j.cgh.2015.01.002] [PMID: 25595794]

[66] Gillespie C, Goode C, Hackett C, Andreyev HJ. The clinical needs of patients with chronic gastrointestinal symptoms after pelvic radiotherapy. Aliment Pharmacol Ther 2007; 26(4): 555-63.
[http://dx.doi.org/10.1111/j.1365-2036.2007.03405.x] [PMID: 17661759]

[67] Francois A, Milliat F, Guipaud O, Benderitter M. Inflammation and immunity in radiation damage to the gut mucosa. Bio Med Res Int 2013; 2013: 123241.
[http://dx.doi.org/10.1155/2013/123241] [PMID: 23586015]

[68] Andreyev HJ, Wotherspoon A, Denham JW, Hauer-Jensen M. Defining pelvic-radiation disease for the survivorship era. Lancet Oncol 2010; 11(4): 310-2.
[http://dx.doi.org/10.1016/S1470-2045(10)70026-7] [PMID: 20149738]

[69] Hoggan BL, Cameron AL. Systematic review of hyperbaric oxygen therapy for the treatment of non-neurological soft tissue radiation-related injuries. Support Care Cancer 2014; 22(6): 1715-26.
[http://dx.doi.org/10.1007/s00520-014-2198-z] [PMID: 24794980]

[70] Mallick S, Madan R, Julka PK, Rath GK. Radiation induced cystitis and proctitis - prediction, assessment and management. Asian Pac J Cancer Prev 2015; 16(14): 5589-94.
[http://dx.doi.org/10.7314/APJCP.2015.16.14.5589] [PMID: 26320421]

[71] Ghorbanzadeh-Moghaddam A, Gholamrezaei A, Hemati S. Vitamin D deficiency is associated with

the severity of radiation-induced proctitis in cancer patients. Int J Radiat Oncol Biol Phys 2015; 92(3): 613-8.
[http://dx.doi.org/10.1016/j.ijrobp.2015.02.011] [PMID: 25890844]

[72] Kim SH, Kim JH, Jung SH. Late complications after proctectomy in rectal cancer patients who underwent radiotherapy. World J Surg 2014; 38(9): 2471-6.
[http://dx.doi.org/10.1007/s00268-014-2577-0] [PMID: 24791668]

[73] Urban ML, Palmisano A, Nicastro M, Corradi D, Buzio C, Vaglio A. Idiopathic and secondary forms of retroperitoneal fibrosis: a diagnostic approach. Rev Med Interne 2015; 36(1): 15-21.
[http://dx.doi.org/10.1016/j.revmed.2014.10.008] [PMID: 25455951]

[74] Khezri A, Berman HL, Rosenstein ED, Kramer N. Spontaneous resolution of apparent radiation associated retroperitoneal fibrosis. J Clin Rheumatol 2011; 17(8): 436-8.
[http://dx.doi.org/10.1097/RHU.0b013e31823a4e54] [PMID: 22089993]

[75] Cheng J, Pei HH, Sun J, Xie QX, Li JB. Radiation-induced hepatitis B virus reactivation in hepatocellular carcinoma: A case report. Oncol Lett 2015; 10(5): 3213-5.
[PMID: 26722314]

[76] Thompson A, Adamson A, Bahl A, *et al.* Guidelines for the diagnosis, prevention and management of chemical- and radiation-induced cystitis. J Clin Urol 2014; 7: 25-35.
[http://dx.doi.org/10.1177/2051415813512647]

[77] Dave CN, Chaus F, Chancellor MB, Lajness M, Peters KM. Innovative use of intravesical tacrolimus for hemorrhagic radiation cystitis. Int Urol Nephrol 2015; 47(10): 1679-81.
[http://dx.doi.org/10.1007/s11255-015-1098-6] [PMID: 26347076]

[78] Hampel C, Neisius A, Thomas C, Thüroff JW, Roos F. [Vesicovaginal fistula. Incidence, etiology and phenomenology in Germany]. Urologe A 2015; 54(3): 349-58.
[http://dx.doi.org/10.1007/s00120-014-3679-x] [PMID: 25784445]

[79] Rodriguez-Wallberg KA, Karlström PO, Rezapour M, *et al.* Full-term newborn after repeated ovarian tissue transplants in a patient treated for Ewing sarcoma by sterilizing pelvic irradiation and chemotherapy. Acta Obstet Gynecol Scand 2015; 94(3): 324-8.
[http://dx.doi.org/10.1111/aogs.12568] [PMID: 25545009]

[80] Xing ZW, Jiang EH, Du JY, *et al.* Long-term follow-up of the genital organs and eye lenses in three cases of acute radiation sickness from a 60Co radiation accident in China. Health Phys 2015; 108(1): 1-7.
[http://dx.doi.org/10.1097/HP.0000000000000163] [PMID: 25437514]

[81] Arrivé L, Chang YC, Hricak H, Brescia RJ, Auffermann W, Quivey JM. Radiation-induced uterine changes: MR imaging. Radiology 1989; 170(1 Pt 1): 55-8.
[http://dx.doi.org/10.1148/radiology.170.1.2909120] [PMID: 2909120]

[82] Geng C, Moteabbed M, Seco J, *et al.* Dose assessment for the fetus considering scattered and secondary radiation from photon and proton therapy when treating a brain tumor of the mother. Phys Med Biol 2016; 61(2): 683-95.
[http://dx.doi.org/10.1088/0031-9155/61/2/683] [PMID: 26716718]

[83] Zur M, Shai A, Leviov M, *et al.* Short-term complications of intra-operative radiotherapy for early breast cancer. J Surg Oncol 2016; 113(4): 370-3.
[http://dx.doi.org/10.1002/jso.24157] [PMID: 26751138]

[84] Incrocci L, Hop WC, Wijnmaalen A, Slob AK. Treatment outcome, body image, and sexual functioning after orchiectomy and radiotherapy for Stage I-II testicular seminoma. Int J Radiat Oncol Biol Phys 2002; 53(5): 1165-73.
[http://dx.doi.org/10.1016/S0360-3016(02)02849-3] [PMID: 12128117]

[85] Magli A, Giangreco M, Crespi M, *et al.* Erectile dysfunction after prostate three-dimensional conformal radiation therapy. Correlation with the dose to the penile bulb. Strahlenther Onkol 2012;

188(11): 997-1002.
[http://dx.doi.org/10.1007/s00066-012-0227-8] [PMID: 23053160]

[86] Darzy KH. Radiation-induced hypopituitarism. Curr Opin Endocrinol Diabetes Obes 2013; 20(4): 342-53.
[http://dx.doi.org/10.1097/MED.0b013e3283631820] [PMID: 23807607]

[87] Leong N, Pai H, Morris WJ, *et al.* Rectal ulcers and recto-prostatic fistulas following I-125 low dose rate prostate brachytherapy. J Urol 2016; pii:S0022-5347(16)00034-3.

[88] Bolan PJ, Arentsen L, Sueblinvong T, *et al.* Water-fat MRI for assessing changes in bone marrow composition due to radiation and chemotherapy in gynecologic cancer patients. J Magn Reson Imaging 2013; 38(6): 1578-84.
[http://dx.doi.org/10.1002/jmri.24071] [PMID: 23450703]

[89] Zou Q, Hong W, Zhou Y, *et al.* Bone marrow stem cell dysfunction in radiation-induced abscopal bone loss. J Orthop Surg 2016; 11: 3.
[http://dx.doi.org/10.1186/s13018-015-0339-9] [PMID: 26739584]

[90] Moravan MJ, Olschowka JA, Williams JP, OBanion MK. Brain radiation injury leads to a dose- and time-dependent recruitment of peripheral myeloid cells that depends on CCR2 signaling. J Neuroinflamm 2016; 13: 30.
[http://dx.doi.org/10.1186/s12974-016-0496-8] [PMID: 26842770]

[91] Trip AK, Sikorska K, van Sandick JW, *et al.* Radiation-induced dose-dependent changes of the spleen following postoperative chemoradiotherapy for gastric cancer. Radiother Oncol 2015; 116(2): 239-44.
[http://dx.doi.org/10.1016/j.radonc.2015.07.036] [PMID: 26253953]

[92] Dalinka MK, Haygood TM. Radiation changes. In: Resnick D, Ed. Diagnosis of Bone and Joint Disorders. Philadelphia, Pa: Saunders 1995; pp. 3276-308.

[93] Howland WJ, Loeffler RK, Starchman DE, Johnson RG. Postirradiation atrophic changes of bone and related complications. Radiology 1975; 117(3 Pt 1): 677-85.
[http://dx.doi.org/10.1148/117.3.677] [PMID: 1188119]

[94] Paling MR, Herdt JR. Radiation osteitis: a problem of recognition. Radiology 1980; 137(2): 339-42.
[http://dx.doi.org/10.1148/radiology.137.2.7433664] [PMID: 7433664]

[95] Dawson WB. Growth impairment following radiotherapy in childhood. Clin Radiol 1968; 19(3): 241-56.
[http://dx.doi.org/10.1016/S0009-9260(68)80001-7] [PMID: 5677640]

[96] Farzin M, Molls M, Kampfer S, *et al.* Optic toxicity in radiation treatment of meningioma: a retrospective study in 213 patients. J Neurooncol 2016; 127(3): 597-606.
[http://dx.doi.org/10.1007/s11060-016-2071-7] [PMID: 26852221]

[97] Sychev YV, McInnis CP, Francis CE. Abducens ocular neuromyotonia as a delayed complication of oropharyngeal carcinoma treated with radiation. Head Neck 2016; 38 (Suppl. 1): E2428-31.
[http://dx.doi.org/10.1002/hed.24370] [PMID: 26836222]

[98] Yock TI, Yeap BY, Ebb DH, *et al.* Long-term toxic effects of proton radiotherapy for paediatric medulloblastoma: a phase 2 single-arm study. Lancet Oncol 2016; 17(3): 287-98.
[http://dx.doi.org/10.1007/s11060-016-2071-7] [PMID: 26830377]

[99] Trifiletti DM, Lee CC, Schlesinger D, Larner JM, Xu Z, Sheehan JP. Leukoencephalopathy after stereotactic radiosurgery for brain metastases. Int J Radiat Oncol Biol Phys 2015; 93(4): 870-8.
[http://dx.doi.org/10.1016/j.ijrobp.2015.07.2280] [PMID: 26530756]

[100] Lee LY, Chen SC, Chen WC, Huang BS, Lin CY. Postradiation trismus and its impact on quality of life in patients with head and neck cancer. Oral Surg Oral Med Oral Pathol Oral Radiol 2015; 119(2): 187-95.
[http://dx.doi.org/10.1016/j.oooo.2014.10.003] [PMID: 25487985]

CHAPTER 3

Iatrogenic Immunopathology

Ioan Jung and **Simona Gurzu***

Department of Pathology, University of Medicine and Pharmacy, Tirgu-Mures, Romania

Abstract: This chapter covers the general aspects regarding the mechanisms of the four specific branches of iatrogenic immunopathology: iatrogenic immunodeficiencies, iatrogenic-induced lymphoproliferative diseases, hypersensitivity-induced lesions and immunopathology of transplantation. Understanding the four types of hypersensitivity reactions is mandatory for understanding the details of drug-induced lesions in organs. Mechanisms and complications of transplantation of solid organs are shown in detail.

Keywords: Adverse drug reaction, Bone marrow, Graft-versus-host disease, Host-versus-graft disease, Hypersensitivity reactions, Iatrogenic, Immunopathology, Lymphoid tissue, Lymphoproliferative disease, Rejection, Transplant.

INTRODUCTION

Iatrogenic immunopathology refers to four types of lesions: iatrogenic immunodeficiencies, iatrogenic-induced lymphoproliferative diseases, hypersensitivity-induced lesions and immunopathology of transplantation.

IATROGENIC IMMUNODEFICIENCIES

These lesions can be caused by medications, irradiation, splenectomy, surgical interventions or iatrogenic viral infections.

Drug-Induced Immunosuppression

Of all medical drugs, cytotoxic substances, steroids and immunomodulators are best known for inducing immunosuppression. Details of drug-induced bone marrow suppression are presented in Chapter 12.

Cytotoxic Drugs, which are prescribed in oncotherapy and to patients with autoimmune diseases, first attack cells with rapid turnover (bone marrow cells,

* **Corresponding author Simona Gurzu:** Department of Pathology, University of Medicine and Pharmacy, Tirgu-Mures, Romania; Tel: 0040-745-673550; Fax: 0040-372-653250; E-mail: simonagurzu@yahoo.com

lymphoid tissue, hair follicles, *etc.*) and immunocompetent cells. Then, a decrease of the immunoglobulin synthesis rate is followed by immunodeficiency. Usually, T-cells are more resistant than B-cells. B-cell-related humoral response is abolished in early phases, followed by a decrease of T-cells-associated cellular immunity [1].

Corticosteroids are frequently used in clinical practice due to their rapid anti-inflammatory and immunosuppressive effects. They cause a decrease in the number of T-cells and, in direct contrast to cytotoxic drugs, cellular immunity is suppressed to a greater extent than is the humoral response. Immunoglobulin (Ig) synthesis is also inhibited [1].

Immunosuppressive Therapy which is especially used in transplanted recipients and patients with autoimmune disorders (*e.g.,* rheumatoid arthritis, systemic lupus erythematosus), is known to induce immunodeficiency. Primarily related to T-cells, the risk of Epstein-Barr virus (EBV) infection is increased in these patients [2, 3]. The *anti-lymphocyte serum* decreases cellular immunity and can induce anaphylaxis and/or serum sickness. *Cyclosporine* has a direct renal and hepatotoxic effect. *Calcineurin inhibitors* promote infection with oncogenic viruses, such as human papilloma virus (HPV) and herpes human virus 8 (HHV8), or exert a direct oncogenic effect. In some cases, development of lymphoproliferative disorders and tumors, such as skin cancer or Kaposi's sarcoma, were reported (*e.g.,* at two months after the initiation of immunosuppressive therapy for Wegener's granulomatosis) [4 - 6]. *Mycophenolate mofetil*, used in patients undergoing solid organ or bone marrow transplantation, can induce GI lesions in the first six months after therapy begins. Side effects include nausea, vomiting, erosions/ulcers, inflammatory bowel disease (IBD)-like disorders, colitis, abdominal pain and diarrhea. It is not nephrotoxic, like cyclosporine and tacrolimus, does not cause hyperlipidemia, as sirolimus does, and induces leukopenia less frequently than does azathioprine [7].

Radiation-Induced Immunodeficiency

Similar to the case of immunosuppressive drugs, the most radiosensitive tissues are those with high turnover, including bone marrow and lymphoid tissues, especially after irradiation of the lymph nodes (*e.g.,* Hodgkin's lymphoma). A second tumor can occur early or very late following radiotherapy (*e.g.,* sarcoma after radiotherapy for oral squamous cell carcinoma arising 16 months after completion of radiotherapy) [1, 8]. Details of radiotherapy-induced lesions are presented in Chapter 2.

Post-Splenectomy Immunodeficiency

Splenectomy is a contributing factor to infections, the most commonly involved agents being pyogenic cocci (*e.g., Streptococcus pneumoniae*) and Gram-negative bacteria. The risk of infection is higher in younger patients and those with disorders of the monocyte-macrophage system. The median time for developing an infection is about six months, ranging from one month to 50 years after splenectomy. A severe complication of patients with asplenia is progressive septicemia with fulminant and even fatal evolution. Purpura fulminans may be associated [1, 9].

Postoperative Immunodeficiency

For invasive or minimally invasive surgical techniques, the risk of postoperative fistulae, abscess formation, secondary peritonitis or sepsis should be taken into account, even in the era of modern medicine [10]. A report from 2016 revealed that, after percutaneous cholecystectomy, the risk of postoperative abscess was about 23% and the 30-day mortality rate was 9% [11]. Even following hernia repair, the risk of mesh infection remains because the foreign material acts as a biofilm and encourages bacteria proliferation [12].

Iatrogenic Viral Infection

Although rare today, infection with HIV, hepatitis viruses (HCV, HBV) or human T-cell lymphotropic virus 1 (HTLV-1) can be transmitted through blood transfusions and other parenteral exposure, or by using improperly sterilized medical equipment. In epidemic areas, the main risk factors are intramuscular/intravenous injections and contaminated blood, transplanted organs or medical and dental instruments [13 - 15].

IATROGENIC LYMPHOPROLIFERATIVE DISORDERS

These disorders can occur in transplant recipients but immunosuppressant therapy (cyclosporine, methotrexate, corticosteroids, tacrolimus, infliximab, azathioprine, calcineurin inhibitors, *etc.*) can also induce lymphoproliferative diseases [3, 5, 6]. A large range of lesions, from lymphoid hyperplasia to atypical lymphoproliferative disorders and malignant lymphomas, can be considered as iatrogenic disorders [1].

The lymph nodes, spleen and/or bone marrow can be affected and EBV infection can be involved. Post-transplant lymphoproliferative disease is a distinct lesion that is described below in the sub-chapter about transplantation, together with the EBV-related pathomechanism of its development [2].

The Society for Hematopathology classifies lymphoproliferative disorders according to five groups [1, 3, 16]:

Early Lesions: reactive plasma cells hyperplasia, infectious mononucleosis-like lymphohistiocytic hyperplasia, *etc*.

Polymorphic Lymphoproliferative Disorders: Monoclonal or polyclonal lesions.

Monomorphic Lymphoproliferative Disorders: B- and T-cell non-Hodgkin's lymphomas, such as large B-cell lymphomas (immunoblastic, centroblastic and anaplastic lymphoma), Burkitt's/Burkitt's-like lymphoma, T-cell lymphomas (large T-cell anaplastic lymphoma and peripheral T-cell lymphoma) and NK-cell lymphoma.

Plasmacytoma-Like Lesions: plasmacytoid lymphoma and multiple myeloma.

T-Cell-Rich Large B-Cell Lymphoma/Hodgkin's Disease-Like Lesions.

HYPERSENSITIVITY-INDUCED LESIONS

Type I Immediate Hypersensitivity or Anaphylactic Reaction

This is an IgE-mediated dose-independent ADR that can induce systemic or localized disorders.

Systemic Reactions refer to drug-induced anaphylactic shock. Several drugs present anaphylactic properties, including serum, vaccines, enzymes (*e.g.*, L-asparaginase), hormones, antibiotics (*e.g.*, penicillin), sulfonamides, local anesthetics, salicylates, polysaccharides, contrast substances, bromsulphthalein, *etc*. Immunoallergic complications have recently been reported regarding fluindione, a vitamin K antagonist with a prolonged half-life. Clinically, bronchoconstriction, glottic edema, hypotension and collapse are characteristic [1, 17, 18].

Localized Reactions refer to cutaneous atopic lesions, such as contact dermatitis, eczema/urticaria, atopic asthma, allergic conjunctivitis, Quincke's edema, *etc*. Iatrogenic asthma can be induced by several drugs, including adrenergic aerosols, aspirin, angiotensin-converting enzyme (ACE) inhibitors and non-steroidal anti-inflammatory drugs (NSAIDs), such as indomethacin or mefenamic acid, tetrazines, *etc*. Angioedema is produced through a bradykinin-mediated or, more rarely, a histamine-related reaction. Urticaria and Quincke's edema occur independently or as components of anaphylactic shock. Allergic contact dermatitis can be induced by gels, creams, latex, *etc*. [1, 17, 19 - 21].

Type II Hypersensitivity or Cytotoxic Reaction

This type of hypersensitivity is IgG- or IgM-mediated and is characterized by binding of the antibodies (*e.g.,* drugs) to the cell membrane. As a consequence, the cell is destroyed by activating complement or promoting phagocytosis. B-cel--related humoral immunity is most strongly affected. The following iatrogenic lesions can be induced: incompatible blood transfusion (hemolysis, hemolytic anemia), iatrogenic lupus, post-vaccination inflammations, autoimmune disorders, *etc.* [1, 17]. Cytotoxic reactions to injected drugs, such as NSAIDs, can induce cutaneous vasculitis and/or necrosis [22].

Type III Hypersensitivity or Immune Complex-Mediated Reaction

This type of hypersensitivity is IgG-mediated and is characterized by the formation of immune complexes (antigen-antibody) within the blood flow. These complexes are stored within the vascular walls or basal membranes, inducing autoimmune lesions like vasculitis, glomerulonephritis, *etc.* It is a dose-independent ADR that can induce systemic or localized reactions.

Systemic Reactions include serum sickness, vasculitis and glomerulonephritis. Serum sickness occurs at about 10 days after passive immunization and is characterized by urticaria, arthralgia, vasculitis and, infrequently, glomerulonephritis. Iatrogenic-induced glomerulonephritis is primarily a chronic autoimmune disorder that can occur in patients with humoral immunity deficiencies. NSAIDs-related immune-mediated aseptic meningitis can also emerge [1, 17, 23].

Localized Reactions are primarily the Arthus reaction, which is an immune-mediated localized vasculitis characterized by necrosis of the skin or subcutaneous tissue that occurs between six and 24 hours after injection of a serum recognized by the human body [1, 17].

Type IV or Delayed Hypersensitivity Reaction

This type of hypersensitivity is mediated by CD4 and/or CD8 T-lymphocytes and their products (interleukin-2, interferon-gamma, cytokines, *etc.*). This reaction can cause delayed contact dermatitis (contact hypersensitivity), vaccine-associated granulomatous inflammation and transplant rejection [1, 17, 21, 24].

In cutaneous processes, the delayed hypersensitivity reaction is developed in two phases: sensitization and elicitation. In the first phase, the antigen-specific effector T-cells are induced in the draining lymph nodes by antigen-captured cutaneous dendritic cells that migrate from the skin. In the second phase, the dendritic cells activate the effector T-cells, inducing an antigen-specific inflammation [24].

An example of this type IV reaction is the Mantoux test, also known as the tuberculin reaction. Intradermal injection of tuberculin is followed by the T-cel--mediated occurrence of localized cutaneous erythema, between 24 and 72 hours after injection. Under the microscope, perivascular lymphohistiocytic infiltrate is characteristic. This is usually a self-limited process, but epithelioid granulomas can occur at several weeks after injection [1, 17].

Latex-related contact dermatitis is difficult to differentiate from "latex allergy", but this differentiation is essential for its treatment [21, 24]. Regarding the pathomechanism of allergic diseases in the genital area, type IV reactions, such as contact dermatitis, are more common than type I allergies [25].

Besides vaccines, several other drugs can interact with immune receptors, inducing delayed sensitivity through T-cell stimulation. The clinical features are generalized maculopapular reactions with identification of CD4 positive cytotoxic T-cells in the epidermis. In some cases, severe cutaneous syndromes can be induced [26]. Details of cutaneous ADRs (CU-ADRs) are presented in Chapter 13.

IMMUNOPATHOLOGY OF TRANSPLANTATION

Before discussing the iatrogenic aspects of transplantation, it is worth mentioning some specific ***definitions*** [27, 28]:

Donor = a person who is used as a source of biological material (blood, tissue or organ).

Recipient = a person who receives biological material.

Graft = human tissue/organ used for transplantation.

Transplantation = transfer of tissue from one part of the body to another, or from a donor to a recipient.

Autotransplantation (autograft, autoplasty, autologous graft) = transplantation of tissue from one part of an individual to another of the same individual (*e.g.,* skin, bone).

Isogenic/syngeneic transplantation = tissue/organ transplantation between genetically identic (syngeneic) persons (*e.g.,* uniovular twins).

Allotransplantation/homotransplantation (allograft, homograft) = transplant of an organ or tissue between genetically different members of the same species (including *cadaveric donor transplantation*).

Xenotransplantation/heterotransplantation (xenograft, heterograft) = transplant between two different species (from an animal to a human being).

Rejection = an immune-mediated response of the human recipient, whereby the graft is attacked by the immune system components of the recipient. Autotransplantation and isogenic transplantation usually present good tolerance, while graft rejection is more common in cases of homotransplantation and xenotransplantation.

Host-versus-graft disease = graft rejection as a result of the immune cells of the recipient attacking the donor's organ. This is more common following solid organ transplantation.

Graft-versus-host disease = attack of the host's tissues by the sensitized lymphocytes of the donor tissue. This is more common in immunosuppressive patients and following bone marrow transplantation.

Harvest injury of the graft = ischemia-related graft injury occurring between the time of removal of the organ from the donor and the cooling process.

Mechanisms of Graft Tolerance – General Data

The *major histocompatibility antigen* complex, also known as *human leukocyte antigen (HLA) genes,* is responsible for the tolerance or rejection of the allograft and xenograft. The HLAs are proteins located on bone marrow cells that initiate the onset of the immune response. Regarding the lymphocytes, T-cells are involved in the process of transplantation and B-cells, especially plasma cell synthesized antibodies, are their close immune partners. To ensure good tolerance, it is necessary to match the HLA genes of the donor and the recipient. Lack of immunologic similarity can induce a T-cell-mediated (or, more rarely, a B-cell antibodies-mediated) acute or chronic rejection. Besides proper donor selection, rejection can be avoided by using immunosuppressive drugs and/or anti-lymphocyte serum. The graft tolerance rate is approximately 85% for the kidney and heart, 75% for the liver and 70% for the lung and pancreas. Host-*versus*-graft and graft-*versus*-host diseases are well understood based on the mechanisms involved in graft rejection [1, 29, 30].

Host-*Versus*-Graft Disease

This disease is most commonly involved in the transplantation of solid organs, such as the heart, kidney, liver, lung and pancreas. The classification of the rejection depends on its timing [1, 31]:

Hyperacute Rejection occurs within the first two to three days following transplantation and is the result of rapid synthesis of anti-graft antibodies. Both T- and B-cells are involved in this rejection.

Acute Cellular (Antibody-Mediated) Rejection occurs in the first two to three months following transplantation and is a T-cell-mediated rejection. The bioptic specimens reveal a rich inflammatory infiltrate within graft parenchyma that is predominantly represented by the CD8 positive suppressor T-lymphocytes. The risk of rejection depends on the amount of inflammatory infiltrate and the size of the graft injured areas. Immunosuppressive drugs can successfully decrease the risk of rejection.

Acute Vascular Rejection occurs in first two to three months following transplantation and is mediated by both T- and B-cells. It is characterized by vascular lesions. Under the microscope, a stepwise evolution is seen: endothelial swelling is followed by accumulation of inflammatory infiltrate. It is first subendothelially located and then presents intramural and transmural disposition. The arteritis-like lesions can be complicated by the formation of hyaline thrombi and, finally, intimal cell proliferation and fibrinoid necrosis. These vascular injuries cannot be cured using immunosuppressive drugs.

Chronic Rejection is the final step of cellular/vascular rejection and occurs between one and two years following transplantation. It is mediated by both T- and B-cells. This type of rejection is observed in patients whose acute antibody-mediated rejection was suppressed using immunosuppressive drugs, allowing the patient to survive for a period of time but, later, intraparenchymatous fibrosis or fibrosis of the vascular wall with further ischemia emerges.

Graft-*Versus*-Host Disease

This disease is most commonly involved in bone marrow transplantation, but can also occur in lung transplant recipients. The main risk factor is the immunosuppressive status of the recipient. In these patients, the immune attack of the donor's cells against the host induces severe clinical symptoms, such as fever, weight loss, maculopapular and/or erythematous cutaneous eruptions, hepatosplenomegaly, anemia, diarrhea and bronchiolitis obliterans in children. It is a life-threatening condition that can sometimes be cured with immunosuppressive drugs [1, 32].

Post-Transplant Lymphoproliferative Disease

This is a potentially lethal complication, with a 50% mortality rate, that can emerge after solid organ (usually heart or lung) or bone marrow transplantation. It occurs in approximately 10% of recipients and can lead to EBV infection. In normal conditions, EBV is stored in circulating B-lymphocytes and is controlled by EBV-specific cytotoxic T-lymphocytes with a role in preserving immunity. Post-transplantation, immunosuppressive drugs decrease the number of T-cells and can induce abnormal proliferation of EBV-infected B-cells, leading to tumorigenesis. Infusion of *ex vivo* T-cells has been recommended for such patients [2].

Heart Transplant-Related Lesions

Before transplantation, graft survival is estimated based on a risk score assigned to the recipient and the donor. For the recipient, a shorter survival time is predicted when body mass index (BMI) is higher than 30, mean pulmonary artery pressure is higher than 30, serum creatinine levels are higher than 1.5 mg/dL, bilirubin levels are greater than 1.5 mg/dL and when a non-continuous flow left ventricle assist device is used. For the donor, graft survival time is predicted on the basis of age and whether a period of ischemia exceeds four hours [33].

Post-transplantation, correct postoperative care includes multiple ECGs, clinical and biochemical evaluation, and periodic endomyocardial biopsies: weekly for the first four weeks, biweekly for the next four weeks, monthly for the next six months, and then every other month for one year [31]. The following iatrogenic lesions may be encountered [1]:

Harvest Injuries or Perioperative Ischemic Myocyte Injuries refer to ischemia-related disorders of myocytes, without the presence of inflammatory infiltrate. This is primarily a transient functional disorder but, in severe and/or long-term ischemia, graft survival can be impacted [31].

Hyperacute Rejection is microscopically characterized by the presence of intraparenchymatous inflammatory infiltrate and vascular lesions: hemorrhages and infrequent microthrombi formation.

Acute Cellular Rejection is the most common type of heart rejection. It is graded according to the criteria of the International Society for Heart and Lung Transplantation. Interstitial myocarditis is the predominant lesion. Upon biopsy, the severity of the coagulative myocyte necrosis is graded as 0 (absent), 1 (mild-focal), 2 (moderate) or 3 (severe-confluent). This grading system is correlated with short-term survival, but not with the rate of one-year post-transplantation survival [31].

Acute Vascular Rejection is very rarely seen. The vascular changes include endothelial swelling, endothelial cells leukocyte adhesion, thrombosis and vasculitis [31].

Chronic Rejection is characterized by coronary sclerosis and/or interstitial myocardial fibrosis. Subendocardial inflammatory infiltrate, with a "sheet-like" arrangement, is one of the regular findings in such cases. The most recent experimental studies have proven that cannabidiol, a non-psychoactive constituent of marijuana with anti-inflammatory properties, could limit the severity of T-cel--mediated chronic autoimmune interstitial myocarditis [34].

Postoperative Multisystem Organ Failure (MSOF) is a complication that can emerge a short time after any complex surgical procedure. The main clinical symptoms/disorders are acute pancreatitis with jaundice (Fig. **3-1**) and septic shock.

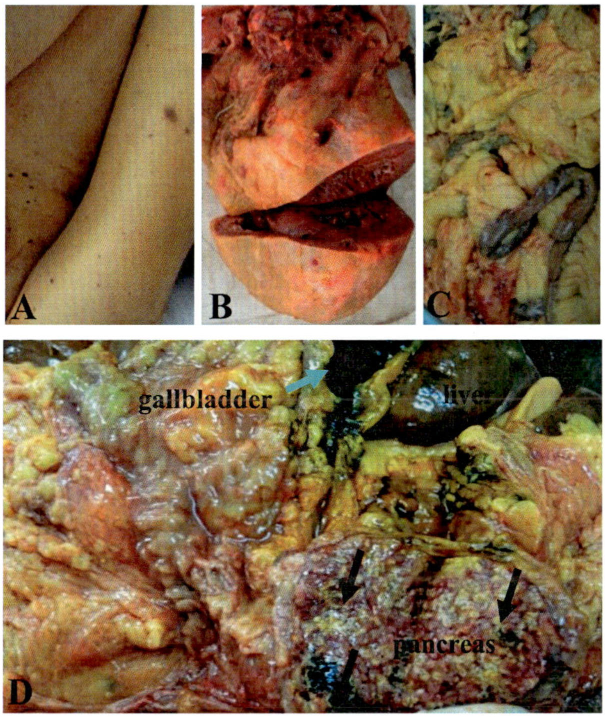

Fig. (3-1). In a patient who died in the first week following heart transplantation, generalized jaundice is seen on the skin (A) and internal organs (B-D). Heart (B), mesenterium (C, D) and liver (D) are impregnated with bilirubin and the bile is black-green stained (D). The patient died as a result of a postoperative MSOF involving fulminant acute pancreatitis (arrows) with hemorrhagic and areas of steatonecrosis (D).

Opportunistic Infections such as toxoplasma-induced myocarditis, can be a post-transplant complication as a result of immunosuppression. Infections with methicillin-resistant *Staphylococcus aureus*, cytomegalovirus (CMV), Nocardia and fungi, such as Blastomyces dermatitidis, have also been reported [1, 35].

Malignancies should be taken into account regarding heart transplant recipients. In the first 10 years following transplantation, a malignant tumor is developed in approximately 39% of recipients. Skin cancer and lymphoproliferative disorders are more commonly found in children, while lymphoma and HCC (Fig. **3-2**) are more common in adult recipients. Other malignant tumors, such as lung cancer, bladder and prostate carcinoma and carcinomas of the oral cavity and GI tract, can also occur [1, 36].

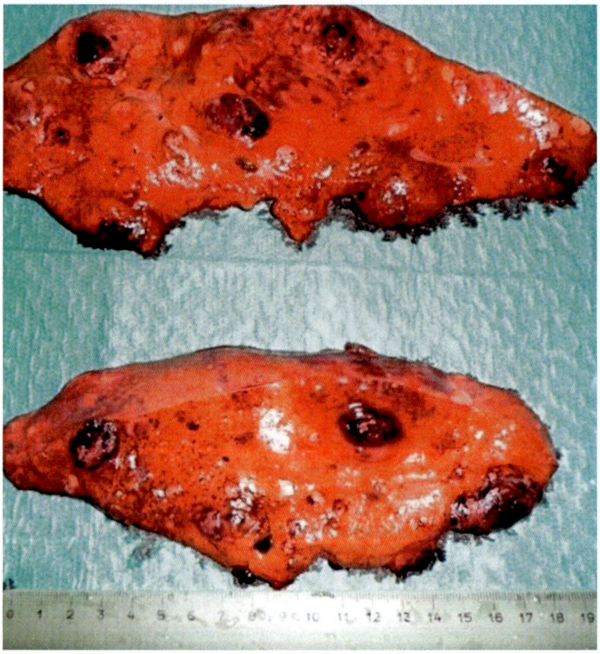

Fig. (3-2). Multicentric HCC in a heart transplant recipient.

Kidney Transplant-Related Lesions

The success of renal transplantation depends on donor-specific antibodies against HLA that strongly influence the hyper acute and acute cellular rejection rate. To avoid this inconvenience, desensitization using immune globulin and rituximab or bortezomib (a proteasome inhibitor that depletes plasma cells) are proposed. Although the five-year graft survival rate for renal transplantation is greater than 90%, graft rejections still occur, with the following particularities [1, 6, 30, 37 - 40]:

Harvest Injuries refer to ischemia-related renal tube disorders. These involve tubular dilation and dystrophic lesions of the epithelium lining. The main consequences are functional disorders, both with and without anuria and hypo-anuria. Transient tube injuries are seen in 50% of patients and prolonged anuria occurs in one third of these. In such cases, the status of the donor or preexistent lesions of the host (infections, tubular necrosis, thrombotic microangiopathy, *etc.*) are responsible for harvest injuries.

Hyperacute Rejection is microscopically characterized by intraparenchymatous inflammatory infiltrate, hemorrhages and vascular thrombi.

Acute Cellular (Tubulointerstitial) Rejection is the most common type of renal rejection. The renal tubes are more affected than are the glomeruli. The rate of acute cellular rejection is higher in patients receiving desensitization therapy for donor-specific antibodies (9% *versus* 5% in non-desensitized patients).

Acute Vascular Rejection is characterized by intimal or transmural arteritis with subsequent renal ischemia. Both cellular and humoral immune mechanisms are involved. The lesions do not usually respond to glucocorticoid pulse therapy. Anti-CD3 (muromonab) and anti-CD20 (rituximab) antibodies, OKT3 and anti-thymocyte globulin show better results. The severity of acute vascular rejection is greater than that of cellular rejection, especially in cases involving fibrinoid necrosis of the vascular wall. The one-year graft survival rate is approximately 75-87% in the absence of graft rejection or presence of acute cellular rejection, 58-65% in cases of vascular rejection with endarteritis, and only 1% in associated fibrinoid necrosis. The corresponding five-year survival rates are 73% (no rejection), 71% (acute cellular rejection) and 34% (vascular rejection).

Chronic Rejection is a severe lesion responsible for renal failure in fewer than 8% of transplanted patients. The interstitium, renal tubes and glomeruli are affected and large fibrotic areas are seen under the microscope.

Opportunistic Infections such as polyoma virus-associated nephropathy (nephritis) and visceral leishmaniasis, can be a post-transplant complication resulting from immunosuppression. Chronic urinary infections are detected in more than 13% of recipients.

Malignancies are an important post-transplant cause of mortality. In Asian countries, urothelial carcinoma is the most common type of malignant tumor following renal transplant, occurring at a median interval of 17-20 months after transplantation. The incidence of urothelial carcinoma is 3.0% after three years of graft survival, increasing to 7.2% at six years and 17.5% at 10 years. In Western countries, non-melanoma skin cancer and lymphoproliferative disorders are more common. These differences could be the result of using aristolochic acid-rich Chinese herbal medications, seemingly increasing the risk of urothelial carcinoma. However, this risk is also increased by the use of analgesics or calcineurin inhibitors, and is higher in females and elderly patients. The incidence of viral-related malignancies, such as HHV8-induced Kaposi's sarcoma and HPV-induced cancer (cervical, anal, vulvar, vaginal, penile, head and neck), is also increased [37].

Liver Transplant-Related Lesions

In patients undergoing hepatic transplantation, improper suture for hepatic artery anastomosis can lead to hepatic artery thrombosis and hyperacute rejection in 5% of cases [41]. Early biliary complications occur in 10-37% of patients, relating to anastomotic/non-anastomotic strictures, bile leak, biliary drain complications, papillary dysfunctions/stenosis, ischemic type biliary lesions and a mortality rate of 2-7% [42].

Acute cellular rejection is the most prevalent type of graft rejection. Under the microscope, periportal inflammation is predominant. *Acute vascular rejection* is rare and can display hemorrhagic necrosis. ***Chronic rejection*** is also rare and is characterized by progressive cholestasis [1].

Several ***other lesions*** can occur, such as recurrent hepatitis, functional cholestasis, stenosis of the inferior cava vein (Budd-Chiari syndrome), ascites, *etc.* In patients with pre-transplant hepatitis, the risk of recurrent or de novo hepatitis in the hepatic draft should be attentively estimated, especially in patients with high levels of serum hepatitis antigens [1].

The risk of candidemia is higher in abdominal organ than in thoracic organ transplantation. Viruses, such as CMV and EBV, and multidrug-resistant Gram-negative pathogens, such as beta lactamase-producing Enterobacteriaceae and carbapenem-resistant Klebsiella pneumoniae, can be responsible for post-transplant infections [43]. Invasive Aspergillus infections occur in 5-42% of liver transplant recipients [44].

In patients receiving liver or renal transplantation, post-transplant immuno-suppression can induce cutaneous disorders, such as infections and risk of *malignant lesions* [45]. The risk of lymphoproliferative disorders and skin cancer following a liver transplant is 10 to 30 times higher than that of the general population, while the risk of colorectal cancer is 2.5 times higher. Other solid tumors, such as HHV8-related Kaposi's sarcoma (especially in endemic areas, such as Italy and Saudi Arabia) and HPV-related cervical cancer, can occur at a median interval of six years after transplantation. Increased risk of kidney, pancreatic, breast, prostate and brain cancer has not been proven [6, 46].

Lifelong immunosuppression increases the risk of post-transplant metabolic alterations. Dyslipidemia, high atherogenic risk and changes in carbohydrate metabolism have been reported in patients receiving mammalian target of rapamycin (mTOR) inhibitors, anti-calcineurins and/or corticosteroids [6, 47].

Food allergies can arise following solid organs transplantation, especially in liver recipients, but can also be a complication for heart, lung, kidney or intestine transplants. Children are more predisposed than adults to developing this post-transplant complication [48].

Lung Transplant-Related Lesions

The main risk, in the case of lung transplantation, is that of early infections. ***Opportunistic infections*** with CMV, herpes virus (HV) or Pneumocystis carinii can be responsible for the emergence of interstitial pneumonia. Post-transplant aspergillosis can also be detected, sometimes with a tumor-like aspect, during chest radiographic examination (aspergilloma) [49].

Other post-transplant complications are pneumothorax in the native lung, chylothorax and ascites [50]. In children, bronchiolitis obliterans can emerge as an indicator of a possible graft-*versus*-host immune response. This is known as *bronchiolitis obliterans syndrome* and is characterized by functional pulmonary changes that do not require histological confirmation. Forced expiratory volume (FEV) and forced expiratory flow (FEF) are, respectively, 10-19% and 25% decreased from the baseline [32].

Acute cellular rejection is microscopically characterized by the presence of rich inflammatory infiltrate within the alveolar septa and perivascular areas, along with associated bronchitis/bronchiolitis. Hemorrhages, necrosis and hyaline membranes (ARDS) occur in severe forms of acute rejection. Acute vascular rejection is rare. In children, the reported post-transplant survival rate is 96.6%, 93.1% and 82.8% at one, three and 12 months, respectively [49].

The main challenge in patients receiving lung transplantation is ***chronic rejection***. This is microscopically characterized by perivascular fibrosis. In children, the median post-transplant survival period is about 59 months (ranging from zero to 159 months) [49]. In adults, the recently reported survival rate for Japanese patients with lymphangioleiomyomatosis who received lung transplantations was 86.7%, 82.5%, 73.7% and 73.7% at one, three, five and 10 years, respectively. However, these rates were better than those for patients undergoing transplants for other etiologies, and also than those recorded in the registry of the International Society for Heart and Lung Transplantation [50].

Post-transplant malignancies are relatively rare (9% of recipients) and primarily relate to thoracic malignancies that are more common in smokers. Lymphoproliferative disorders, cutaneous and non-cutaneous solid tumors (gynecological and GI tract malignancies, prostate, kidney, brain and breast cancer) have also been reported. The mean interval of cancer occurrence is about 52 months following transplantation [51]. Unusual pulmonary allograft Kaposi's sarcoma was reported in patients with HHV8 infection [46].

Bone Marrow Transplant-Related Lesions

A proper evaluation of bone marrow or hematopoietic stem cells transplantation can be offered based on bone marrow aspiration. Success is characterized by the following smear characteristics [1]:

First Day: presence of adipocytes and scattered inflammatory cells, without hematopoietic precursors.

First Week: scattered erythroblasts and myeloblasts.

Second Week: clusters of hematopoietic precursors.

Third Week: hematopoietic cells with features between young and mature cells.

Bone marrow rejection is a non-specific reaction of the human body under which bone marrow smears reveal a progressive loss of hematogenous cells, edema, hemorrhages, necroses and lymphoplasmacytosis, and formation of non-specific granulomas. The most common complications of bone marrow transplantations are opportunistic infections and graft-*versus*-host disease [1, 52].

Acute Graft-Versus-Host Disease

The main histological feature of this disease is presence of rich perivascular inflammatory infiltrate but, in severe cases, the following manifestations are associated [1, 32, 53, 54]:

Skin Lesions which can be classified according to four degrees of severity. Grade I relates to vacuolization of the epidermal basal cells and minimal perivascular lymphocyte infiltrate in the dermis, associated with rash. In grades II and III, presence of apoptotic keratinocytes is characteristic, while necrosis and bullae can be seen in grade IV (Fig. **3-3**). Mucosal lesions can be associated.

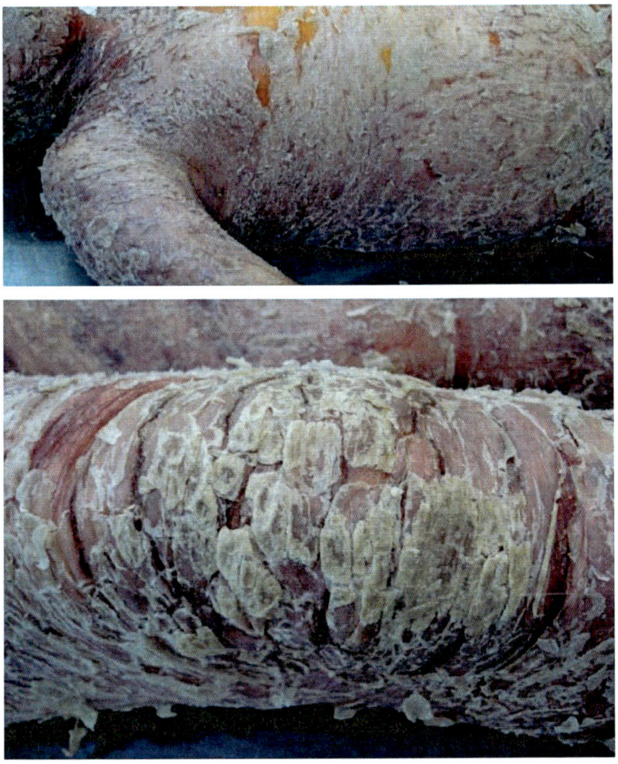

Fig. (3-3). Generalized grade IV cutaneous lesions resulting from graft-*versus*-host disease in a patient who died following bone marrow transplantation.

GI Tract Lesions which are the first sign of bone marrow rejection in 30-60% of cases. The clinical symptoms are diarrhea, vomiting, abdominal pain and infrequent functional ileus. Morphological lesions are similar to those produced by radio- or chemotherapy. Ulcerations and necroses predominantly occur in the mouth, esophagus, stomach and small intestine. Colonic lesions are classified according to four degrees of severity: grade I – focal crypt necroses; grade II – crypt abscesses; grade III – multi-crypt necroses; and grade IV – epithelial denudation. These can mimic ulcerative colitis.

Liver Disorders which occur in later stages and relate to cholestasis and high serum transaminases levels. Under the microscope, cholestasis and degenerative changes to the intrahepatic bile ducts are characteristic. Epithelial bile duct regeneration can be associated with reactive cytologic atypia. The hepatocytes can present a ballooning aspect with infrequent necrosis.

Lung Injuries which are more common in children. After hematopoietic stem cells transplantation, bronchiolitis obliterans can be an indicator of graft-*versus*-

host disease. The functional characteristics are similar to those reported regarding lung transplantation, but lesions are not as common. For this reason, other graft-*versus*-host diseases involving restrictive lung disorders, such as scleroderma, bronchiolitis obliterans organizing pneumonia and myositis, should be ruled out before establishing the diagnosis of post-transplant bronchiolitis. Moreover, spirometry is not feasible in young children.

Renal Disorders which, following allogenic hematopoietic stem cells transplantation, are rare complications characterized by nephritic syndrome, which can occur at a median time interval of 20.5 months (ranging from three to 174 months) after transplantation. Under the microscope, membranous glomerulonephritis and minimal change disease are the predominant lesions. Corticosteroids and immunosuppressive drugs induce remission in 59.1% and 81.3% of patients with membranous glomerulonephritis and minimal change disease, respectively.

Chronic Graft-Versus-Host Disease

This is a multiorganic syndrome that usually occurs approximately 100 days after bone marrow transplantation. The following manifestations can be encountered [1, 55]:

Skin Lesions occur between three and four months after transplantation and can be localized or generalized. These lesions can mimic autoimmune and collagen diseases. Scleroderma-like lesions (atrophy of epidermis, dermal hyalinosis, *etc.*) and other manifestations, such as lichenoid or vitiligoid patterns with nail dystrophy, can also occur. *Permanent alopecia of the scalp,* also known as *anagen effluvium,* is a rare complication that can be induced by high doses of chemotherapeutics (mainly busulfan and cyclophosphamide), but can also be a dose-independent ADR. In some cases, it can be a clinical manifestation of chronic graft-*versus*-host disease of an unknown mechanism. The frontoparietal and temporal areas are especially affected. Under the microscope, this condition can have a non-scarring (several miniaturized follicles/vellus hair and few normal hair follicles) or scarring (concentric fibrosis around the follicles and lichenoid inflammatory infiltrate) pattern.

GI Tract Lesions refer to fibrosis of the submucosa and serosa layers associated with perivascular hyalinization. Desquamative esophagitis is associated.

Liver Disorders relate to progressive bile duct degeneration and atrophy, cholestasis, fibrosis of the portal spaces and perivascular hyalinization.

Other Lesions

Opportunistic Infections are frequent complications, occurring in half of recipients. They can be produced by viruses (EBV infection, HV-induced cutaneous lesions or conjunctivitis, *etc.*), bacteria (*e.g.*, nocardiosis), parasites (*e.g.*, leishmaniasis) or fungi [39, 52, 56, 57]. GI inflammation following bone marrow transplantation can be the consequence of acute graft-*versus*-host disease or a result of super infection by opportunistic organisms. Viral enteritis is common [54]. Septicemia following bone marrow transplantation is difficult to manage [58]. Delayed infections are primarily produced through T-cell-related cellular immunity disorders [56].

Malignancies mainly refer to EBV-induced lymphoproliferative disorders and lymphomas. Secondary aggressive malignant neuroendocrine tumors were also reported [57].

Other Complications occurring following bone marrow transplantation include ADRs and other autoimmune processes, such as neuromyelitis optica. Plasmapheresis can reduce their consequences [52].

CONFLICT OF INTEREST

The authors confirm that this chapter content has no conflict of interest.

ACKNOWLEDGEMENTS

Declared none.

REFERENCES

[1] Jung J, Ed. Patologie iatrogenă. Tîrgu-Mureş, Romania: University Press 2006.

[2] McAulay KA, Haque T, Crawford DH. Tumour necrosis factor gene polymorphism: a predictive factor for the development of post-transplant lymphoproliferative disease. Br J Cancer 2009; 101(6): 1019-27.
[http://dx.doi.org/10.1038/sj.bjc.6605278] [PMID: 19738620]

[3] Sekiguchi Y, Shimada A, Ichikawa K, *et al.* Epstein-Barr virus-positive multiple myeloma developing after immunosuppressant therapy for rheumatoid arthritis: a case report and review of literature. Int J Clin Exp Pathol 2015; 8(2): 2090-102.
[PMID: 25973110]

[4] Deschênes I, Dion L, Beauchesne C, de Brum-Fernandes A. Kaposis sarcoma following immune suppressive therapy for Wegeners granulomatosis. J Rheumatol 2003; 30(3): 622-4.
[PMID: 12610826]

[5] Alobaid A, Torlakovic E, Kongkham P. Primary central nervous system immunomodulatory therapy-induced lymphoproliferative disorder in a patient with ulcerative colitis: a case report and review of the literature. World Neurosurg 2015; 84(6): 2074.e15-.
[http://dx.doi.org/10.1016/j.wneu.2015.07.009] [PMID: 26171889]

[6] Carenco C, Faure S, Ursic-Bedoya J, Herrero A, Pageaux GP. Solid, non-skin, post-liver transplant tumors: Key role of lifestyle and immunosuppression management. World J Gastroenterol 2016; 22(1): 427-34.
[http://dx.doi.org/10.3748/wjg.v22.i1.427] [PMID: 26755888]

[7] Calmet FH, Yarur AJ, Pukazhendhi G, Ahmad J, Bhamidimarri KR. Endoscopic and histological features of mycophenolate mofetil colitis in patients after solid organ transplantation. Ann Gastroenterol 2015; 28(3): 366-73.
[PMID: 26126799]

[8] Marchitto G, Marci V, Berrone M, Pentenero M. Early arising sarcoma after adjuvant radiotherapy for oral squamous cell carcinoma. J Oral Maxillofac Surg 2015; pii:S0278-2391:01592-X

[9] Theilaccker C, Ludewig K, Serr A, *et al.* Overwhelming post-splenectomy infection: a prospective multicenter cohort study. Clin Infect Dis 2015; pii: civ1195.

[10] van Ruler O, Boermeester MA. [Surgical treatment of secondary peritonitis: A continuing problem. German version]. Chirurg 2016; 87(1): 13-9.
[http://dx.doi.org/10.1007/s00104-015-0115-8] [PMID: 26689581]

[11] Furtado R, Le Page P, Dunn G, Falk GL. High rate of common bile duct stones and postoperative abscess following percutaneous cholecystostomy. Ann R Coll Surg Engl 2016; 98(2): 102-6.
[http://dx.doi.org/10.1308/rcsann.2016.0004] [PMID: 26741665]

[12] Narkhede R, Shah NM, Dalal PR, Mangukia C, Dholaria S. Postoperative mesh infection-still a concern in laparoscopic era. Indian J Surg 2015; 77(4): 322-6.
[http://dx.doi.org/10.1007/s12262-015-1304-x] [PMID: 26702240]

[13] Patel P, Borkowf CB, Brooks JT, Lasry A, Lansky A, Mermin J. Estimating per-act HIV transmission risk: a systematic review. AIDS 2014; 28(10): 1509-19.
[http://dx.doi.org/10.1097/QAD.0000000000000298] [PMID: 24809629]

[14] Hogan C, Iles J, Frost EH, *et al.* Epidemic history and and iatrogenic transmission of blood-borne viruses in mid-20th century Kinshasa. J Infect Dis 2016; 214(3): 353-60.
[http://dx.doi.org/10.1093/infdis/jiw009] [PMID: 26768251]

[15] Miller FD, Elzalabany MS, Hassani S, Cuadros DF. Epidemiology of hepatitis C virus exposure in Egypt: Opportunities for prevention and evaluation. World J Hepatol 2015; 7(28): 2849-58.
[http://dx.doi.org/10.4254/wjh.v7.i28.2849] [PMID: 26668697]

[16] Harris NL, Ferry JA, Swerdlow SH. Posttransplant lymphoproliferative disorders: summary of Society for Hematopathology Workshop. Semin Diagn Pathol 1997; 14(1): 8-14.
[PMID: 9044505]

[17] Gurzu S, Jung I. Basic Concepts of Pathology. Tîrgu-Mureş, Romania: University Press 2011.

[18] Ngo S, Benhamou Y, Armengol G, *et al.* [Agranulocytosis related to fluindione: A case report]. Rev Med Interne 2016; 37(1): 58-61.
[http://dx.doi.org/10.1016/j.revmed.2015.05.013] [PMID: 26096756]

[19] Braire-Bourrel M, Augey F, Doutre MS. Drugs-induced urticaria and angioedema. Rev Prat 2015; 65(7): 972-6.
[PMID: 26619738]

[20] Goossens RA. Allergic contact dermatitis from the vehicle components of topical pharmaceutical products. Immunol Allergy Clin North Am 2014; 34(3): 663-670, ix-x.
[http://dx.doi.org/10.1016/j.iac.2014.04.010] [PMID: 25017683]

[21] Burkhart C, Schloemer J, Zirwas M. Differentiation of latex allergy from irritant contact dermatitis. Cutis 2015; 96(6): 369-371, 401.
[PMID: 26761937]

[22] Kılıç İ, Kaya F, Özdemir AT, Demirel T, Çelik İ. Nicolau syndrome due to diclofenac sodium

(Voltaren®) injection: a case report. J Med Case Reports 2014; 8: 404. [http://dx.doi.org/10.1186/1752-1947-8-404] [PMID: 25471251]

[23] Mutarelli EG, Adoni T. Iatrogenic meningitis. Arq Neuropsiquiatr 2013; 71(9B): 659-60. [http://dx.doi.org/10.1590/0004-282X20130145] [PMID: 24141499]

[24] Honda T, Kabashima K. Novel concept of iSALT (inducible skin-associated lymphoid tissue) in the elicitation of allergic contact dermatitis. Proc Jpn Acad Ser B Phys Biol Sci 2016; 92(1): 20-8. [http://dx.doi.org/10.2183/pjab.92.20] [PMID: 26755397]

[25] Eubel J, Diepgen TL, Weisshaar E. [Allergic diseases in the genital area]. Hautarzt 2015; 66(1): 45-52. [http://dx.doi.org/10.1007/s00105-014-3561-1] [PMID: 25532902]

[26] Pickler WJ, Adam J, Watkins S, Wuillemin N, Yun J, Yerly D. Int Arch Allergy Immunol 2015; 168: 13-24. [http://dx.doi.org/10.1159/000441280] [PMID: 26524432]

[27] http://medical-dictionary.thefreedictionary.com. Accessed at 16th of January 2016.

[28] http://www.merriam-webster.com/dictionary. Accessed at 16th of January 2016.

[29] https://en.wikipedia.org/wiki. Accessed at 16th of January 2016.

[30] Yang CY, Lee CY, Yeh CC, Tsai MK. Renal transplantation across the donor-specific antibody barrier: Graft outcome and cancer risk after desensitization therapy. J Formos Med Assoc 2015; pii: S0929-6646(15)00377-0.

[31] Fyfe B, Loh E, Winters GL, Couper GS, Kartashov AI, Schoen FJ. Heart transplantation-associated perioperative ischemic myocardial injury. Morphological features and clinical significance. Circulation 1996; 93(6): 1133-40. [http://dx.doi.org/10.1161/01.CIR.93.6.1133] [PMID: 8653833]

[32] Yu J. Postinfectious bronchiolitis obliterans in children: lessons from bronchiolitis obliterans after lung transplantation and hematopoietic stem cell transplantation. Korean J Pediatr 2015; 58(12): 459-65. [http://dx.doi.org/10.3345/kjp.2015.58.12.459] [PMID: 26770220]

[33] Trivedi JR, Cheng A, Ising M, Lenneman A, Birks E, Slaughter MS. Heart transplant survival based on recipient and donor risk scoring: a unos database analysis. ASAIO J 2016; 62(3): 297-301. [http://dx.doi.org/10.1097/MAT.0000000000000337] [PMID: 26771395]

[34] Lee WS, Erdelyi K, Matyas C, *et al.* Cannabidiol limits Tcell-mediated chronic autoimmune myocarditis: implications to autoimmune disorders and organ transplantation. Mol Med 2016 In press. [http://dx.doi.org/10.2119/molmed.2016.00007] [PMID: 26772776]

[35] Yousuf T, Kramer J, Kopiec A, *et al.* In search for equilibrium: immunosuppression *versus* opportunistic infection. J Clin Med Res 2016; 8(2): 175-7. [http://dx.doi.org/10.14740/jocmr2439w] [PMID: 26767088]

[36] Lateef N, Basit KA, Abbasi N, Kazmi SM, Ansari AB, Shah M. Malignancies after heart transplant. Exp Clin Transplant 2016; 14(1): 12-6. [http://dx.doi.org/10.6002/ect.2015.0214] [PMID: 26643469]

[37] Wu MJ, Lian JD, Yang CR, *et al.* High cumulative incidence of urinary tract transitional cell carcinoma after kidney transplantation in Taiwan. Am J Kidney Dis 2004; 43(6): 1091-7. [http://dx.doi.org/10.1053/j.ajkd.2004.03.016] [PMID: 15168390]

[38] Pendón-Ruiz de Mier V, Navarro Cabello MD, Martínez Vaquera S, *et al.* Incidence and long-term prognosis of cancer after kidney transplantation. Transplant Proc 2015; 47(9): 2618-21. [http://dx.doi.org/10.1016/j.transproceed.2015.08.043] [PMID: 26680052]

[39] Komitopoulou A, Tzenou T, Baltadakis J, Apostolidis J, Karakasis D, Harhalakis N. Is leishmaniasis an unusual suspect of infection in allogeneic transplantation? Transpl Infect Dis 2014; 16(6): 1012-8. [http://dx.doi.org/10.1111/tid.12316] [PMID: 25412926]

[40] Shimizu T, Tanabe T, Shirakawa H, Omoto K, Ishida H, Tanabe K. Acute vascular rejection after renal transplantation and isolated v-lesion. Clin Transplant 2012; 26 (Suppl. 24): 2-8. [http://dx.doi.org/10.1111/j.1399-0012.2012.01673.x] [PMID: 22747468]

[41] Coelho GR, Leitao AS Jr, Cavalcante FP, *et al.* Continuous *versus* interrupted suture for hepatic artery anastomosis in liver transplantation: differences in the incidence of hepatic artery thrombosis. Transplant Proc 2008; 40(10): 3545-7. [http://dx.doi.org/10.1016/j.transproceed.2008.06.066] [PMID: 19100434]

[42] Kienlein S, Schoening W, Andert A, Kroy D, Neumann UP, Schmeding M. Biliary complications in liver transplantation: Impact of anastomotic technique and ischemic time on short- and long-term outcome. World J Transplant 2015; 5(4): 300-9. [http://dx.doi.org/10.5500/wjt.v5.i4.300] [PMID: 26722658]

[43] Kritikos A, Manuel O. Bloodstream infections after solid organ transplantation. Virulence 2016; 7(3): 329-40. [http://dx.doi.org/10.1080/21505594.2016.1139279] [PMID: 26766415]

[44] Wiltberger G, Schmelzle M, Schubert S, *et al.* Invasive cardiac aspergillosis after orthotopic liver transplantation. Z Gastroenterol 2014; 52(8): 813-7. [http://dx.doi.org/10.1055/s-0034-1366647] [PMID: 25111721]

[45] Fernandes S, Carrelha AS, Marques Pinto G, Nolasco F, Barroso E, Cardoso J. Patologia dermatológica em doentes transplantados hepáticos e renais referenciados à consulta de dermatologia e venereologia. Acta Med Port 2013; 26(5): 555-63. [PMID: 24192095]

[46] Nannini N, Rebusso A, Lunardi F, *et al.* Asymptomatic pulmonary allograft Kaposi Sarcoma: A case report. Exp Clin Transplant 2016 In press. [http://dx.doi.org/10.6002/ect.2015.0133] [PMID: 26767437]

[47] Zimmermann A, Zobeley C, Weber MM, Lang H, Galle PR, Zimmermann T. Changes in lipid and carbohydrate metabolism under mTOR- and calcineurin-based immunosuppressive regimen in adult patients after liver transplantation. Eur J Intern med 2016 29: 104-9. [http://dx.doi.org/10.1016/j.ejim.2015.12.022] [PMID: 26775180]

[48] Needham JM, Nicholas SK, Davis CM. Food allergies developing after solid organ transplant. Pediatr Transplant 2015; 19(8): 827-35. [http://dx.doi.org/10.1111/petr.12613] [PMID: 26767488]

[49] Schmid FA, Inci I, Bürgi U, *et al.* Favorable outcome of children and adolescents undergoing lung transplantation at a European adult center in the new era. Pediatr Pulmonol 2016; 51(11): 1222-8. [http://dx.doi.org/10.1002/ppul.23383] [PMID: 26773327]

[50] Ando K, Okada Y, Akiba M, *et al.* Lung transplantation for lymphangioleiomyomatosis in Japan. PLos One 2016; 11:e 0146749.

[51] Ordóñez Dios IM, Montoro Ballesteros F, Vaquero Barrios JM, Cobos Ceballos MJ, Redel Montero J, Santos Luna F. Analysis of the incidence of noncutaneous neoplasia after lung transplantation and its impact on prognosis. Transplant Proc 2015; 47(9): 2659-60. [http://dx.doi.org/10.1016/j.transproceed.2015.10.013] [PMID: 26680065]

[52] Baumer FM, Kamihara J, Gorman MP. Neuromyelitis optica in an adolescent after bone marrow transplantation. Pediatr Neurol 2015; 52(1): 119-24. [http://dx.doi.org/10.1016/j.pediatrneurol.2014.07.007] [PMID: 25444090]

[53] Beyar-Katz O, Kruzel Davila E, Zuckerman T, *et al.* Adult nephrotic syndrome after hematopoietic stem cell transplantation: renal pathology is the best predictor of response to therapy. Biol Blood Marrow Transplant 2016; 22(6): 975-81. [http://dx.doi.org/10.1016/j.bbmt.2015.12.014] [PMID: 26740372]

[54] Jones B, Kramer SS, Saral R, *et al.* Gastrointestinal inflammation after bone marrow transplantation:

graft-*versus*-host disease or opportunistic infection? AJR Am J Roentgenol 1988; 150(2): 277-81. [http://dx.doi.org/10.2214/ajr.150.2.277] [PMID: 3276085]

[55] Basilio FM, Brenner FM, Werner B, Rastelli GJ. Clinical and histological study of permanent alopecia after bone marrow transplantation. An Bras Dermatol 2015; 90(6): 814-21. [http://dx.doi.org/10.1590/abd1806-4841.20154013] [PMID: 26734861]

[56] Perko R, Kang G, Sunkara A, Leung W, Thomas PG, Dallas MH. Gamma delta T cell reconstitution is associated with fewer infections and improved event-free survival after hematopoietic stem cell transplantation for pediatric leukemia. Biol Blood Marrow Transplant 2015; 21(1): 130-6. [http://dx.doi.org/10.1016/j.bbmt.2014.09.027] [PMID: 25445640]

[57] Tamura S, Ishida H, Naito T, *et al.* Secondary neuroendocrine tumor after allogeneic bone marrow transplantation. Pediatr Int 2015; 57(6): 1178-81. [http://dx.doi.org/10.1111/ped.12720] [PMID: 26711919]

[58] Matsumoto K, Yamamoto W, Ohgusa E, *et al.* Disseminated *Cunninghamella bertholletiae* infection with septic pulmonary embolism after allogeneic bone marrow transplantation. Transpl Infect Dis 2014; 16(2): 304-6. [http://dx.doi.org/10.1111/tid.12190] [PMID: 24593246]

CHAPTER 4

Iatrogenic Pathology of the Cardiovascular System

Simona Gurzu* and **Ioan Jung**

Department of Pathology, University of Medicine and Pharmacy, Tirgu-Mures, Romania

Abstract: This chapter includes a synthesis of data regarding cardiovascular-related lesions induced by medical drugs or radiotherapy, and also relates to the specific injuries that can be caused by diagnostic and/or therapeutic interventions. The effects of chemotherapeutics and non-chemotherapeutic drugs on the myocardium are analyzed in detail, with a focus on anthracycline-induced cardiovascular effects in children. Some of the disorders are illustrated using representative pictures taken during autopsies. Although a common technique, insertion of prosthetic grafts can lead to complications, such as thrombosis, aberrant neointimal hyperplasia or dehiscence. Percutaneous vascular intervention complications can be related to the catheter or to the intervention itself. The differences between in-stent restenosis and postoperative thrombosis are also presented. The final part of this chapter is dedicated to open heart surgical intervention complications.

Keywords: Adverse drug reaction, Anthracyclines, Arrhythmia, Cardiovascular, Hypersensitive cardiomyopathy, Hypovolemia, Myocarditis, Neointimal hyperplasia, Open heart surgery, Percutaneous intervention, Prosthetic graft, Stenosis, Stent, Torsade de pointes, Vasculitis.

INTRODUCTION

Cardiovascular-related iatrogenic lesions can be induced by medical drugs (ADRs), radiotherapy performed to treat mediastinal or lung tumors (see Chapter 2), or diagnostic and therapeutic procedures. The specific ADRs and iatrogenic consequences of diagnostic and therapeutic procedures are presented in this chapter.

DRUG-INDUCED LESIONS

Chemotherapeutic Drugs

Hypersensitive-mediated cardiomyopathy and toxic myocarditis are the most

* **Corresponding author Simona Gurzu:** Department of Pathology, University of Medicine and Pharmacy, Tirgu-Mures, Romania; Tel: 0040-745-673550; Fax: 0040-372-653250; E-mail: simonagurzu@yahoo.com

severe chronic complications of antineoplastic therapy, especially in patients treated with *anthracyclines* (Table **4-1**). A 10-fold higher risk of developing heart failure has been reported in doxorubicin users when compared to healthy patients [1]. Anthracyclines-induced mitochondrial DNA damage is more severe in patients below the age of four and above the age of 65 [1, 2]. Their combination with cardiolipins in the internal membranes of mitochondria leads to depletion of adenosine triphosphate (ATP) and decreased myocardial contractility. Then, mitochondrial edema produces necrosis of cardiomyocytes and subsequent myocarditis and myocardial sclerosis [1, 2]. It is a cumulative lifetime dose-dependent mechanism.

In children, an average dose of 300 mg anthracyclines/m^2 is considered to produce clinical heart failure within about seven years. In some cases, heart transplantation is required approximately nine years after cancer diagnosis. Long-term monitoring of cardiotoxicity (echocardiography at 3, 6, 12, 36, 60 and 84 months after completion of treatment), identification and normalization of ejection fraction, and treatment of heart failure can increase life expectancy in these patients. At the same time, drugs to treat anti-anthracycline cardiac-induced lesions, such as dexrazoxane, can be simultaneously prescribed in adult patients but are not yet approved for children. ACE inhibitors can also be used for myocardial protection. A decrease of the left ventricular ejection fraction of over 10% below the lower value is an indicator for cessation of anthracycline-based therapy. In children, severe heart failure emerges as a result of anthracycline-induced cardiomyopathy, and cardiac transplantation offers a 50% chance of 10-year survival. This is the only therapeutic option in such cases [1].

Alkylating drugs, such as cyclophosphamide, can induce endothelial lesions and subsequent intramural hematomas and edema, but myocarditis and pericarditis have also been reported within two weeks of drug administration (Table **4-1**). However, in most cases, only transient arrhythmia presents [1].

Table 4-1. Cardiovascular-related ADRs induced by antineoplastic drugs. Data from references [1 - 7].

Type of ADR	Drugs
Angina	Anthracyclines, cyclophosphamide, 5-fluorouracil (5-FU)
Arrhythmia	Cyclophosphamide, anthracyclines (ventricular/supraventricular arrhythmia), 5-FU, lithium
Tachycardia	Anthracyclines (sinus tachycardia)
Torsade de pointes (polymorphic ventricular tachycardia) – QT prolongation or long QT syndrome	Anthracyclines

(Table 4-1) contd.....

Type of ADR	Drugs
Alterative myocarditis/ Myocardial fibrosis – toxic effect	Anthracyclines (daunorubicin, doxorubicin, epirubicin, idarubicin, mitoxantrone), 5-FU, cyclophosphamide, isophosphamide
Cardiomyopathy	Lithium, anthracyclines (congestive cardiomyopathy and left ventricular hypertrophy)
Pericarditis/endocarditis	Anthracyclines, cyclophosphamide
Vasculitis/thrombosis	Cyclophosphamide, vaccines

Other chemotherapeutics known to induce cardiovascular disorders are *5-F--based agents* that can cause contraction of the coronary vessels with subsequent myocardial ischemia and arrhythmias [1]. Intravenous administration of 5-FU induces more severe cardiotoxicity as compared to oral fluoropyrimidine, such as capecitabine [4, 5]. However, even in cases of oral administration of capecitabine combined with oxaliplatin (XELOX or CAPOX regimens), long-term use at high doses induces cardiotoxicity in 1-18% of cases [5 - 7]. Angina is the most common consequence, but myocardial infarction and lethal myocardial fibrosis (Fig. **4-1**) occur in 11% of patients with capecitabine-induced cardiotoxicity [5 - 7].

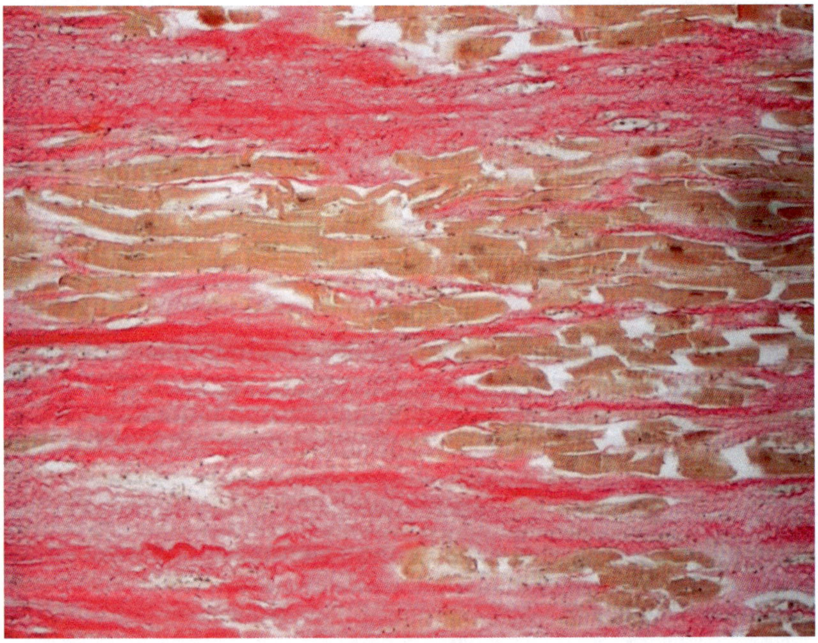

Fig. (4-1). Chemotherapy-induced lethal cardiotoxicity. The 36-year-old female received capecitabine and oxaliplatin, and subsequently developed diffuse myocardial fibrosis, emphasized in red with Van Gieson's stain. Ob. 4x.

Non-Chemotherapeutic Drugs

Antirabic vaccine, noradrenaline overdose and other agents, such as *amphetamine-containing weight-loss pills,* are known to induce myocarditis. In our department, three young females of ages ranging from 30 to 35 years, all long-term users of weight loss pills, presented in the emergency department with symptoms suggesting myocarditis. Two of these patients died suddenly.

Alpha blockers, used for the treatment of benign prostate hyperplasia, can produce palpitations, extrasystoles, long QT syndrome with a risk of torsade de pointes, angina exacerbation, postural hypotension and potentially life-threatening ventricular arrhythmias [8]. For this reason, anti-prostatic hyperplasia drugs should not be sold without a medical prescription and measurement of the QT interval is necessary in long-term users. In elderly males with cardiac disorders, the use of such drugs should be taken into account when making a proper diagnosis and devising a therapeutic regimen.

Drug-induced long QT syndrome can also occur in patients taking fluoroquinolones, antihistamines or antiarrhythmic drugs class IA (disopyramide, procainamide) or class III administered orally (amiodarone) or intravenously (ibutilide, almokalant). Simultaneous use of an antiarrhythmic drug class I/III and second generation antihistamines is not permitted. At the same time, antiarrhythmic drugs should not be used in conjunction with tricyclic depressants.

Table 4-2. Vascular disorders induced by non-chemotherapeutic drug. Data from references [1 - 10].

Type of ADR	Drugs
Vasodilation, hypovolemia	Thiopental (anesthetic barbiturate), iodinated intravenous contrast, osmotic agents (mannitol), Kayexalate® (sodium polystyrene sulfonate) – used to treat chronic renal failure and decreases kalemia
Cold extremities	Beta blockers (atenolol, propranolol, metoprolol, pindolol, alprenolol), diuretics
Peripheral edema	Corticosteroids, beta blockers (atenolol)
Vasculitis/thrombosis	Sulfonamides, aspirin, phenylbutazone, penicillin, augmentin (amoxicillin with clavulanate), chlorpromazine, promethazine, thioridazine, lithium, amitriptyline, cytotoxic drugs (cyclophosphamide), serum sickness, procainamide, hydralazine, iodine, bromocriptine (anti-prolactin drug), etomidate (anesthetic drug), estrogen, tamoxifen
TTP	Sulfonamides, penicillin, serum sickness
Polyarteritis nodosa	Sulfonamides, corticosteroids, thiouracil, phenylbutazone, thiazides
Hypercholesterolemia	Vitamin D overdose
Atherosclerosis	Progesterone (gestagens)

TTP = Thrombotic thrombocytopenic purpura.

Aside from the drugs listed in Tables **4-2** and **4-3**, cardiovascular iatrogenic disorders can also be produced by antimicrobials (erythromycin, clarithromycin, fluoroquinolones), antifungals (ketoconazole, itraconazole), antimalarials (quinine, halofantrine), neuroleptics (phenothiazine, thioridazine, chlorpromazine, haloperidol), antipsychotics (sertindole, pimozide), prokinetics (cisapride), antispasmodics (terodiline), *etc*. Insulin stimulates intramyocardial lipid storage and ventricular hypertrophy, increasing the severity of diabetic cardiomyopathy [9, 10].

Table 4-3. Cardiac disorders induced by non-chemotherapeutic drugs. Data from references [1-10].

Type of ADR	Drugs
Angina exacerbation	Alpha blockers
Arrhythmia	Digitalis (and calcium), beta-adrenergics, quinine, tricyclic antidepressants (amitriptyline, doxepin, desipramine, imipramine, clomipramine)
Long QT syndrome/torsade de pointes	Fluoroquinolones (sparfloxacin), antihistamines (terfenadine, astemizole), bepridil, prenylamine, droperidol, alpha blockers
Hypotension/hypertension	Glucocorticoids, sympathomimetics, sulfonamides (sulfadiazine), neuroleptics/antidepressant drugs (imipramine, doxepin, promethazine), cyclosporine, bromocriptine (anti-prolactin drug), intravenous anesthetics (propofol, ketamine), inhalational anesthetics (enflurane, isoflurane, desflurane), contraceptive pills
Bradycardia/ tachycardia	Neuroleptic/antidepressant drugs (imipramine, clomipramine, reserpine), barbiturates (thiopental) inhalational anesthetics (desflurane), depolarizing myorelaxants (succinylcholine)
Pericarditis	Emetine, procainamide, hydralazine, isoniazid, minoxidil
Endocarditis	Corticosteroids, antibiotics
Alterative myocarditis/fibrosis	Penicillin, sulfonamides, amphetamines, methyldopa, antirabic vaccination
Interstitial myocarditis/fibrosis	Penicillin, ampicillin, tetracycline, streptomycin, cephalosporin, sulfonamides, methyldopa, digitalis, procainamide, phenylbutazone, amitriptyline, theophylline, furosemide, reserpine, spironolactone, diclofenac, indomethacin, isoniazid, allopurinol
Cardiomyopathy	Emetine, phenothiazines, isoproterenol, chloroquine (antimalarial, antiretroviral in HIV infection, antirheumatic)
Myocardial hypertrophy/fatty change	Insulin
Heart failure	Chlorpromazine, imipramine, amitriptyline, progesterone, drugs used for penile erectile dysfunctions, especially in association with nitrates (sildenafil, tadalafil, vardenafil)

IATROGENIC LESIONS DURING DIAGNOSTIC AND THERAPEUTIC PROCEDURES

Insertion of Prosthetic Grafts

Prosthetic cardiovascular grafts are fabricated using synthetic polymers (*e.g.*, polytetrafluoroethylene [ePTFE], polyethylene terephthalate [Dacron®], polyurethane, polycarbonate-urethane), metal, plastic, biopolymers/biomaterials (*e.g.*, polyglycolic acid, polyhydroxyalkanoates, polycaprolactone) or nanocomposites. They are usually larger than 6 mm, with the exception of the new generation of tissue-engineered vascular prostheses, which allow for the synthesis of smaller grafts with high porosity [11].

Graft insertion is followed by a local inflammatory reaction, ultimately leading to graft incorporation with newly formed connective tissue lined with neointima. This is a stepwise process that comprises three phases [11 - 14]:

The ***proliferative phase*** occurs in the first two weeks following graft insertion and is primarily characterized by proliferation of granulation tissue that penetrates within the prosthetic wall of the metallic or plastic network. The newly synthesized extracellular matrix then promotes formation of the neointima on the inner graft surface.

The ***graft endothelialization phase*** occurs between 10 days and one month following graft insertion. The attached endothelial cells originate from the circulating pluripotent bone marrow-derived mesenchymal cells. The complete endothelialization is followed by vascular remodeling.

The ***stabilizing phase*** occurs during the subsequent six months and involves the formation of a connective tissue-embedded prosthetic graft that incorporates myofibroblasts and smooth muscle fibers. The biodegradable scaffolds degrade after about four weeks and, within six months, are completely absorbed and replaced by an extracellular matrix that incorporates collagen and elastin fibers.

Graft endothelialization is mandatory for controlling thrombosis, excessive inflammation and intimal thickening. Neointimal hyperplasia, which can occur during the second phase of incorporation, can induce early restenosis, especially in small vessels. During the third phase, formation of irregularly dispensed connective tissue can be a cause of late in-stent luminal restenosis. Other incorporation-related complications are the following: thrombosis with/without vascular occlusion (most common between days four and seven), prosthetic aneurysmal dilatation, dehiscence, graft rupture and perivascular hemorrhage [11 - 14]. These graft-related complications are presented in detail in the following sub-chapters.

Thrombosis, dehiscence and infections are major complications occurring after open vascular repair with Dacron or ePTFE prostheses (Fig. **4-2**). Dacron wrapping of aortic dissection or aneurysm can also be followed by dissection/rupture of the subjacent artery segments (Fig. **4-3**), probably as a result of tissue ingrowth [11]. Perioperative rupture of the tube and thrombosis are associated with a mortality rate of approximately 32% [15, 16]. In one of our cases, a 70-year-old male was hospitalized with severe generalized atherosclerosis and rupture of the abdominal aneurysm localized at the aortic bifurcation. A Dacron tube was inserted to replace the distal abdominal aorta and common iliac arteries (Fig. **4-4**), but lethal thrombosis occurred two days after surgery [17].

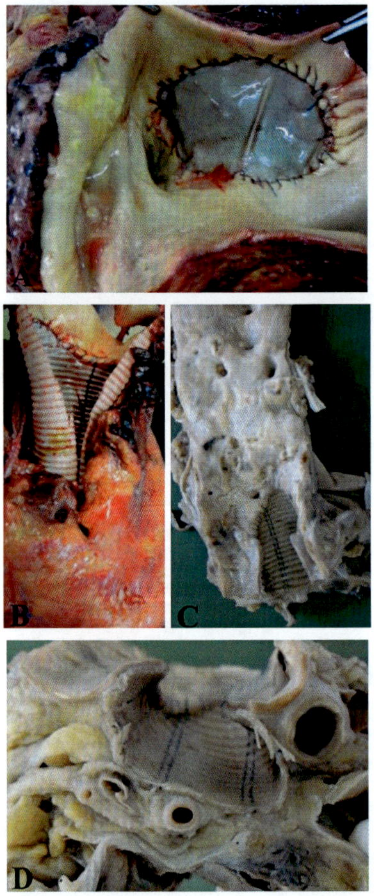

Fig. (4-2). Insertion of Dacron devices – autopsy findings. A – Dacron mesh used for aortoplasty, in a patient with aortic aneurysm who died due to myocardial infarction; B – Dacron tube used for aortoplasty, in a patient with severe atherosclerosis and dissection of ascending aorta who died due to hemorrhagic shock; C, D – Dacron tube used for aortofemoral bypass, in a patient with generalized obstructive atherosclerosis who died due to myocardial infarction.

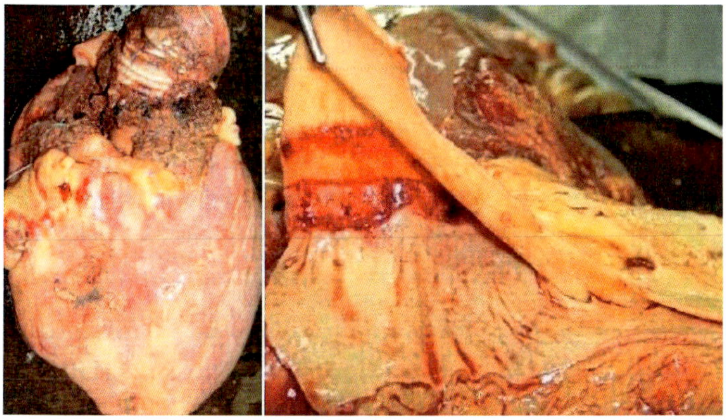

Fig. (4-3). Insertion of a Dacron tube for aortoplasty in a patient with severe atherosclerosis and dissection of the ascending aorta (left). The patient died as a result of subsequent dissection of the abdominal aorta (right) and hemorrhagic shock.

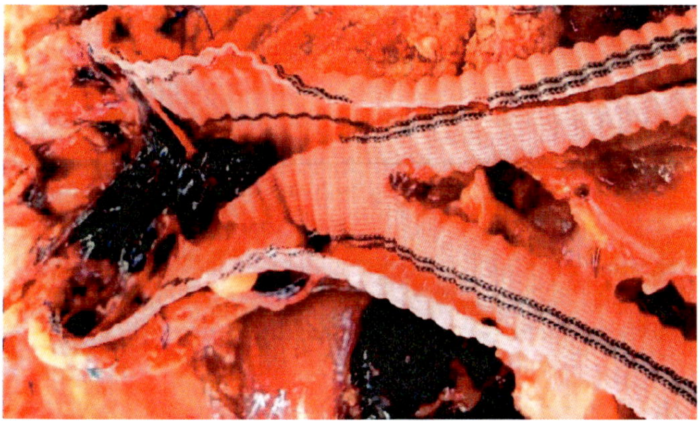

Fig. (4-4). Insertion of a Dacron tube for aortoplasty and replacement of common iliac arteries in a patient with aneurysm of the abdominal aorta and severe atherosclerosis. The patient died due to thrombotic complications.

The late rupture of abdominal aortic aneurysm after endovascular repair occurs in 0.9% of cases, after a median time of 37 months, primarily due to graft-related endoleaks [16]. Only 45% of ePTFE grafts are patented as femoropopliteal bypass grafts at five years [11].

Following percutaneous atrial septal defect closure using Dacron grafts, postoperative arrhythmias have been reported in 5.8% of patients. Device embolization (0.8% of cases), thrombosis (1.2%) and central retinal artery occlusion are infrequent complications. The mortality rate is about 1% and post-percutaneous fixing of the septal defect's surgical closure is necessary in another 1.2% of cases [18, 19].

PERCUTANEOUS VASCULAR INTERVENTIONS

Percutaneous coronary interventions (PCIs) refer to diagnostic angiography, balloon angioplasty and stent implantation. They are commonly used in departments of interventional cardiology and are performed through cardiac catheterization *via* femoral or, more rarely, radial arteries. Percutaneous coronary angioplasty (PTCA) is performed for balloon dilatation or stent implantation in patients with obstructive arterial lesions [20].

The conceptual description of coronary angioplasty was first put forth in 1964 by Dotter and Judkins, who originally used an implantable prosthetic device. In 1977, Gruentzig and Myler performed the first coronary angioplasty followed by balloon angioplasty, while in 1979 Hartzler performed the same on a patient with acute myocardial infarction. The second important moment was marked in 1986 when Sigwart and Puel realized the first stent implantation in a human coronary artery. In 1994, the FDA approved the use of stents for vascular dilatation after failed balloon angioplasty [21].

In the period leading up to 1999, the bare metal stent (BMS) was progressively replaced by various drug eluting stents (DESs), first with sirolimus, then with everolimus, taxol, pimecrolimus and dual pimecrolimus-paclitaxel [21, 22].

The latest stent types approved by the European Medicines Agency (EMA), in 2011, are the so-called bioresorbable vascular scaffolds (BVSs) [21]. BVS is made up of several types of alloy, such as magnesium, poly-L-lactic acid, poly--lactic acid, tyrosine polycarbonate or poly-salicylic acid, and, by comparison with the BMS, the BVS is thicker (80 *vs.* 150-200 μm) [20, 23]. Some of the BVSs are paclitaxel, everolimus or sirolimus and the resorption time is between one and three years, with minimal lumen loss, ranging from 0-0.64 mm [23]. BVSs were used in approximately 30 cases in 2011, and the number of PTCA cases involving BVS increased to 13,000 in 2014. The newest BVS is the novolimus-eluting stent, with a thickness of 100 μm [23].

Aside from coronary arteries, percutaneous angiography/angioplasty is also used for stent insertion in femoral arteries, carotid arteries or for other obstructive arterial lesions [24]. Bifurcation stents are also known to be used in daily practice.

Percutaneous graft insertion can be followed by catheter- or patient-related complications. These are most commonly periprocedural vascular lesions, but systemic complications have also been reported [25]. No absolute indications are known for coronary angiography or carotid endarterectomy, but special attention should be paid to diabetics, patients with morbid obesity, cardiomyopathy or severe brain ischemia. Acute renal failure has been reported in 2% of cases and the post-angiography mortality rate is approximately 0.08% [26].

A. Catheter-Related Vascular Lesions

Peri-PCI vascular lesions occur in about 0.7-1.7% of cases [27, 28]. Over recent decades, a significant decrease of this rate was observed, dropping from 1.7% in 1998 to 0.2% in 2007. After PTCA, the complication rate decreases from 3.1% to 1% [29]. In the first month following PTCA, local delivery of pro-angiogenic substances, such as vascular endothelium growth factor (VEGF-A), seems to reduce the risk of thrombosis [12, 13]. The VEGF-A-eluting stents have not been proven to accelerate neointimal formation or to decrease the risk of in-stent restenosis [30]. DESs with everolimus or other substances have been proven to significantly reduce neointimal proliferation [22].

1. *Vascular Lesions at the Place Of Insertion of the Catheter*

After the femoral approach, hematoma following sheath removal emerges in 90% of patients, usually without consequence (Fig. **4-5**). Hematoma occurs more commonly following puncture above the inguinal ligament and can be prevented using manual compression for 20-30 minutes after catheter removal [25, 31]. Although rare, large hematomas can produce compression of vessels and nerves, leading to further periprocedural deep vein thrombosis and neuropathies, such as meralgia paresthetica [32].

Femoral pseudoaneurysm, also known as periarterial pulsating hematoma or sprue aneurysm, is reported in 0.42-3.7% of cases. It involves, most frequently, the superficial femoral artery, due to its smaller caliber as compared to the common femoral artery, and lack of underlying bone (low access). Pseudoaneurysm can be a consequence of lacking manual compression [25, 31].

Other rare local complications are arteriovenous fistulae (0.25-1%) and iliac artery dissection [33]. Femoral thrombosis/embolism can occur in 0.25-0.42% of cases, primarily in females with DM or peripheral arterial disease. It can induce limb ischemia, white painful foot, and sensory and motor disorders [34]. The rate of complications depends on the type of catheter, intervention and anticoagulant therapy. Obesity increases the risk of acute complications [31].

The most common chronic complication of catheter-related arterial injuries is femoral neuralgia syndrome. It was reported in about 30% of patients in the 1990s [35], but is rare nowadays. Chronic ischemia-induced neuralgia of the internal saphenous nerve following catheterization of the femoral artery was reported in one recently published case [36].

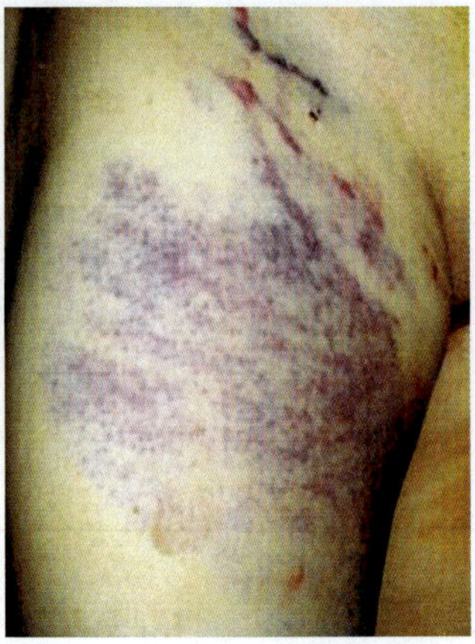

Fig. (4-5). Subcutaneous hematoma at the site of insertion of the catheter for transfemoral PCI.

2. *Vascular Lesions during Catheter Advancement*

In hypertensive patients with severe generalized atherosclerosis who underwent PCI, dissection or perforation of the abdominal aorta with subsequent hemoperitoneum or retroperitoneal hematoma was reported in fewer than 0.8% of cases. The risk is higher in patients receiving antiplatelet or anticoagulant therapy [37].

Although rare, dissection or rupture by the catheter of the ascending aorta can be fatal. Rupture of the guidewire or direct aortic involvement following dissection of the coronary artery can lead to the formation of a periaortic hematoma with subsequent hemopericardium. In one of our cases, percutaneous stent implantation into the femoral artery *via* the subclavian artery was followed by aortic root perforation and cardiac tamponade, as a result of the abnormally detached guidewire (Fig. **4-6**), probably due to a manufacturing defect [17].

In patients with aortic coarctation who have undergone endovascular therapy, aortic rupture has been reported in 23 cases published since 2015. Periprocedural aortic aneurysm has also been reported following angioplasty (0-13%), BMS (0-5%) and DES insertion (<1%) [38].

Stent insertion *via* carotid endarterectomy can predispose the patient to arterial dissection, embolization and thrombosis. In one recently published case regarding a 78-year-old woman who underwent carotid endarterectomy combined with coronary artery bypass grafting, rupture of the internal carotid artery at the distal tip of the stent was observed. To save the life of the patient, insertion of a prosthetic graft was performed *via* a small saphenous vein [24].

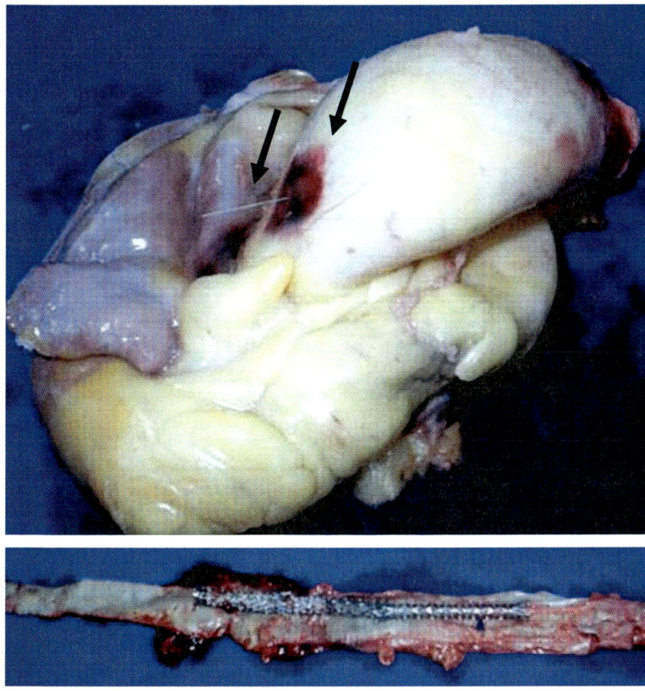

Fig. (4-6). The guidewire detached (top) during implantation of a BMS into the femoral artery (bottom) *via* the subclavian artery, followed by perforation of the ascending aorta (top). The patient died as a result of cardiac tamponade.

In patients with atrial fibrillation, percutaneous radio frequency catheter ablation can be successfully performed. During ventricular or right heart catheterization, cardiac perforation, damage to the aortic valves and thermal esophageal lesions have been reported [39].

3. ***PCI-Related Lesions of the Coronary Arteries***

The most common PCI-related complications are coronary artery perforation, dissection or restenosis, in-stent restenosis and thrombosis. Other rare lesions are coronary artery-left ventricular fistulae, stent displacement, intraventricular stent loss, *etc.*

- Coronary artery perforation

The incidence of coronary artery perforation significantly decreased from 3% during the 1990s to 0.3-0.6% in the 2000s [40 - 42]. Based on the size and extent of perforation, Ellis's angiographic classification (1994) identifies four types of perforations [43, 44]:

- Type I: incomplete perforation of the vascular wall, with formation of an intramural crater and without extravasation of the contrast medium (20%).
- Type II: complete perforation with extravasation limited to the pericardium or myocardium (39%).
- Type III: severe extravasation with frank or delayed tamponade (41%).
- Type IV: prominent extravasation into the heart chambers (<0.8%).

The risk of coronary artery perforation is higher in female patients (due to their narrower vessels) and hypertensive patients, but also in patients with severe coronary sclerosis and calcified areas larger than 10 mm [42]. Aggressive arterial handling or debulking in a fully-anticoagulated patient can also cause perforation. Rupture is more common in cases of insertion of stents with a hydrophilic or stiff guidewire or in cases of use of an oversized balloon. Distal rupture of the guidewire has rarely been observed [43]. The risk of tamponade is 0.4%, 3.3% and 45.7% for patients of Ellis's perforation classes I, II, and III, respectively [42].

- Coronary artery dissection

PCI-related coronary artery dissection has been reported with an incidence of 0.75-39%. The highest risk of dissection was observed in patients with severe coronary sclerosis, ST-elevation or associated myocardial infarction. Anticoagulant therapy, implantation of short stents and a dissection flap thickness larger than 0.31 mm are also risk factors of dissection [45, 46].

Based on the size and aspect of the angiography-detected luminal filling defect, six types of coronary dissections have been proposed by the National Heart, Lung and Blood Institute (NHLBI) [47]:

- Type A: minimal luminal narrowing (minor radiolucent area).
- Type B: formation of a false lumen (double lumen).
- Type C: contrast medium seen as an "extraluminal cap".
- Type D: spiral luminal filling defect ("barber shop pole").
- Type E: new persistent filling defect within the lumen.
- Type F: total luminal occlusion without distal anterograde flow, with retrograde spread into the aorta (Fig. **4-7**).

The coronary dissection types A and B occurs in 58% of cases and are clinically benign lesions. In patients with dissection types C-F, luminal obstruction is associated with myocardial infarction and/or cardiogenic shock. Open bypass surgery is thus necessary to save the patient's life [17, 45, 47].

In 60.8% of patients with PCI-related aortic dissection, the entry point is a coronary artery dissection [48]. The right coronary artery is more frequently involved (84.2%) with no difference between the use of BMS or DES [45, 47].

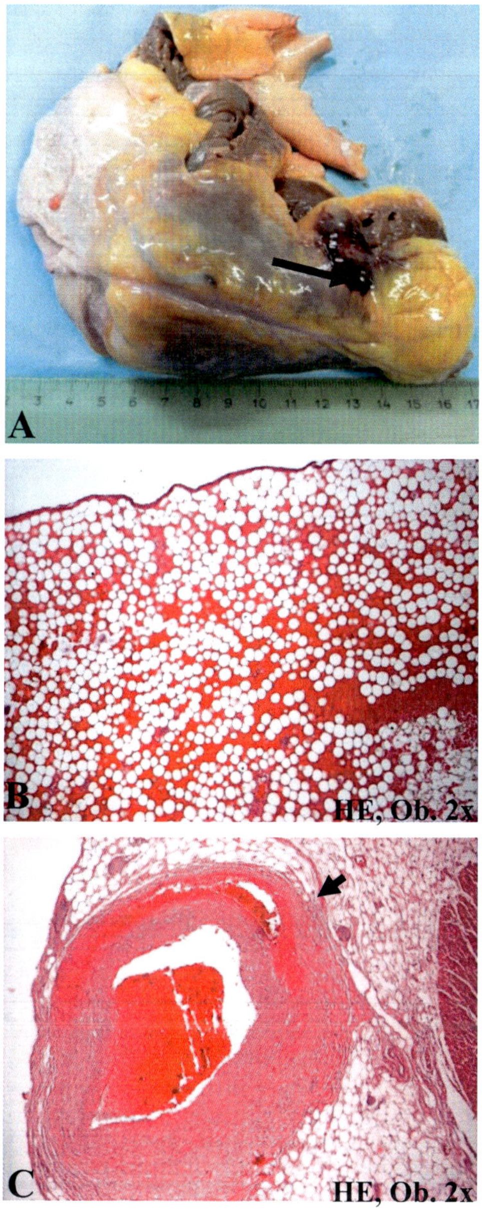

Fig. (4-7). Subepicardial hematoma (A, B) in a 74-year-old female with type F coronary artery dissection (C) after coronary angiography. The patient died as a result of cardiac tamponade.

• Coronary artery restenosis

Vascular restenosis occurs in 40-50% of cases and secondary angioplasty is necessary in 20-30% of restenotic cases. The process begins with damage to the intima and atherosclerotic plaques during stent insertion. Then, negative connective tissue remodeling occurs during the second phase of stent incorporation. This is followed by excessive connective tissue formation during the stabilizing process, inducing enlargement of the preexisting atherosclerotic plaques. In contrast, positive remodeling produces excessive coronary artery dilatation [14].

• In-stent restenosis

A stenosis greater than 50% is the result of excessive neointimal hyperplasia (the second phase of stent incorporation) followed by irregular connective tissue formation during the stabilizing period. After implantation of a BMS in-stent, restenosis occurs in 25% of patients and has been long considered as "the Achilles' tendon of PCI". The discovery of a DES that inhibits neointimal growth was thought to avoid this complication [12, 49]. However, after DES insertion, in-stent restenosis is still reported in 3-20% of patients [49]. The sirolimus DES insertion can be associated with a focal (≤10 mm length) stenosis, but this can also be diffuse (>10 mm) after paclitaxel DES [50].

In-stent restenosis remains the most common post-PTCA complication requiring coronary artery bypass grafting or coronary endarterectomy with/without stent removal. Removal of the atheromatous core within the restenosed DES is more difficult than for BMS [49]. Implantation of BVS has recently been suggested for patients with BMS/DES in-stent restenosis [51].

To reduce the risk of restenosis, normal BMI and normal blood pressure is required at the time of PCI (<140/90 mm Hg), and small DES lengths are indicated [52]. Little is known about the mechanism of late in-stent restenosis, which can occur at one year after PTCA and is more severe for DES than BMS [53].

• Thrombosis

After balloon dilatation, coronary artery thrombosis occurs in 5-10% of cases. The main cause is rupture of the atherosclerotic plaques with/without subsequent coronary dissection [14]. The thrombosis can be acute (periprocedural, first day after PCI), subacute (second day to one month), late (one month to one year) or very late (more than one year) [54].

In-stent thrombosis is very rare. For both BMS and BVS implantation, the reported incidence of acute/subacute thrombosis is about 1% [51]. It is mainly caused by stent malposition, improper stent expansion and inadequate antiplatelet therapy. Nickel allergies have also been reported to induce BMS-related thrombosis [55]. Very late thrombosis is more common after DES implantation than after BMS. This thrombosis can be a neoatherosclerosis complication. Its genesis is caused by poor and incompetent regenerated endothelium, which presents poorly formed cell junctions, reduced expression of antithrombotic molecules and decreased nitric oxide production [53, 56].

- Coronary artery aneurysm

A true aneurysm is defined as a vascular dilatation above 20% that occurs following PCI. The reported incidence rate is 0.3-3.9%, which is slightly higher following BMS than DES [57]. Glucocorticoids increase the risk of aneurysm formation. The following three types of post-PCI aneurysms are described in the literature [58, 59]:

- Type I: acute aneurysm – occurs between three and four weeks after stent implantation, presenting fast growth and frequently associated pericarditis.
- Type II: sub acute to chronic aneurysm – occurs after six months following stent implantation, can be asymptomatic or associated with angina.
- Type III: mycotic aneurysm – has been reported for both DES and BMS implantations. Fever and systemic disorders (bacteremia) are associated with this type.
    - Coronary artery pseudoaneurysm

This is a complication of coronary artery dissection attributable to mechanical trauma during catheter advancement. Its occurrence is caused by thrombolytic therapy. Spontaneous closure and very late thrombosis of the false aneurysm have been reported between one and 11 years following angioplasty [60].

B. Other complications of percutaneous vascular interventions

- *Allergy* - usually caused by medications used for anesthesia, can lead to asthmatiforme crisis, vasopressor syncope, anaphylactic shock, *etc.* [61].
- *Heparin-induced thrombocytopenia* – an immune-mediated lesion that can emerge a few days following intervention. Its incidence is approximately 1-3%. Procoagulant/pro-inflammatory agents can cause thrombosis [55].
- *Infections* – the peripuncture gateway is the most common source of infections that can lead to septicemia. The incidence is below 1% and the agent involved is usually *Staphylococcus aureus*. In PTCA, the critical period of occurrence of positive blood cultures is between the first hours (18% of patients) to 12 hours

(12%) after angioplasty. Most cases are asymptomatic [62].

- *Cholesterol crystals embolism* – emboli are released from the injured atheromas in about 2% of patients. It is usually an asymptomatic process, but finger cyanosis can be associated, primarily following femoral/radial puncture. Retinal atheroembolism has been infrequently reported following coronarography [63].
- *Nephropathy* – contrast-induced tubular/interstitial nephropathy – defined as rising serum creatinine level of ≥ 0.5 mg/dL (25% above the baseline value) or a ≥ 25% drop in the estimated glomerular filtration rate after contrast administration – occurs in 3-30% of cases, representing one third of in-hospital acute kidney injuries [64, 65]. Risk factors are DM, preexisting chronic renal dysfunction and older age. Regards the contrast agent, large volume and high osmolar contrast substances are more prone to inducing allergy (3.1% of cases), as compared to low (0.7%) or iso-osmolar agents (<0.5%) [64]. In kidney transplant recipients with stable kidney function prior to hypo-osmolar iodinated intravascular contrast administration, the reported incidence of acute contrast-induced nephropathy is 5.64% [65]. In most cases, this relates to a mild type nephropathy that is reversible within seven days, but in severe forms hemodialysis might be necessary.
- *Periprocedural myocardial infarction* – PCI-related myocardial infarction occurs with an incidence of 0.05-0.07%, rising even higher in cases of multiple stents implantation [66]. After carotid endarterectomy, the risk of myocardial infarction is about 0.8% and depends on the patient's age, history of coronary artery disease, peripheral artery disease and restenosis. The risk is slightly higher for carotid angioplasty and stenting, associated with a risk of 0.7% [67].
- *Arrhythmia* – bradycardia occurs in 3.5% of patients and post-PCI tachyarrhythmia affects approximately 0.1% of patients [68].
- *Cerebrovascular disorders* – PCI-related stroke is reported in 0.23-0.44% of cases, being caused by microemboli, broken atheromas or air embolism [69]. Carotid angioplasty and stenting are associated with higher risks of periprocedural stroke and death as compared to carotid endarterectomy [67].

OPEN HEART SURGERY

A. Postoperative Complications

During open heart surgery, extracorporeal circulation *can induce severe hypoxia* with subsequent brain hypoxic lesions and/or *severe hemolysis* with acute renal failure. *Hypoxia-related hemorrhagic subendocardial necrosis* (Fig. **4-8**) can induce ventricular fibrillation. Focal necrosis is not lethal.

Postoperative fibrinous pericarditis is a common complication that is usually without clinical consequences.

Stone heart syndrome is an ischemic irreversible myocardial contraction that occurs, though rarely, as a complication of cardiac surgery. *Myocardial stunning* (*neurogenic stunned myocardium*) is an ischemia-induced decreasing of left ventricular myocardial contraction [70].

Coronary artery-ventricular fistulae have been reported in 0.22% of patients who have undergone open heart surgery. The left ventricle is primarily involved, but communication with the right ventricle, right atrium, pulmonary artery and coronary sinus can also occur. The main consequence is myocardial ischemia with postoperative ST segment depression or T wave abnormalities detected on the ECG [71].

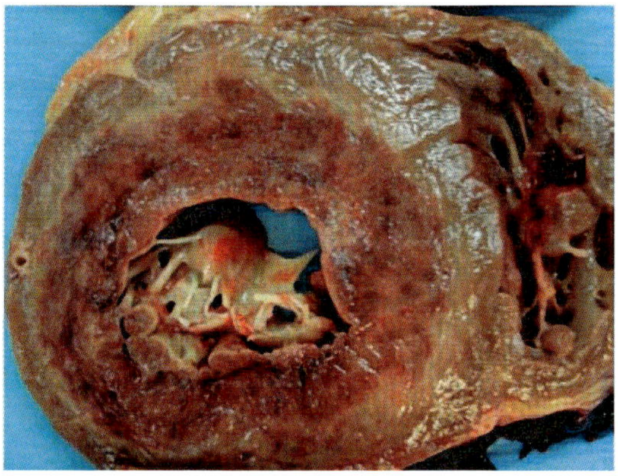

Fig. (4-8). Left ventricle diffuse subendocardial hemorrhagic necrosis following open heart surgery. The patient died as a result of cardiogenic shock.

B. Prosthetic Valve Replacement

The implantation of *glutaraldehyde-fixed biological valves* can be complicated by dystrophic calcification, valvular deformities or stenosis and functional disorders. The development of decell techniques, space filler and detoxification of porcine valves have been experimentally tested [72].

The implantation of *mechanical valves* can be followed by infection, thrombosis, embolism and dehiscence (between the valve and the anulus fibrosus) with further paravalvular leakage and/or perivalvular prosthetic regurgitation. Closure of the paravalvular leak can be performed percutaneously using specific devices [73].

During *mitral valve replacement,* the coronary sinus can be damaged [74]. Left ventricular rupture has been reported in 0.7% of patients who have undergone mitral valve replacement, with 50-67% of these leading to in-hospital death [75]. Based on their location, three types of ventricular ruptures that can occur after mitral valve replacement are known [76, 77]:

- Type I: rupture located in the atrioventricular groove. This is the most common type of rupture that occurs in patients with calcified mitral valve annulus or bacterial endocarditis with mitral valve annular abscess. It can be caused by resection of the posterior leaflet and chordae, placement of subannular sutures for valvular replacement and improper inspection of the left ventricular posterior wall after surgical replacement.
- Type II: rupture located at the base of the papillary muscles. This type is a consequence of excessive resection of the posterior papillary muscles.
- Type III: rupture of the posterior left ventricular wall. This type of trauma is extremely rare and can occur after implantation of large valves.

Aortic valve replacement can be followed by fibrosis of endocardium and aortic intima with subsequent stenosis of the coronary artery orifices and myocardial ischemia [78]. A high risk of heart failure is reported for patients who undergo aortic valve replacement after prior coronary artery bypass surgery with patent left internal thoracic artery. In these cases, the intraoperative injuries of the left internal thoracic artery can lead to inadequate myocardial preservation during the cross-clamp period. This complication can be avoided by controlling the arterial flow through extrathoracic supraclavicular occlusion [79]. Delayed chylopericardium (1500 cc milky fluid in the pericardial cavity) has been reported as a rare complication within four months of aortic bioprosthetic valve replacement [80].

Postoperative invasive hemodynamic monitoring with a pulmonary artery catheter (Swan-Ganz catheter) can induce pulmonary artery rupture and massive lethal pulmonary hemorrhage or pulmonary artery false aneurysm. This can be seen on chest radiographs and CT scans as a lung nodule, usually on the right lung, which should be differentiated from lung tumors – embolization is the treatment of choice [81].

C. Coronary Artery Bypass Grafting

In patients undergoing aortocoronary bypass graft surgery following previous valvular replacement, the risk of acute myocardial infarction and/or left ventricular rupture is increased (Fig. **4-9**). Infarction in other organs, such as the kidney or intestine, can be associated (Fig. **4-10**).

Aortocoronary replacement by the saphenous vein can be followed by graft arterializations and risk of atherosclerosis, due to high-pressure distension. Early graft failure (about one month after surgery) is characterized by intraluminal thrombi that can produce acute myocardial infarction. Late graft failure (venous graft disease), with a recurrence of angina, can be morphometrically detected on the angiography as a thickening of the venous wall due to hypertrophy of the tunica media [82].

In diabetics and patients with symptomatic peripheral arterial disease, use of the saphenous vein should be avoided due to the high risk of painful and delayed wound healing. Wound healing disturbances are also common in obese patients, females, smokers and patients with low preoperative hematocrit levels [83].

Although not common, rhabdomyolysis after a coronary artery bypass graft has been reported as a cause of acute renal failure [84].

Another infrequent postoperative complication is radial nerve injury caused by external compression. It can induce reversible left forearm muscle weakness and flexion of the fingers of the left hand [85]. Post-coronary artery bypass drafting chylothorax has also been reported [86].

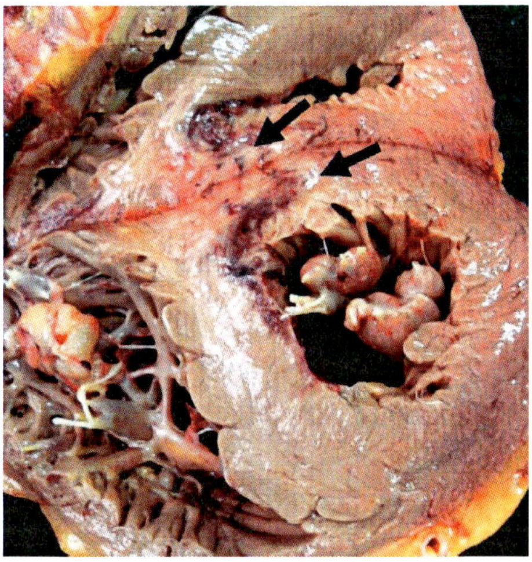

Fig. (4-9). Posteroseptal acute myocardial infarction with ventricular wall rupture in a 70-year-old female who underwent an aortic valve replacement and triple aortocoronary bypass.

D. Myocardial Reperfusion Injury

Reperfusion injury is a worldwide public health issue with increasing incidence. It can occur after major open heart operations (Fig. **4-11**) or after PCI performed for thrombolysis or stent implantation in patients with obstructive coronary sclerosis or acute myocardial infarction [17, 87].

The reperfusion of ischemic myocardium should be performed in the first two to four hours after blood supply deprivation. After this period, necrosis of myocytes and the absence of oxygen induces transformation of xanthine dehydrogenase into xanthine oxidase (oxidative stress). Then, blood supply return will cause the xanthine oxidase-mediated release of superoxides from the damaged myocytes and subsequent expansion of the necrotic area [88]. Local and systemic inflammatory processes are also activated [87].

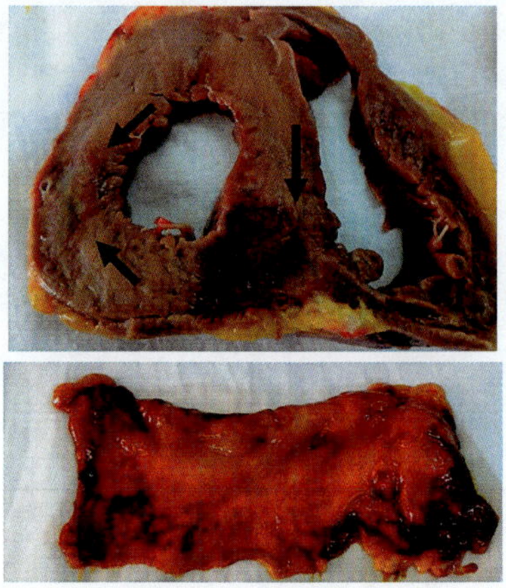

Fig. (4-10). Posteroseptal and lateral acute myocardial infarction (top) and intestinal infarction (bottom) in a 67-year-old male who died two days after a mitral valve replacement and aortocoronary bypass.

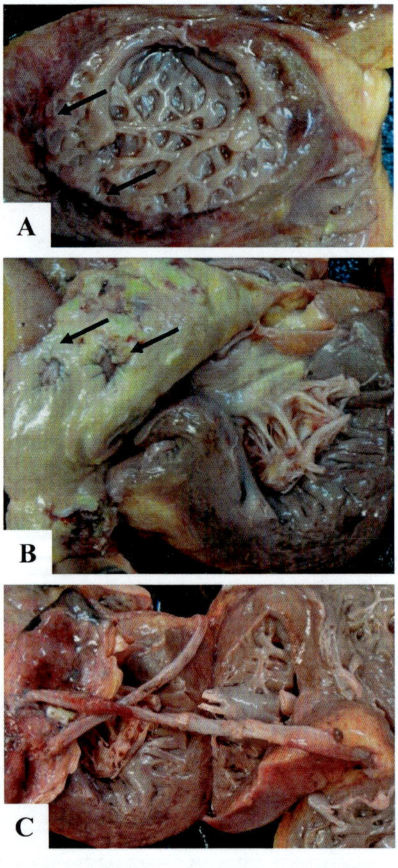

Fig. (4-11). Left ventricle apical subendocardial reperfusion lesions in a 65-year-old obese female who underwent a double aortocoronary bypass.

It is important to note that, during reperfusion, a transient arrhythmia emerges as a result of successful restoration of blood flow. It is induced by the blood inflow-related decrease of the extracellular K^+, due to the enhanced activity of the Na^+ K^+ pump, in turn caused by the intracellular accumulation of Na^+ and depletion of K^+ during the necrotic process. High extracellular levels of K^+ are associated with intracellular Ca^{2+} overload. The result is delayed after depolarization and subsequent transient arrhythmia, which involves premature ventricular contraction, ventricular fibrillation, accelerated idioventricular rhythm, nonsustained ventricular tachycardia and/or bradycardia [89].

Allopurinol is a xanthine oxidase inhibitor thought to reduce the expansion of a necrotic area and the period of transient arrhythmia, both signs of successful reperfusion [89]. New treatments, such as mesenchymal stromal cell therapy, thought to have immunomodulatory, anti-inflammatory and tissue reparative properties, are under review, but no specific therapy for reperfusion lesions has been validated to date [87].

E. Pacemaker Implantation

Pacemaker-related complications are rare and comprise infections, ventricular rupture, endocardium breakage and thrombosis. Malpositioned transvenous permanent pacemakers leading into the left ventricle have also been reported [90]. This is caused by a dilated heart or a patent foramen ovale, but perforation of the septum by the lead is also possible [90]. Although rare, lead misplacement into the left ventricle can be complicated by atrial fibrillation, thrombosis, thromboembolism (37%), perforation of the mitral valve, mitral insufficiency, aortic valve endocarditis, diaphragmatic pacing and loss of capture [90, 91]. Implantation of the ventricular lead into the distal coronary sinus or other cardiac veins can also be unexpected accidents [92].

F. Surgical Correction of Atrioventricular Septal Defects

Septal defects closure is primarily performed with Dacron material, using a single- or two-patch method [93]. In patients with isolated muscular ventricular septal defects, percutaneous closure can be performed, but surgery is still used for perimembranous defects [94]. Although the survival period is quite long (1 year – 80%; 10 years – 78%; 20 years – 65%), the seven-day and one-month mortality rates are approximately 11% and 15%, respectively [95].

The most common postoperative complications are infections (8-21%), pulmonary hypertensive crises (6-10%), moderate or severe valvular regurgitation, valvular stenosis (the mitral valve is most affected), thrombosis, embolism, patch dehiscence, residual shunt, pericardial/pleural effusions, arrhythmias (atrioventricular dissociation, bradyarrhythmia, atrioventricular block), renal failure and respiratory failure [93 - 95]. The major complications are early death, necessity of reoperation or permanent pacemaker implantation, and, in infants, incidental suture of other structures, such as the pulmonary artery, with subsequent pulmonary infarction [94]. The risk of postoperative complications, especially those that involve the mitral valve, is greater in infants with Down's syndrome [93].

OTHER CARDIOVASCULAR THERAPEUTIC PROCEDURES

- ***Intravenous Injections/Perfusions*** The most common complications are thrombosis, thrombophlebitis, hemorrhages and aneurysms, especially after intravenous administration of cytotoxic drugs. Infection of the catheter can lead to septic endocarditis (Fig. **4-12**). Accidental perivenous injection of some drugs, such as thiopental or potassium chloride, can produce tissue necrosis. Intravenous injection of propofol is associated with acute pain that can be avoided by pre-administered ketamine. Antirabic vaccination can induce myocarditis. Acute pulmonary edema can be a consequence of a high level of intravenously injected fluids [88].

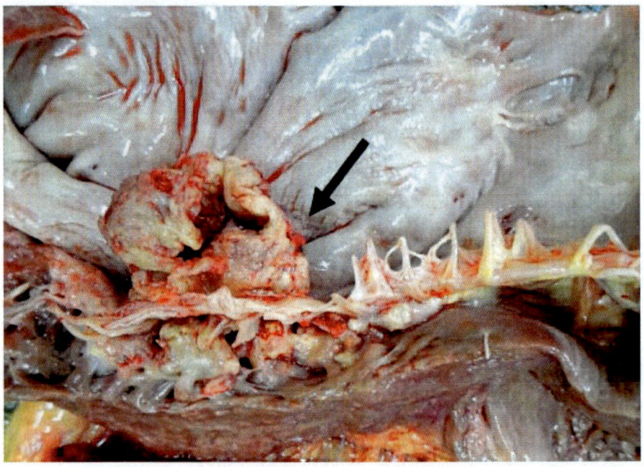

Fig. (4-12). Infective endocarditis in a diabetic patient with sub acute septicemia. The patient died of septic shock.

- ***Intravenous Injection of Contrast Materials*** The most common complications are perivenous artifacts and retrograde flow of contrast material. It has been observed that injection of contrast material into the antecubital vein of the right arm may provide better image quality in head and neck CT scans, as compared to injection into the left arm [88, 96].
- ***Central Vein Puncture*** The rate of periprocedural complications is about 15%.

Central venous catheterization is associated with risk of hematoma, necrosis of the surrounding tissues, arterial puncture, sepsis and embolism (air, gas or a malpositioned catheter). During puncture, other surrounding structures, such as the carotid artery, vagus nerve, phrenic nerve or cervical plexus, can be damaged, inducing Claude Bernard-Horner syndrome. Pneumothorax, hemothorax and chylothorax can be consequence of technical errors or occur following subclavian vein puncture [97].

- ***External Cardiac Massage*** The most common cardiovascular lesions that occur after cardiopulmonary resuscitation are vascular or myocardial rupture by fractured ribs (Fig. **4-13**) [98]. Following PCI, stent distortion, compression or displacement and additional vascular injuries can emerge [99].

  After major cardiac interventions, the rate of postoperative cardiac arrest is 0.7-2.9%. According to the European Resuscitation Council (ERC), defibrillation or pacing is recommended in these patients before external cardiac compression is attempted [100].

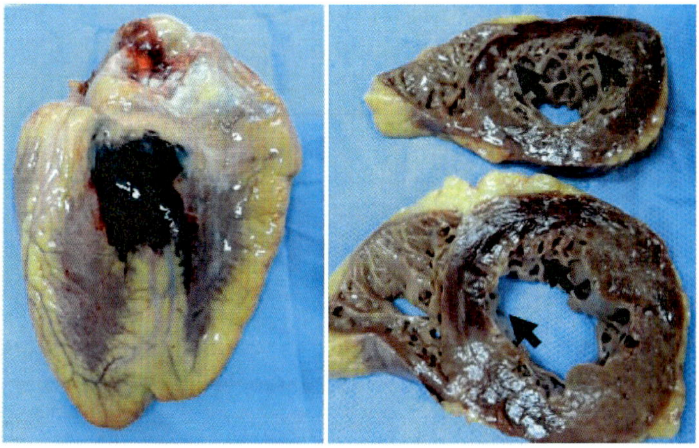

Fig. (4-13). Subepicardial hematoma following external cardiopulmonary resuscitation with ribs fractures (left) in a patient with double stent implantation, performed for acute extended anteroseptal myocardial infarction (right). The patient died as a result of cardiogenic shock.

CONFLICT OF INTEREST

The authors confirm that this chapter content has no conflict of interest.

ACKNOWLEDGEMENTS

Declared none.

REFERENCES

[1] Kucharska W, Negrusz-Kawecka M, Gromkowska M. Cardiotoxicity of oncological treatment in children. Adv Clin Exp Med 2012; 21(3): 281-8.

[PMID: 23214190]

[2] Nitiss KC, Nitiss JL. Twisting and ironing: doxorubicin cardiotoxicity by mitochondrial DNA damage. Clin Cancer Res 2014; 20(18): 4737-9.
[http://dx.doi.org/10.1158/1078-0432.CCR-14-0821] [PMID: 24916696]

[3] www.rhombnet.com. Accessed August 25, 2015.

[4] Overman MJ, Varadhachary GR, Kopetz S, *et al.* Phase II study of capecitabine and oxaliplatin for advanced adenocarcinoma of the small bowel and ampulla of Vater. J Clin Oncol 2009; 27(16): 2598-603.
[http://dx.doi.org/10.1200/JCO.2008.19.7145] [PMID: 19164203]

[5] Gurzu S, Jung I, Comsulea M, Kadar Z, Azamfirei L, Molnar C. Lethal cardiotoxicity, steatohepatitis, chronic pancreatitis, and acute enteritis induced by capecitabine and oxaliplatin in a 36-year-old woman. Diagn Pathol 2013; 8: 150.
[http://dx.doi.org/10.1186/1746-1596-8-150] [PMID: 24041405]

[6] Manojlovic N, Babic D, Stojanovic S, Filipovic I, Radoje D. Capecitabine cardiotoxicity case reports and literature review. Hepatogastroenterology 2008; 55(85): 1249-56.
[PMID: 18795667]

[7] Y-Hassan S, Tornvall P, Törnerud M, Henareh L. Capecitabine caused cardiogenic shock through induction of global Takotsubo syndrome. Cardiovasc Revasc Med 2013; 14(1): 57-61.
[http://dx.doi.org/10.1016/j.carrev.2012.10.001] [PMID: 23218901]

[8] Lepor H, Lepor NE, Hill LA, Trohman RG. The QT interval and selection of alpha-blockers for benign prostatic hyperplasia. Rev Urol 2008; 10(2): 85-91.
[PMID: 18660858]

[9] Jankovic D, Winhofer Y, Promintzer-Schifferl M, *et al.* Effects of insulin therapy on myocardial lipid content and cardiac geometry in patients with type-2 diabetes mellitus. PLoS One 2012; 7(12): e50077.
[http://dx.doi.org/10.1371/journal.pone.0050077] [PMID: 23226508]

[10] Feleke E, Lyngstam O, Råstam L, Rydén L. Complaints of cold extremities among patients on antihypertensive treatment. Acta Med Scand 1983; 213(5): 381-5.
[http://dx.doi.org/10.1111/j.0954-6820.1983.tb03755.x] [PMID: 6136158]

[11] Ravi S, Chaikof EL. Biomaterials for vascular tissue engineering. Regen Med 2010; 5(1): 107-20.
[http://dx.doi.org/10.2217/rme.09.77] [PMID: 20017698]

[12] Muller KM, Offner FA, Bohle RM. 2008.

[13] Van Belle E, Tio FO, Couffinhal T, Maillard L, Passeri J, Isner JM. Stent endothelialization. Time course, impact of local catheter delivery, feasibility of recombinant protein administration, and response to cytokine expedition. Circulation 1997; 95(2): 438-48.
[http://dx.doi.org/10.1161/01.CIR.95.2.438] [PMID: 9008462]

[14] Michaelides A. Percutaneous transluminal coronary angioplasty 2010.

[15] Kuralay E, Oz BS, Cingöz F, *et al.* Perpendicular insertion of Dacron patch for aortoplasty in adult coarctation of aorta to increase circular elasticity. J Card Surg 2003; 18(3): 257-9.
[http://dx.doi.org/10.1046/j.1540-8191.2003.02040.x] [PMID: 12809401]

[16] Antoniou GA, Georgiadis GS, Antoniou SA, *et al.* Late rupture of abdominal aortic aneurysm after previous endovascular repair: a systematic review and meta-analysis. J Endovasc Ther 2015; 22(5): 734-44.
[http://dx.doi.org/10.1177/1526602815601405] [PMID: 26286073]

[17] Gurzu S, Lostun A, Egyed-Zsigmond E, *et al.* Diagnostic errors in non-iatrogenic and iatrogenic cardiovascular deaths analyzed in 838 autopsies. Exp Clin Cardiol 2014; 20: 3920-31.

[18] Jeon JP, Cho YD, Han MH. Intra-arterial thrombolysis of central retinal artery occlusion following

percutaneous atrial septal defect closure. Catheter Cardiovasc Interv 2015. [http://dx.doi.org/10.1002/ccd.26100] [PMID: 26153142]

[19] Atashband A, Lakkis N. First comprehensive analysis of outcomes in adult patients after percutaneous closure of isolated secundum atrial septal defects. Cardiovasc Hematol Agents Med Chem 2015; 13(1): 63-9. [http://dx.doi.org/10.2174/187152571301150730115936] [PMID: 26245662]

[20] Onuma Y, Serruys PW, Muramatsu T, *et al.* Incidence and imaging outcomes of acute scaffold disruption and late structural discontinuity after implantation of the absorb Everolimus-Eluting fully bioresorbable vascular scaffold: optical coherence tomography assessment in the ABSORB cohort B Trial (A Clinical Evaluation of the Bioabsorbable Everolimus Eluting Coronary Stent System in the Treatment of Patients With De Novo Native Coronary Artery Lesions). JACC Cardiovasc Interv 2014; 7(12): 1400-11. [http://dx.doi.org/10.1016/j.jcin.2014.06.016] [PMID: 25523532]

[21] Iqbal J, Gunn J, Serruys PW. Coronary stents: historical development, current status and future directions. Br Med Bull 2013; 106: 193-211. [http://dx.doi.org/10.1093/bmb/ldt009] [PMID: 23532779]

[22] Berg R, Aragon J, Royter V, *et al.* Pimecrolimus and dual pimecrolimus-paclitaxel eluting stents decrease neointimal proliferation in a porcine model. Catheter Cardiovasc Interv 2007; 70(6): 871-9. [http://dx.doi.org/10.1002/ccd.21299] [PMID: 17932889]

[23] Gogas BD. Bioresorbable scaffolds for percutaneous coronary interventions 2014. [http://dx.doi.org/10.5339/gcsp.2014.55]

[24] Illuminati G, Caliò FG, Pizzardi G, Vietri F. Internal carotid artery rupture caused by carotid shunt insertion. Int J Surg Case Rep 2015; 14: 89-91. [http://dx.doi.org/10.1016/j.ijscr.2015.07.030] [PMID: 26255001]

[25] Tavakol M, Ashraf S, Brener SJ. Risks and complications of coronary angiography: a comprehensive review. Glob J Health Sci 2012; 4(1): 65-93. [PMID: 22980117]

[26] Bryniarski KL, Zabojszcz M, Dębski G, *et al.* Knowledge of chronic total occlusion among Polish interventional cardiologists. Postepy Kardiol Interwencyjnej 2015; 11(2): 89-94. [http://dx.doi.org/10.5114/pwki.2015.52280] [PMID: 26161099]

[27] Babu SC, Piccorelli GO, Shah PM, Stein JH, Clauss RH. Incidence and results of arterial complications among 16,350 patients undergoing cardiac catheterization. J Vasc Surg 1989; 10(2): 113-6. [http://dx.doi.org/10.1016/0741-5214(89)90342-X] [PMID: 2788227]

[28] Manuel-Rimbau E, Lozano P, Gómez A, Bethencourt A, Gómez FT. Lesiones vasculares yatrogénicas tras cateterismo cardíaco. Rev Esp Cardiol 1998; 51(9): 750-5. [http://dx.doi.org/10.1016/S0300-8932(98)74818-3] [PMID: 9803801]

[29] Applegate RJ, Sacrinty MT, Kutcher MA, *et al.* Trends in vascular complications after diagnostic cardiac catheterization and percutaneous coronary intervention *via* the femoral artery, 1998 to 2007. JACC Cardiovasc Interv 2008; 1(3): 317-26. [http://dx.doi.org/10.1016/j.jcin.2008.03.013] [PMID: 19463320]

[30] Swanson N, Hogrefe K, Javed Q, Malik N, Gershlick AH. Vascular endothelial growth factor (VEGF)-eluting stents: *in vivo* effects on thrombosis, endothelialization and intimal hyperplasia. J Invasive Cardiol 2003; 15(12): 688-92. [PMID: 14660819]

[31] Kacila M, Vranic H, Hadzimehmedagic A, Sehovic S. The frequency of complications of pseudoaneurysm: Diagnostic and therapeutic interventions. Med Arh 2011; 65: 78-81. [PMID: 21585178]

[32] Butler R, Webster MW. Meralgia paresthetica: an unusual complication of cardiac catheterization *via* the femoral artery. Catheter Cardiovasc Interv 2002; 56(1): 69-71. [http://dx.doi.org/10.1002/ccd.10149] [PMID: 11979538]

[33] Scheinert D, Ludwig J, Steinkamp HJ, Schröder M, Balzer JO, Biamino G. Treatment of catheter-induced iliac artery injuries with self-expanding endografts. J Endovasc Ther 2000; 7(3): 213-20. [http://dx.doi.org/10.1177/152660280000700308] [PMID: 10883959]

[34] Samal AK, White CJ. Percutaneous management of access site complications. Catheter Cardiovasc Interv 2002; 57(1): 12-23. [http://dx.doi.org/10.1002/ccd.10179] [PMID: 12203921]

[35] Hallett JW Jr, Wolk SW, Cherry KJ Jr, Gloviczki P, Pairolero PC. 1990.

[36] Gross C, Lecocq J, Ribaud J, Vautravers P, Bareiss P. [An unusual complication of coronarography: neuralgia of the internal saphenous]. Rev Neurol (Paris) 2003; 159(2): 212-4. [PMID: 12660577]

[37] Chan YC, Morales JP, Reidy JF, Taylor PR. Management of spontaneous and iatrogenic retroperitoneal haemorrhage: conservative management, endovascular intervention or open surgery? Int J Clin Pract 2008; 62(10): 1604-13. [http://dx.doi.org/10.1111/j.1742-1241.2007.01494.x] [PMID: 17949429]

[38] Tretter JT, Jones TK, McElhinney DB. Aortic wall injury related to endovascular therapy for aortic coarctation. Circ Cardiovasc Interv 2015; 8(9): e002840. [http://dx.doi.org/10.1161/CIRCINTERVENTIONS.115.002840] [PMID: 26291468]

[39] Rolf S, Boldt LH, Parwani AS, *et al.* Findings and outcome of fluoroscopic visualization of the oesophageal course during catheter ablation of atrial fibrillation. Europace 2011; 13(6): 796-802. [http://dx.doi.org/10.1093/europace/eur046] [PMID: 21398313]

[40] Gruberg L, Pinnow E, Flood R, *et al.* Incidence, management, and outcome of coronary artery perforation during percutaneous coronary intervention. Am J Cardiol 2000; 86(6): 680-682, A8. [http://dx.doi.org/10.1016/S0002-9149(00)01053-5] [PMID: 10980224]

[41] Dippel EJ, Kereiakes DJ, Tramuta DA, *et al.* Coronary perforation during percutaneous coronary intervention in the era of abciximab platelet glycoprotein IIb/IIIa blockade: an algorithm for percutaneous management. Catheter Cardiovasc Interv 2001; 52(3): 279-86. [http://dx.doi.org/10.1002/ccd.1065] [PMID: 11246236]

[42] Shimony A, Joseph L, Mottillo S, Eisenberg MJ. Coronary artery perforation during percutaneous coronary intervention: a systematic review and meta-analysis. Can J Cardiol 2011; 27(6): 843-50. [http://dx.doi.org/10.1016/j.cjca.2011.04.014] [PMID: 21862280]

[43] Witzke CF, Martin-Herrero F, Clarke SC, Pomerantzev E, Palacios IF. The changing pattern of coronary perforation during percutaneous coronary intervention in the new device era. J Invasive Cardiol 2004; 16(6): 257-301. [PMID: 15155997]

[44] Ellis SG, Ajluni S, Arnold AZ, *et al.* Increased coronary perforation in the new device era. Incidence, classification, management, and outcome. Circulation 1994; 90(6): 2725-30. [http://dx.doi.org/10.1161/01.CIR.90.6.2725] [PMID: 7994814]

[45] Zidi M, Nallet O, Esteve JB, Michaud P, Cattan S. [Extensive iatrogenic coronary dissection during coronary angioplasty: a series of 19 consecutive patients]. Ann Cardiol Angeiol (Paris) 2010; 59(5): 306-10. [http://dx.doi.org/10.1016/j.ancard.2010.08.012] [PMID: 20887973]

[46] Bouki KP, Sakkali E, Toutouzas K, *et al.* Impact of coronary artery stent edge dissections on long-term clinical outcome in patients with acute coronary syndrome: an optical coherence tomography study. Catheter Cardiovasc Interv 2015; 86(2): 237-46. [http://dx.doi.org/10.1002/ccd.25855] [PMID: 25620191]

[47] Rogers JH, Lasala JM. Coronary artery dissection and perforation complicating percutaneous coronary intervention. J Invasive Cardiol 2004; 16(9): 493-9.
[PMID: 15353832]

[48] Núñez-Gil IJ, Bautista D, Cerrato E, *et al.* Incidence, management, and immediate- and long-term outcomes after iatrogenic aortic dissection during diagnostic or interventional coronary procedures. Circulation 2015; 131(24): 2114-9.
[http://dx.doi.org/10.1161/CIRCULATIONAHA.115.015334] [PMID: 25888682]

[49] Nishigawa K, Fukui T, Takanashi S. Off-pump coronary endarterectomy with stent removal for in-stent restenosis in the left anterior descending artery. Interact Cardiovasc Thorac Surg 2015; 21(5): 594-7.
[http://dx.doi.org/10.1093/icvts/ivv210] [PMID: 26273070]

[50] Tsigkas GG, Karantalis V, Hahalis G, Alexopoulos D. Stent restenosis, pathophysiology and treatment options: a 2010 update. Hellenic J Cardiol 2011; 52(2): 149-57.
[PMID: 21478125]

[51] Moscarella E, Varricchio A, Stabile E, *et al.* Bioresorbable vascular scaffold implantation for the treatment of coronary in-stent restenosis: results from a multicenter Italian experience. Int J Cardiol 2015; 199: 366-72.
[http://dx.doi.org/10.1016/j.ijcard.2015.07.002] [PMID: 26241643]

[52] Tocci J, Barbato E, Coluccia R, *et al.* Blood Pressure Levels at the Time of Percutaneous Coronary Revascularization and Risk of Coronary In-Stent Restenosis. Am J Hypertens 2015; hpv131.
[PMID: 26271109]

[53] Zhang BC, Karanasos A, Regar E. OCT demonstrating neoatherosclerosis as part of the continuous process of coronary artery disease. Herz 2015; 40(6): 845-54.
[http://dx.doi.org/10.1007/s00059-015-4343-y] [PMID: 26259732]

[54] Vencatesan S. www.drsvenkatesan.co.in. Accessed at 4th of July 2015.

[55] Konishi T, Yamamoto T, Funayama N, *et al.* Stent thrombosis caused by metal allergy complicated by protein S deficiency and heparin-induced thrombocytopenia: a case report and review of the literature. Thromb J 2015; 13: 25.
[http://dx.doi.org/10.1186/s12959-015-0055-z] [PMID: 26207097]

[56] Otsuka F, Finn AV, Yazdani SK, Nakano M, Kolodgie FD, Virmani R. The importance of the endothelium in atherothrombosis and coronary stenting. Nat Rev Cardiol 2012; 9(8): 439-53.
[http://dx.doi.org/10.1038/nrcardio.2012.64] [PMID: 22614618]

[57] Aoki J, Kirtane A, Leon MB, Dangas G. Coronary artery aneurysms after drug-eluting stent implantation. JACC Cardiovasc Interv 2008; 1(1): 14-21.
[http://dx.doi.org/10.1016/j.jcin.2007.10.004] [PMID: 19393139]

[58] Zhang F, Qian JY, Ge JB. Rapid development of late stent malapposition and coronary aneurysm following implantation of a paclitaxel-eluting coronary stent. Chin Med J (Engl) 2007; 120(7): 614-6.
[PMID: 17442215]

[59] Jindal RK, George R, Singh B. Giant coronary aneurysm following drug-eluting stent implantation presenting as fever of unknown origin. J Invasive Cardiol 2007; 19(7): 313-4.
[PMID: 17620677]

[60] Babunashvili AM. [A case of spontaneous closure of left main coronary artery false aneurysm and stent thrombosis 11 years after coronary artery stenting]. Kardiologiia 2008; 48(7): 87-92.
[PMID: 18789035]

[61] Finder RL, Moore PA. Adverse drug reactions to local anesthesia. Dent Clin North Am 2002; 46(4): 747-757, x.
[http://dx.doi.org/10.1016/S0011-8532(02)00018-6] [PMID: 12436829]

[62] Ramsdale DR, Aziz S, Newall N, Palmer N, Jackson M. Bacteremia following complex percutaneous coronary intervention. J Invasive Cardiol 2004; 16(11): 632-4.
[PMID: 15550732]

[63] Rousseau A, de Monchy I, Barreau E, *et al.* Retinal emboli in cholesterol crystal embolism 2013.
[http://dx.doi.org/10.1155/2013/421352]

[64] Murphy SW, Barrett BJ, Parfrey PS. Contrast nephropathy. J Am Soc Nephrol 2000; 11(1): 177-82.
[PMID: 10616853]

[65] Haider M, Yessayan L, Venkat KK, Goggins M, Patel A, Karthikeyan V. Incidence of contrast-induced nephropathy in kidney transplant recipients. Transplant Proc 2015; 47(2): 379-83.
[http://dx.doi.org/10.1016/j.transproceed.2015.01.008] [PMID: 25769577]

[66] Pasceri V, Patti G, Nusca A, Pristipino C, Richichi G, Di Sciascio G. Randomized trial of atorvastatin for reduction of myocardial damage during coronary intervention: results from the ARMYDA (Atorvastatin for Reduction of MYocardial Damage during Angioplasty) study. Circulation 2004; 110(6): 674-8.
[http://dx.doi.org/10.1161/01.CIR.0000137828.06205.87] [PMID: 15277322]

[67] Boulanger M, Cameliere L, Felgueiras R, *et al.* 2015.

[68] Chen J, Gao L, Yao M, Chen J. Ventricular arrhythmia onset during diagnostic coronary angiography with a 5F or 4F universal catheter. Rev Esp Cardiol 2008; 61(10): 1092-5.
[http://dx.doi.org/10.1157/13126050] [PMID: 18817686]

[69] Dukkipati S, ONeill WW, Harjai KJ, *et al.* Characteristics of cerebrovascular accidents after percutaneous coronary interventions. J Am Coll Cardiol 2004; 43(7): 1161-7.
[http://dx.doi.org/10.1016/j.jacc.2003.11.033] [PMID: 15063423]

[70] Schmitt JP, Schröder J, Schunkert H, Birnbaum DE, Aebert H. Role of apoptosis in myocardial stunning after open heart surgery. Ann Thorac Surg 2002; 73(4): 1229-35.
[http://dx.doi.org/10.1016/S0003-4975(02)03401-X] [PMID: 11996268]

[71] Demirkilic U, Ozal E, Bingol H, *et al.* Surgical treatment of coronary artery fistulas: 15 years experience. Asian Cardiovasc Thorac Ann 2004; 12(2): 133-8.
[http://dx.doi.org/10.1177/021849230401200211] [PMID: 15213080]

[72] Lim HG, Kim GB, Jeong S, Kim YJ. Development of a next-generation tissue valve using a glutaraldehyde-fixed porcine aortic valve treated with decellularization, α-galactosidase, space filler, organic solvent and detoxification. Eur J Cardiothorac Surg 2015; 48(1): 104-13.
[http://dx.doi.org/10.1093/ejcts/ezu385] [PMID: 25315752]

[73] Osken A, Aydin E, Akdemir R, Gunduz H. Percutaneous closure of an aortic prosthetic paravalvular leak with device in a patient presenting with heart failure. Heart Views 2015; 16(2): 56-8.
[http://dx.doi.org/10.4103/1995-705X.159221] [PMID: 26240734]

[74] Evora PR, Ribeiro PJ, Menardi AC, Vicente WV, Rodrigues AJ. Coronary sinus iatrogenic lesion during repeated mitral valve replacement: case report of an immediate transmitral annulus repair. Rev Bras Cir Cardiovasc 2003; 18: 186-8.
[http://dx.doi.org/10.1590/S0102-76382003000200013]

[75] Yamaguchi A. Left ventricular rupture following mitral valve replacement. Kyobu Geka 2015; 68(8): 596-602.
[PMID: 26197900]

[76] Treasure RL, Rainer WG, Strevey TE, Sadler TR. Intraoperative left ventricular rupture associated with mitral valve replacement. Chest 1974; 66(5): 511-4.
[http://dx.doi.org/10.1378/chest.66.5.511] [PMID: 4430201]

[77] Sersar SI, Jamjoom AA. Left ventricular rupture post mitral valve replacement. Clin Med Cardiol 2009; 3: 101-13.

[PMID: 20508770]

[78] Funada A, Mizuno S, Ohsato K, *et al.* Three cases of iatrogenic coronary ostial stenosis after aortic valve replacement. Circ J 2006; 70(10): 1312-7. [http://dx.doi.org/10.1253/circj.70.1312] [PMID: 16998265]

[79] Kuralay E, Cingöz F, Günay C, *et al.* Supraclavicular control of patent internal thoracic artery graft flow during aortic valve replacement. Ann Thorac Surg 2003; 75(5): 1422-8. [http://dx.doi.org/10.1016/S0003-4975(02)04989-5] [PMID: 12735556]

[80] Mundra V, Savage EB, Novaro GM, Asher CR. Delayed chylous pericardial effusion after aortic valve replacement. Tex Heart Inst J 2011; 38(4): 431-2. [PMID: 21841877]

[81] Matsuyama T, Fukada Y, Endo Y, *et al.* Massive pulmonary hemorrhage during cardiac operation; report of a case. Kyobu Geka 2015; 68(7): 535-7. [PMID: 26197831]

[82] Perek B, Malinska A, Stefaniak S, *et al.* Predictive factors of late venous aortocoronary graft failure: ultrastructural studies. PLoS One 2013; 8(8): e70628. [http://dx.doi.org/10.1371/journal.pone.0070628] [PMID: 23940610]

[83] Düsterhöft V, Bauer M, Buz S, Schaumann B, Hetzer R. Wound-healing disturbances after vein harvesting for CABG: a randomized trial to compare the minimally invasive direct vision and traditional approaches. Ann Thorac Surg 2001; 72(6): 2038-43. [http://dx.doi.org/10.1016/S0003-4975(01)03047-8] [PMID: 11789790]

[84] Sudarsanan S, Omar AS, Pattath RA, Al Mulla A. Acute kidney injury associated with rhabdomyolysis after coronary artery bypass graft: a case report and review of the literatures. BMC Res Notes 2014; 7: 152. [http://dx.doi.org/10.1186/1756-0500-7-152] [PMID: 24636137]

[85] Fernández de Caleya D, Duarte J, Lozano A, Torrente N. [Radial nerve injury caused by external compression during the dissection of the internal mammary artery in coronary surgery]. Rev Esp Anestesiol Reanim 1992; 39(6): 371-3. [PMID: 1293655]

[86] Hoskote SS, Devarapally SR, Dasgupta R, Pang Y, Shapiro JM. Fatal pulmonary embolism complicating a postoperative chylothorax despite adequate thromboprophylaxis. Blood Coagul Fibrinolysis 2013; 24(8): 887-9. [http://dx.doi.org/10.1097/MBC.0b013e3283626266] [PMID: 23751608]

[87] Rowart P, Erpicum P, Detry O, *et al.* Mesenchymal stromal cell therapy in ischemia/reperfusion injury. J Immunol Res 2015; 2015: 602597.

[88] Jung J, Ed. Patologie iatrogenă. Tîrgu-Mureş, Romania: University Press 2006.

[89] Libby P, Bonow RO, Mann DL, Zipes DP, Eds. Braunwald's Heart Disease: A text book of cardiovascular medicine. 8th ed., Saunders Hardcover 2007.

[90] Zaher MF, Azab BN, Bogin MB, Bekheit SG. Inadvertent malposition of a permanent pacemaker ventricular lead into the left ventricle which was initially missed and diagnosed two years later: a case report. J Med Case Reports 2011; 5: 54. [http://dx.doi.org/10.1186/1752-1947-5-54] [PMID: 21306607]

[91] Van Erckelens F, Sigmund M, Lambertz H, Kreis A, Reupcke C, Hanrath P. Asymptomatic left ventricular malposition of a transvenous pacemaker lead through a sinus venosus defect: follow-up over 17 years. Pacing Clin Electrophysiol 1991; 14(6): 989-93. [http://dx.doi.org/10.1111/j.1540-8159.1991.tb04147.x] [PMID: 1715075]

[92] Meyer JA, Millar K. Malplacement of pacemaker catheters in the coronary sinus. Recognition and clinical significance. J Thorac Cardiovasc Surg 1969; 57(4): 511-8. [PMID: 5774628]

[93] Tumanyan MR, Filaretova OV, Chechneva VV, Gulasaryan RS, Butrim IV, Bockeria LA. Repair of complete atrioventricular septal defect in infants with down syndrome: outcomes and long-term results. Pediatr Cardiol 2015; 36(1): 71-5.
[http://dx.doi.org/10.1007/s00246-014-0966-7] [PMID: 25099029]

[94] Saurav A, Kaushik M, Mahesh Alla V, *et al.* Comparison of percutaneous device closure *versus* surgical closure of peri-membranous ventricular septal defect: A systematic review and meta-analysis. Catheter Cardiovasc Interv 2015; 86(6): 1048-56.
[http://dx.doi.org/10.1002/ccd.26097] [PMID: 26257085]

[95] Boening A, Scheewe J, Heine K, *et al.* Long-term results after surgical correction of atrioventricular septal defects. Eur J Cardiothorac Surg 2002; 22(2): 167-73.
[http://dx.doi.org/10.1016/S1010-7940(02)00272-5] [PMID: 12142181]

[96] You SY, Yoon DY, Choi CS, *et al.* Effects of right- *versus* left-arm injections of contrast material on computed tomography of the head and neck. J Comput Assist Tomogr 2007; 31(5): 677-81.
[http://dx.doi.org/10.1097/RCT.0b013e318038d8fb] [PMID: 17895776]

[97] Saxena P, Shankar S, Kumar V, Naithani N. Bilateral chylothorax as a complication of internal jugular vein cannulation. Lung India 2015; 32(4): 370-4.
[http://dx.doi.org/10.4103/0970-2113.159579] [PMID: 26180388]

[98] Tattoli L, Maselli E, Romanelli MC, Di Vella G, Solarino B. Complete cardiac rupture associated with closed chest cardiac massage: case report and review of the literature. J Forensic Sci 2014; 59(2): 564-7.
[http://dx.doi.org/10.1111/1556-4029.12340] [PMID: 24749147]

[99] Haas NA, Happel CM, Jategaonkar S, *et al.* Compression, distortion and dislodgement of large caliber stents in congenital heart defects caused by cardiopulmonary resuscitation: a case series and review of the literature. Clin Res Cardiol 2014; 103(9): 719-25.
[http://dx.doi.org/10.1007/s00392-014-0706-2] [PMID: 24700361]

[100] Ley SJ. Standards for resuscitation after cardiac surgery. Crit Care Nurse 2015; 35(2): 30-7.
[http://dx.doi.org/10.4037/ccn2015652] [PMID: 25834006]

CHAPTER 5

Iatrogenic Pathology of the Lungs and Airways

Ioan Jung and **Simona Gurzu**[*]

Department of Pathology, University of Medicine and Pharmacy, Tirgu-Mures, Romania

Abstract: This chapter includes a synthesis of data regarding the lesions of the lungs and airways that can be induced by medical drugs or diagnostic and/or therapeutic interventions. Drug-induced lesions are difficult to identify and mainly relate to laryngeal or pulmonary edema, hypersensitivity pneumonitis and diffuse alveolar damage with hyaline membranes. In patients taking anticoagulants, the occurrence of spontaneous hemothorax or aberrant thromboembolism should also be taken into account. Diagnostic procedures that involve the airways are sometimes, though rarely, followed by complications that include post intubation croup, ulcerations or granulomas, but infrequent iatrogenic tracheal rupture and injuries to cranial nerves are also reported. Mechanical ventilation and hyperbaric oxygen therapy can be followed by pulmonary edema, interstitial emphysema or pneumothorax. In preterm babies, Wilson-Mikity syndrome and intraventricular brain hemorrhage can occur following oxygen therapy. All of these data are examined in detail in this chapter.

Keywords: Adverse drug reaction, Airways, Anaphylaxis, Aspiration, Croup, edema, Embolism, Hemothorax, Hyaline membranes, Hyperpigmentation, Intra-alveolar hemorrhage, Lung, Pneumonia, Pneumothorax, Respiratory distress syndrome, Wilson-Mikity syndrome.

DRUG-INDUCED LESIONS

The ADRs of the lungs and airways are caused by enzymatic deficiencies and can be induced through three basic mechanisms [1]:

- Immune hypersensitivity reactions – can cause anaphylaxis, bronchial asthma and eosinophilic pneumonia, and can be cured with steroids.
- Direct toxicity – drugs that are metabolized in the lungs can induce alveolocapillary damage. These dose-dependent injuries cannot be resolved using steroids.
- Idiosyncrasy – individual susceptibility that is not dose-dependent. This can start as a noncardiogenic pulmonary edema that can be handled with steroids.

[*] **Corresponding author Simona Gurzu:** Department of Pathology, University of Medicine and Pharmacy, Tirgu-Mures, Romania; Tel: 0040-745-673550; Fax: 0040-372-653250; E-mail: simonagurzu@yahoo.com

Up until the 1960s, about 20 drugs were reported to affect the lungs and bronchi [2]. Nowadays, it is known that more than 400 drugs can cause pulmonary disorders and 3-5% of all drugs present pulmonary toxicity [3]. Moreover, 0.03% of all in-hospital deaths seem to be caused by drug-induced pulmonary lesions [2].

The most common ADRs of the lungs and airways (Table **5-1**) are allergies and serum disease that can be associated with ***acute laryngeal edema***. Eighty-four drugs are known to induce anaphylaxis, leading to anaphylactic shock (76.6%), severe systemic reactions (10.5%), acute laryngeal edema (9%), severe bronchospasm (2.1%) and death (1.8%) [4].

Acute pulmonary edema can be a consequence of inhalation of pure oxygen, administration of nitrofurantoin or intravenous perfusions with a high volume of liquid. It is worth mentioning that concomitant administration of steroids causes salt and water retention [5].

The antiarrhythmic amiodarone is considered the most common drug to induce dose-dependent direct toxicity in the lungs (Table **5-1**). Approximately 5-6% of patients treated with amiodarone present lung disorders, from mild ***pneumonia*** to severe lesions, such as ***intra-alveolar hemorrhages*** and ***diffuse alveolar damage with hyaline membranes*** [1, 3, 7].

Other drugs known to induce pulmonary disorders are antibacterial agents, such as nitrofurantoin, and immunosuppressive drugs, such as sirolimus, *etc.* (Table **5-1**) [2, 8].

Drug-induced pulmonary injuries are more frequently found in patients of extreme ages, due to low renal filtration [7]. Some drugs, such as nitrofurantoin, especially affect women, though the cause is yet unknown [3].

Genetic factors influence the reactions of the body. In patients treated with gefitinib, an anti-EGFR agent that is used in patients with non-small cell lung cancer, ***interstitial pneumonia*** is a rare side effect in Europe but quite common in Japan. Similar divergence is reported for bortezomib (used in multiple myeloma and lymphomas) and tacrolimus (an immunosuppressive drug used in bone transplant recipients) – their pulmonary toxicity being more common in Japanese and African-American populations. At the same time, methotrexate-related pulmonary toxicity is more common in patients testing positive for HLA-B40 [3].

Because idiosyncratic reactions are more common than we know, drug-induced lung injury is usually a diagnosis of exclusion. To confirm one's suspicion, nonspecific clinical symptoms (dry cough, subfebrility, dyspnea, wheezing, hypoxemia, chest pain, fatigue, allergic reactions, rash, arthralgia, *etc.*) should be correlated with the presence of alveolar/interstitial/mixed inflammatory foci with asymmetrical distribution, subpleural masses, pleural thickening and effusion, altered lung function (decrease of carbon monoxide diffusing capacity), hematological disturbances (increased CD8+ lymphocytes, neutrophils and eosinophils) and occurrence of foamy macrophages and eosinophils in the bronchoalveolar lavage fluid [2]. The diagnosis of drug hypersensitivity is based on skin tests (72.9% of cases) correlated with laboratory examinations [4].

Table 5-1. ADRs of the lungs and airways according to specific drugs. Data from references [1 - 20].

ADR type	Drugs
Cough, hiccup, laryngospasm, bronchospasm	Thiopental, inhalational anesthetics (desflurane), NSAIDs, beta blockers, mitomycin C (antitumor antibiotic)
Anaphylaxis	Antibiotics (penicillin, cephalosporin, quinolone, *etc.*), muscle relaxants, latex, anesthetic NSAIDs, acetaminophen, iodinated or MRI contrast media, immunotherapy, vaccines
Airway infections	Topiramate (anticonvulsant)
Bronchial dilation	Halothane
Bronchiolitis obliterans	Cyclophosphamide, methotrexate, penicillin
Hyperpigmentation of bronchial mucosa	Busulfan
Iatrogenic bronchial asthma	Aspirin, NSAIDs (indomethacin)
Alveolar hypoventilation	Narcotics, aminoglycosides, corticosteroids
Acute pulmonary edema	Oral corticosteroids and perfusions, amiodarone, nitrofurantoin, narcotics, tocolytics, depolarizing myorelaxants (succinylcholine) used in newborns and infants, biological monoclonal antibodies
Intra-alveolar hemorrhage	Aspirin, anticoagulants, amiodarone, sirolimus (rapamycin)
Eosinophilic (Löffler's) pneumonia	Cytotoxic drugs (bleomycin), antibiotics (penicillin), sulfonamides, nitrofurantoin, methotrexate, phenytoin (anticonvulsant), para-aminosalicylic acid (mesalazine)
Acute fibrinous pneumonia	Amiodarone, aciclovir, decitabine, proton pump inhibitors (PPIs)
Interstitial pneumonia/ lung fibrosis	Cytotoxic drugs (busulfan, bleomycin, methotrexate, procarbazine, cyclophosphamide, chlorambucil, azathioprine), nitrofurantoin, amiodarone, carbamazepine, gleevec, mesalazine, bleomycin, pingyangmycin (bleomycin derivative with sclerosant effect), nitrogen mustard (alkylating drug)
Lipoid pneumonia	Amiodarone or chronic aspiration of nasal drops
Perivascular and peribronchial fibrosis	LSD (lysergic acid diethylamide) – analogs (dose-dependent ADR)
Secondary tuberculosis	Corticosteroids, cytotoxic drugs

(Table 5-1) contd.....

ADR type	Drugs
Vasculitis	Sulfonamides, aspirin, phenylbutazone, penicillin, cytotoxic drugs, serum sickness
Pleuritis	Procainamide, hydralazine, isoniazid
Hemothorax	Anticoagulants, cytotoxic drugs

Spontaneous Hemothorax is an uncommon complication that can occur in patients undergoing anticoagulant therapy. In one of our cases, a 61-year-old woman who had undergone mitral valve replacement was prescribed anticoagulant therapy and discharged. At home, without medical prescription, NSAIDs were taken. Two weeks later, she was hospitalized with severe bradycardia, cough and thoracic pain, and pulmonary X-rays showed bilateral opacity. A blood volume of 3500 ml was drained from the left hemothorax, but the patient died of hemorrhagic shock on the first day following hospitalization. At necropsy, 600 ml of blood was observed in the right hemothorax and 300 ml in the left.

Drug-Induced Acute Respiratory Distress Syndrome (ARDS) has been reported in patients treated with amiodarone, but also with 5-FU-based regimens (Fig. **5-1**). Discontinuation of the drug, application of corticosteroids and supportive measure care is necessary, but a mortality rate of 50% remains in amiodarone users [7, 9].

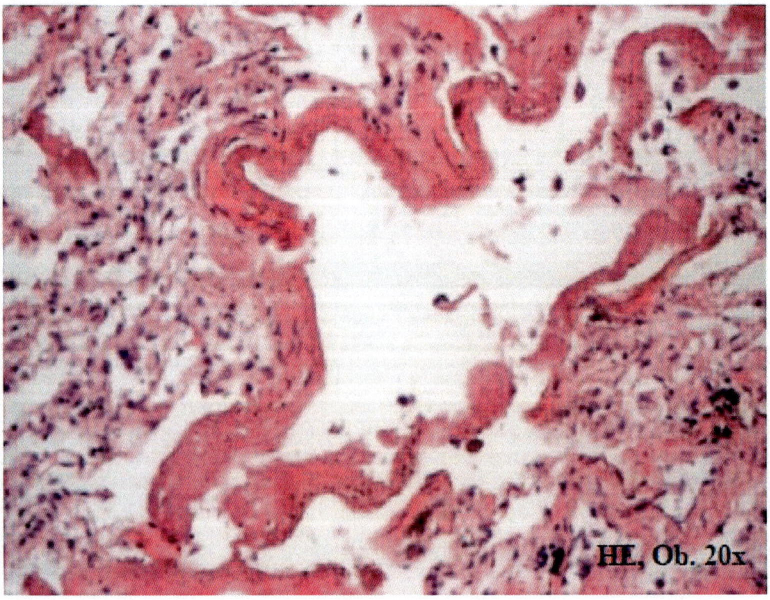

Fig. (5-1). Chemotherapy-associated ARDS with hyaline membranes. This patient received capecitabine and oxaliplatin and presented multiorgan failure syndrome.

In patients with cerebral arteriovenous malformations, ARDS has been reported as a systemic pulmonary complication after endovascular embolization with Onyx-18. The direct toxicity of the copolymer solvent DMSO [$(CH_3)_2SO$], which is partially metabolized in the lung, has been supposed [10].

IATROGENIC PNEUMONIAS

Pneumonias can be induced by drugs, radiation, oxygen therapy, surgical interventions and other medical procedures that affect the patient's immune system.

- ***Interstitial Pneumonia***

The pathomechanism of ADRs-related pneumonia comprises drug-induced proliferation of type-II alveolocytes and fibroblasts. It has recently been observed in patients with ulcerative colitis or Crohn's disease that have been treated with 4-aminosalicylic acid (mesalazine) [11]. Several other drugs (Table **5-1**), radiation and oxygen therapy can also be responsible for the onset of interstitial pneumonia.

- ***Acute Fibrinous and Organizing Pneumonia***

This is a rare but relatively specific iatrogenic lesion, first reported by Basely *et al.* in 2002 [12]. It is characterized by drug-induced proliferation of type II alveolocytes intermingled with fibrin deposits. Amiodarone, proton pump inhibitors (PPIs) and other drugs (Table **5-1**) were found to be its promoters. Microscopically, it is characterized by hyaline membranes and the presence of eosinophils and other inflammatory cells in alveolar septa. Bilateral patchy infiltrate/consolidation can be seen on chest radiography. This can be an acute process, with a high rate of mortality in the first month after onset of symptoms, but sub acute forms that respond to steroids have also been reported [13].

- ***Lipoid Pneumonia***

This is known as the "amiodarone effect" or "cholesterol pneumonia" and can be induced by amiodarone or long-term inhalation of nasal drops with mineral oils [5, 7].

In a representative case published in 1949 by Rossier and Bühlmann, bilateral lipoid pneumonia was reported in a patient with daily nasal inhalation of paraffin-based oil for 20 years. The total volume of nasal drops was estimated to be 64 liters 14].

Lipoid pneumonia is characterized by the formation of intraparenchymatous foci of lipid-laden macrophages admixed with other inflammatory cells and multinucleated giant cells. These foci can generate foreign body granulomas with scarring [5]. The radiological features are non-specific. CT scans can reveal alveolar consolidations of low attenuation values, ground-glass opacities with thickening of intralobular septa (crazy paving pattern) and alveolar nodules [15].

- ***Löffler's Eosinophilic Pneumonia***

This type of pneumonia can be induced by any drugs including antibiotics or organic compounds, such as mesalazine or sulfasalazine (Table **5-1**). In early stages, increased serum level of eosinophils and two microscopic patterns can be seen (type I and II), while lung fibrosis occurs in late stages [2, 5, 16]:

- Type I: bronchopneumonia-like features with intra-alveolar inflammatory exudate rich in eosinophils.
- Type II: intraparenchymatous granulomas centered by fibrinoid necrosis, which is surrounded by fibroblasts, macrophages, epithelioid cells and eosinophils. Sulfasalazine can induce formation of sarcoidosis-like granulomas.

- ***Immunodeficiency-Associated Pneumonia***

This type of pneumonia is a nosocomial infection and can occur in immunosuppressed patients. The proton pump inhibitors (PPIs) are causal factors, even in short-term users [17, 18]. The most common pathogens are *Pneumocystis carinii, Klebsiella pneumoniae*, fungi (*Candida albicans, Aspergillus flavus, Histoplasma capsulatum*) and viruses (*e.g.,cytomegalovirus*) [5].

Pulmonary aspergillosis is microscopically characterized by the presence of branching septate hyphae or a fungus granuloma called aspergilloma (Fig. **5-2**).

Hemorrhagic pneumonia, usually produced by *Staphylococcus*, is very rare and primarily affects infants (Fig. **5-3**) or older adults. It also occurs in HIV-infected patients, although a decreased rate of opportunistic infection has been observed in the antiretroviral therapy era [19].

Klebsiella-related pneumonia primarily affects the upper lobes and should be considered for differential diagnosis of upper lung opacities. In one of our cases, such pneumonia was diagnosed at the autopsy of a 60-year-old immunosuppressed alcoholic male. It was originally confused with delirium tremens, but on the basis of progressive respiratory failure and ground-glass opacity of the right superior pulmonary lobe, revealed in the pulmonary X-rays, a lung tumor was then suspected. The patient died within a few days of admission and Klebsiella-related pneumonia was observed at autopsy (Fig. **5-4**).

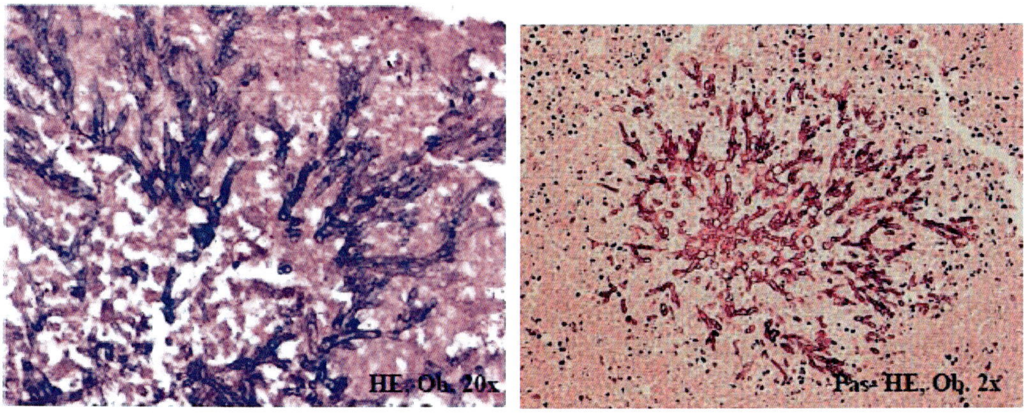

Fig. (5-2). Aspergillus with dichotomous branching septate hyphae (left) and aspergilloma (right), in immunosuppressed patients with pneumonia.

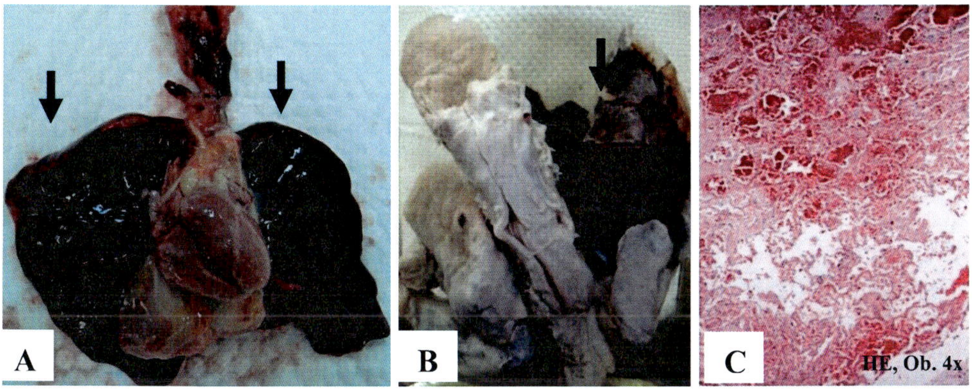

Fig. (5-3). Hemorrhagic pneumonia in immunosuppressed infants. **A.** Bilateral pneumonia. **B.** Pneumonia of the right lung induced by *Staphylococcus aureus*. **C.** Microscopic examination shows rich intra-alveolar hemorrhagic infiltrate.

IMMUNODEFICIENCY-ASSOCIATED TUBERCULOSIS

In immunosuppressed patients, airborne infection with mycobacterium tuberculosis but also reactivated tuberculosis should be considered. Dual infection with *mycobacterium tuberculosis* and other bacteria, such as *Streptococcus pneumoniae*, is also possible [20].

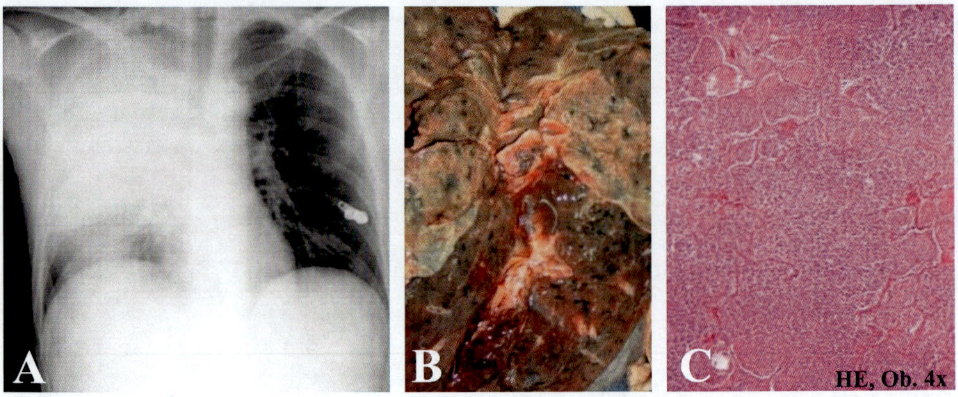

Fig. (5-4). In an immunosuppressed patient, lobar Klebsiella-related pneumonia shows opacity of the upper right lung (**A**). Involvement of the upper lobe (**b**) and abscesses (**c**) were observed at autopsy.

In one of our cases, a 28-year-old male, hospitalized with fever, a high erythrocytes sedimentation rate (ESR) and several adenopathies (laterocervical, supraclavicular and mediastinal), we suspected Hodgkin's lymphoma. The lymph node bioptic specimen did not confirm this suspicion, however. The histopathological diagnosis was "reactive histiocytosis" only. Corticosteroids were prescribed without any improvements. Some weeks later, the chest CT scan revealed mediastinal and paratracheal adenopathies and multiple bilateral nodules in the lung parenchyma. The second lymph node biopsy revealed tuberculous lymphadenitis. This representative case highlights the necessity of a correct differential diagnosis, and reveals that drug-induced immunodeficiency can cause the occurrence of miliary tuberculosis [5].

IATROGENIC PULMONARY EMBOLISM

Iatrogenic pulmonary embolism is a complication rarely encountered in daily diagnosis, yet, at the same time, this embolism is one of the three most commonly undiagnosed illnesses identified at autopsy [21]. The most commonly embolized substances are thrombi, fat and bone marrow. Patients can present non-specific symptoms, and more than 10% of them are asymptomatic [21]. Pulmonary embolism can be related to diagnostic or therapeutic procedures, and can be caused by chemotherapeutics and steroids.

- ***Thromboembolism*** is the most common type of in-hospital embolism and should be suspected in any patient with a previous history of thromboembolism and in those with deep vein thrombosis. The risk is higher in elderly and obese patients, and is caused by immobilization, spinal cord injury, mechanical ventilation and drug-induced sedation [21]. Thromboembolism can also occur soon after surgery, especially that of the head, neck and perineal areas [21, 22]. Sometimes, it can be successfully treated using anticoagulants [23]. Thromboprophylaxis is recommended in intensive care units (ICUs) [21].

The risk of catheter-related thrombosis is associated with the duration of catheterization and the catheter localization. The reported incidence is 10-69% from femoral veins, 40-56% from internal jugular veins and 2-10% from subclavian veins [21]. Drug-related pulmonary thromboembolism is especially commonly reported in oncology departments. Chemotherapeutics are causal factors. Fatal pulmonary thromboembolism can occur in patients with metastatic carcinomas (Figs. **5-5** and **5-6**).

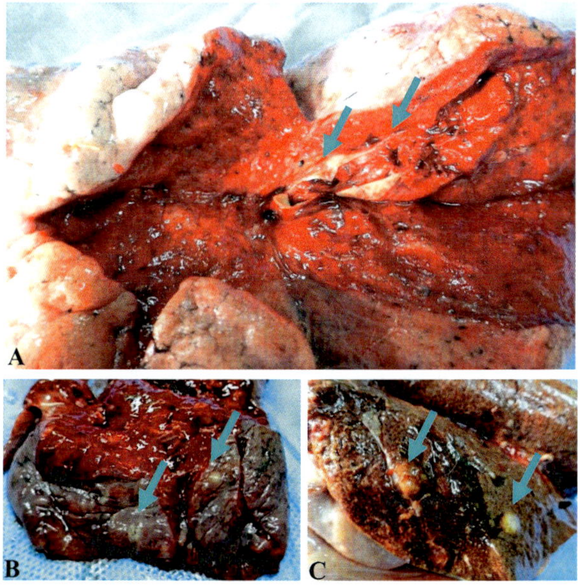

Fig (5-5). Spontaneous fatal pulmonary thromboembolism (**A**) in a patient with a history of gastrectomy and chemotherapy performed on a gastric carcinoma with lung (**B**) and liver metastases (**C**).

- ***Fat embolism*** can be induced by intravenous administration of an oily solution [24]. Prolonged steroid therapy and/or total parenteral nutrition can cause non-traumatic fat embolism [25]. Fat embolism has also been reported as a complication of joint reconstruction surgery [24]. Fat embolism can induce ARDS [26], but bilateral fat pulmonary embolism with hemorrhagic infarction has also been reported [24]. The recent development of aesthetic surgery techniques has led to a changing spectrum of fat embolism. Nowadays, an increasing number of cases involve fat embolism following intramuscular gluteal lipoinjection, and injuries of the gluteal blood vessels are more common. The incidence is not yet known [27].
- ***Bone marrow embolism*** can occur during spine or intraosseous surgical

interventions, after bone marrow transplantation, or as a consequence of cardiopulmonary resuscitation-induced ribs fractures [25]. Pneumothorax, pulmonary dystelectasis and disseminated intravascular coagulation (DIC) can be associated (Fig. **5-7**).

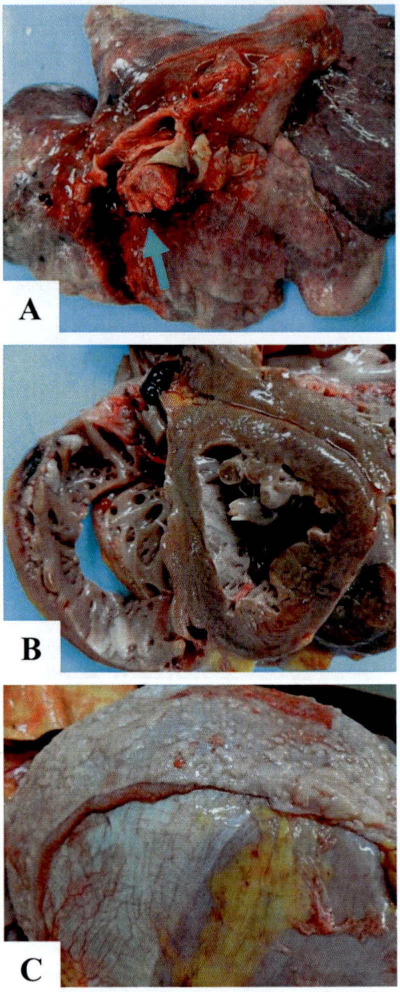

Fig. (5-6). Fatal pulmonary thromboembolism (A) with acute dilatation of the right cardiac ventricle (B) in a young female with a history of hysterectomy, bilateral ovariectomy and oncotherapy performed to treat an ovarian carcinoma with peritoneal carcinomatosis and diaphragmatic metastases (C).

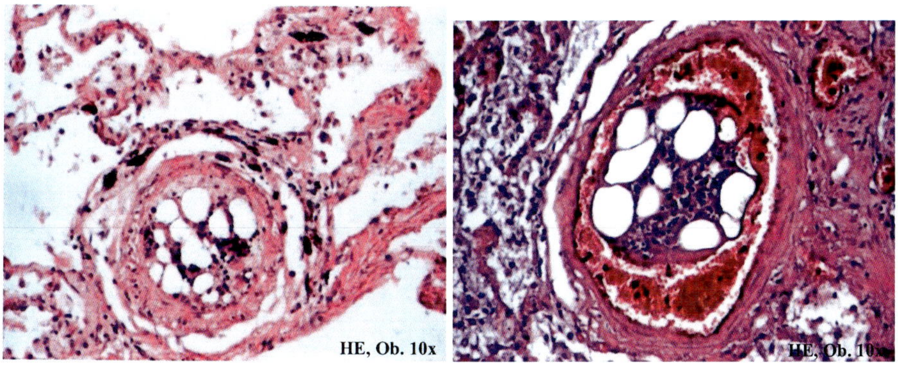

Fig. (5-7). Bone marrow embolism in pulmonary arteries.

• ***Other Unusual Iatrogenic Causes of Pulmonary Embolism***

Septic Emboli can be mobilized in immunocompromised patients, being primarily associated with mycotic septicemia (*e.g.,* septicemia involving the mucormycosis, Cunninghamella bertholletiae, after allogeneic stem cell transplantation) [28].

Bone Cement Embolism has been reported following multiple percutaneous vertebroplasties. It can be seen as nodular opacities on chest radiography. Typical CT scans reveal multiple tubular or branching dense opacities located along the pulmonary arteries, which are more easily visible in CT pulmonary angiography [29, 30].

Sodium Hyaluronate is primarily used as an intra-articular injection for pain relief in patients with knee synovial lesions. Its pulmonary embolization is seen on chest radiography as a bilateral interstitial lesion, with multiple ground-glass opacities [31].

IATROGENIC LESIONS DURING OTHER DIAGNOSTIC AND THERAPEUTIC PROCEDURES

Laryngoscopy, Bronchoscopy And Intubation

In intubated patients, direct compression can induce laryngeal edema, decubitus (pressure) ulcers, necrosis of the laryngeal and tracheal mucosa, rupture of the vocal cords, laryngospasm and bronchospasm (more common in smokers). Ulceronecrotic laryngitis (Fig. **5-8**) primarily emerges after 48 hours of intubation [5]. Postintubation croup with acute stridor is more common in children [32].

In patients intubated for over 90 hours, post intubation ulcerations and granulomas are more severe and can cause predisposition to fistulae [5, 33]. Post-laryngoscopy sore throat is reported in 30% of patients after the use of traditional intubation blade [34]. Laryngeal stenosis and progressive hoarseness can occur weeks or even months after intubation [5, 33].

Iatrogenic tracheal rupture and injuries to cranial nerves (IX, X and XII) are rare complications, but their real incidence is underestimated [35, 36]. Septic cricoid chondronecrosis and retropharyngeal abscess with subsequent mediastinitis are other unusual post intubation lesions [37, 38].

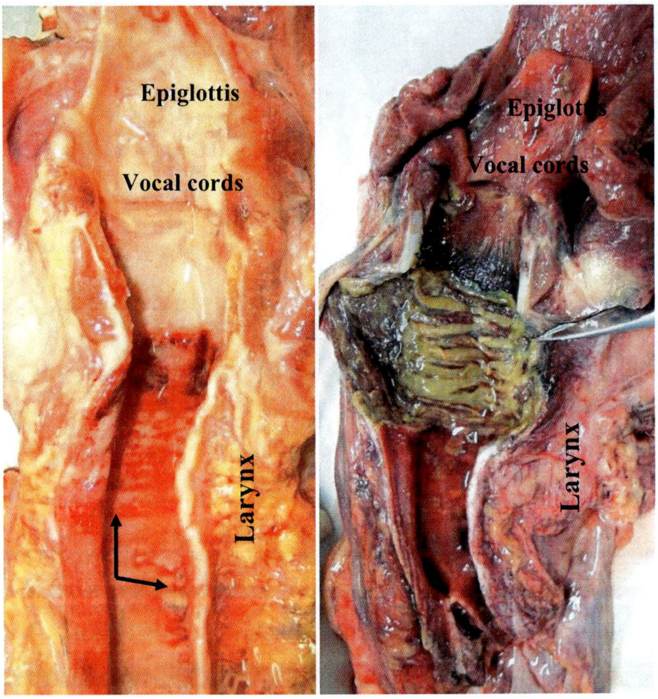

Fig. (5-8). Postintubation laryngotracheitis with decubitus ulcers (left) covered by fibrin (right).

Although widely used to clean the laryngoscope, ortho-phthalaldehyde can predispose the patient to allergic reactions [39].

Artificial teeth, crowns or bridges can be aspirated during endotracheal intubation and can induce severe aspiration pneumonia and even death. These can be removed through bronchoscopy. In one recent paper, aspiration into the right lung of three bridge teeth with spontaneous coughing after six months was presented [40].

Aspiration of saliva, nasopharyngeal secretions or gastric content during general anesthesia can produce atelectasis, bronchopneumonia, pulmonary abscesses, ARDS, pulmonary edema and Mendelson's syndrome (the gastric content induces autodigestion of the pulmonary parenchyma) [5].

Mechanical Ventilation and Hyperbaric Oxygen Therapy

During mechanical ventilation and hyperbaric oxygen therapy, several lesions can occur, such as acute pulmonary edema, ARDS, interstitial emphysema, air embolism, pneumothorax and bronchopneumonia.

- ***Acute Pulmonary Edema***

Hyperbaric oxygen therapy can infrequently induce acute pulmonary edema, especially in patients with low cardiac ejection fractions. The supposed mechanism involves increasing peripheral vasoconstriction and cardiac afterload as a result of induced hyperoxia [41].

- ***Interstitial Emphysema and Air Embolism***

High intrapulmonary pressure induced by mechanical ventilation or external cardiac massage can cause acute pulmonary interstitial emphysema. Air bubbles can be spread through the interstitium in the mediastinal space and the subcutaneous tissue of the neck and thorax. This lesion type can be lethal, especially in children. In some cases, the air can be accumulated in the subpleural space and bullae can be observed (Fig. **5-9**). This air can also enter the veins, leading to air embolism.

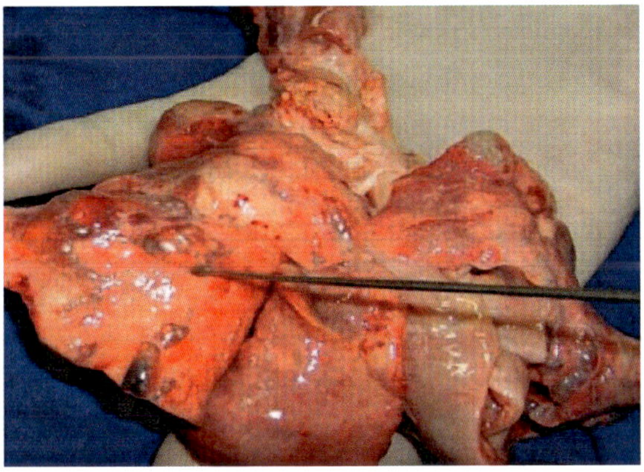

Fig. (5-9). Artificial respiration-induced bilateral interstitial emphysema in a child with Duchenne muscular dystrophy.

- ***Pneumothorax***

In patients receiving hyperbaric oxygen therapy, tension pneumothorax is a rare complication caused by chronic lung diseases, mechanical ventilation and chest trauma [42].

- ***Bronchopneumonia***

This is a life-threatening disorder commonly associated with mechanical ventilation. The prevalent agents (74%) are Gram-negative bacteria, such as *Escherichia coli*, *Pseudomonas*, *Klebsiella* and *Acinetobacter*. In the remaining cases (~20%), Gram-positive bacteria, especially *Staphylococcus aureus* and Streptococcus beta-hemolysis, are involved [43].

Oxygen Therapy in Neonates and Children

Because in many cases long-term or intermittent ventilatory support is required for neonatology and pediatric clinics, non-invasive ventilation through a mask interface is indicated for use rather than invasive ventilation [44]. To avoid tracheostomy and to reduce the rate of complications, a high flow nasal cannula is indicated for neonates [45].

In children receiving mechanical ventilation, the most common complications are acute pulmonary edema, interstitial emphysema, pneumothorax and pneumonia. Neurological disorders, lung fibrosis and other specific lesions can also be induced [5].

In preterm babies who require oxygen inhalation for more than 60 days, nosocomial infections occur in 15% of cases, with a mortality rate of 10-13% [45]. Other specific lesions are Wilson-Mikity syndrome, retinopathy and cerebral hemorrhages.

- ***Wilson-Mikity Syndrome***

This is a rare form of chronic lung disease that occurs in preterm babies (gestational age below 30 weeks and 1000-1500 g birth weight) receiving oxygen therapy, without previous respiratory injuries. Intrauterine infections can be a causal factor. It is characterized by bilateral emphysema diagnosed in the first two to four weeks of life, followed by pulmonary fibrosis. The clinical consequences are recurrent cyanosis, dyspnea, progressive respiratory distress and respiratory failure that persists despite ventilatory support. The mortality rate is approximately 10% [5, 46].

- ***Retinopathy***

Retinopathy can be a consequence of administration of pure oxygen, inducing hypoxia- and VEGF-mediated retinal neoangiogenesis [47]. In adults, it is an acute reversible lesion, but retrolental fibroplasia with/without blindness can occur in preterm babies [5]. There are five stages of oxygen-related retinopathy, with incidence ranging from 69% (stage 0) to 0.1% (stage 5 – total retinal detachment). Approximately 3% of affected babies require surgery [45].

- ***Intraventricular Brain Hemorrhage***

This is an infrequently reported oxygen therapy-related consequence. There are four grades of severity: in preterm babies hospitalized for more than 60 days, its incidence ranges from 75% (grade 0) to 4% (grade 4 – intraparenchymatous hemorrhage) [45].

Acute Lung Injury (ALI)

ALI is a common lesion diagnosed in the ICU that can have several causes, from drug overdoses to oxygen inhalation, open heart surgery to shock [48].

Due to surfactant destruction, the morphological lesions vary from slight to thick hyaline membranes and fibrosis of the alveolar septa. Progressive respiratory failure is associated with a high mortality rate [48 - 50].

Mechanical ventilation may precipitate ALI-induced respiratory failure. The exact mechanism is unknown. On the one hand, thick hyaline membranes also enclose the capillaries, and a high pressure upon the septa can produce vascular rupture. On the other hand, the inhaled oxygen stimulates proliferation of alveolocytes that supplementarily increase the septal thickening. To protect the lung, optimal settings and ventilation modes, it is necessary to use low tidal volume and high positive-end expiratory pressure (PEEP) [48].

Tyrosine kinase inhibitors, such as dasatinib, have shown attenuating lung inflammation and fibrosis in experimental ARDS, independent of etiology, but careful dose monitoring is required [51].

Other Diagnostic Procedures

- ***Percutaneous Transthoracic Needle Biopsy of the Lung***

Periprocedural complications include pneumothorax (8-64%), vascular lesions (hemoptysis, hemothorax, mediastinal and chest wall hemorrhages, intraparenchymatous hemorrhages, arterial bronchial fistulae), air embolisms (a life-threatening complication that occurs in 0.02-0.07% of cases) and malignant seeding of the needle tract with pulmonary or chest wall metastasis [52 - 55].

- ***Barium Swallow For Examination of the Upper GI Tract***

Barium swallow can be followed by barium aspiration during the rapid drinking phase. If the cough reflex does not occur, barium can be aspirated into the trachea, bronchia and lungs. Barium-induced pneumonia can be treated with fibrosis, but is a fatal complication otherwise [56].

Other Therapeutic Procedures

- ***Surgical Interventions of the Head and Neck Area***

Thyroid Surgery– voice alteration (dysphonia) is the result of incidental intraoperative injury of the recurrent laryngeal nerve (a branch of cranial nerve X) and subsequent paralysis of the vocal cords. The incidence is about 46% following total thyroidectomy and 14% after partial resection of the thyroid gland. Spontaneous rehabilitation is seen in 84-92% of patients within six months of surgery. To preserve the anatomical structure and functional integrity of the nerve, use of intraoperative neuromonitoring is suggested [57, 58]. Details regarding thyroid surgery are presented in Chapter 17.

Transcutaneous Injection Laryngoplasty– this technique is frequently used in patients with unilateral vocal cord paralysis, without significant complications [59].

Rhinoplasty– although uncommon, unilateral recurrent laryngeal and hypoglossal (XII) nerve paralysis following rhinoplasty is sometimes reported. This is known as Tapia's syndrome and is characterized by unilateral vocal cord and tongue paralysis within 24-48 hours of surgery. The mechanism probably involves direct compression of the lateral wall of the inferior part of the oropharynx or the superior part of hypopharynx, where the two nerves lie adjacent to one another, during packing of pharynx [36, 60]. Details regarding rhinoplasty are presented in Chapter 21.

Cervical Spine Surgery – this surgery can be followed by late dysphonia, which occurs in 10% of patients within six weeks to three months of surgery [61, 62]. This lesion is considered a result of incidental recurrent nerve injury, but pharyngeal and laryngeal trauma, hematoma, edema, injury of the superior laryngeal nerve and arytenoid cartilage dislocation (frequently misdiagnosed as vocal fold paresis) can be involved in the etiology of postoperative prolonged hoarseness [62]. This is usually a reversible disorder [61].

Tapia's syndrome was recently reported in a 17-year-old male patient with idiopathic scoliosis, following *guidewire-assisted pedicle screw insertion and arthrodesis* at the level of T1-L1, which induced neuropraxia of the recurrent laryngeal nerve and right-side cranial nerve X injury. In this patient, right vocal fold immobility, decreased sensation of the endolarynx and left-side tongue deviation postoperatively emerged [63].

- ***Surgery of Lungs***

Pulmonary artery pseudoaneurysm is a rare but possible lethal complication of ***pulmonary lobectomy*** [64].

Percutaneous Radio Frequency Lung Tumor Ablation can induce air embolism, probably as a result of a bronchovenous fistulae. It is caused by chronic obstructive pulmonary disease and mechanical ventilation. Pleural adhesions prevent pneumothorax and lung collapse, and cause the air embolism [55]. Details regarding lung surgery are presented in Chapter 17.

CONFLICT OF INTEREST

The authors confirm that this chapter content has no conflict of interest.

ACKNOWLEDGEMENTS

Declared none.

REFERENCES

[1] Bedrossian CW. Iatrogenic and toxic injury. In: Dail DH, Hammar SP, Eds. Dail and Hammar's Pulmonary Pathology. New York: Springer-Verlag 1987; pp. 511-34.

[2] Allison A, Zander D. Drug reactions and other iatrogenic pulmonary diseases. In: Zander DS, Farver CF, Eds. Pulmonary pathology. Churchill, Livingstone, Elsevier 2008; pp. 397-415.

[3] Wick JY. Pulmonary insult: understanding drug-induced lung disease. www.pharmacytimes.com. Accessed August 25, 2015.

[4] Renaudin JM, Beaudouin E, Ponvert C, Demoly P, Moneret-Vautrin DA. Severe drug-induced anaphylaxis: analysis of 333 cases recorded by the Allergy Vigilance Network from 2002 to 2010. Allergy 2013; 68(7): 929-37.
[http://dx.doi.org/10.1111/all.12168] [PMID: 23741979]

[5] Jung J, Ed. Patologie iatrogenă. Tîrgu-Mureş, Romania: University Press 2006.

[6] www.pneumotox.com. Accessed August 25, 2013.

[7] Papiris SA, Triantafillidou C, Kolilekas L, Markoulaki D, Manali ED. Amiodarone: review of pulmonary effects and toxicity. Drug Saf 2010; 33(7): 539-58.
[http://dx.doi.org/10.2165/11532320-000000000-00000] [PMID: 20553056]

[8] Ferrozzi F, Schiavi A, Ganzetti A, Bassi P, Campani R. [Pulmonary iatrogenic lesions in chemotherapy: computerized tomography findings]. Radiol Med (Torino) 1998; 96(1-2): 62-7. [PMID: 9819620]

[9] Gurzu S, Jung I, Comsulea M, Kadar Z, Azamfirei L, Molnar C. Lethal cardiotoxicity, steatohepatitis, chronic pancreatitis, and acute enteritis induced by capecitabine and oxaliplatin in a 36-year-old woman. Diagn Pathol 2013; 8: 150. [http://dx.doi.org/10.1186/1746-1596-8-150] [PMID: 24041405]

[10] Tawil I, Carlson AP, Taylor CL. Acute respiratory distress syndrome after onyx embolization of arteriovenous malformation. Crit Care Res Pract 2011; 2011: 918185. [http://dx.doi.org/10.1155/2011/918185]

[11] Auffret M, Béné J, Lambert M, Gautier S. [Mesalazine-related interstitial lung disease: an under-diagnosed effect?]. Therapie 2014; 69(6): 531-2. [http://dx.doi.org/10.2515/therapie/2014205] [PMID: 25320942]

[12] Beasley MB, Franks TJ, Galvin JR, Gochuico B, Travis WD. Acute fibrinous and organizing pneumonia: a histological pattern of lung injury and possible variant of diffuse alveolar damage. Arch Pathol Lab Med 2002; 126(9): 1064-70. [PMID: 12204055]

[13] Hara Y, Shinkai M, Kanoh S, *et al.* Clinico-pathological analysis referring hemeoxygenase-1 in acute fibrinous and organizing pneumonia patients. Respir Med Case Rep 2015; 14: 53-6. [PMID: 26029580]

[14] Rossier PH, Buhlmann A. Eine Oelpneumonie nach jahrelangem Gebrauch von flüssigem Paraffin als Nasentropfen. Schweiz Med Wochenschr 1949; 79(30): 685. [PMID: 18138799]

[15] Lin J, Huang LL, Zhang JW, Ye MH, Feng JX. Endogenous lipoid pneumonia presenting as solitary pulmonary nodule: a case report. Int J Clin Exp Pathol 2015; 8(8): 9727.: 30. [PMID: 26464746]

[16] Mohyuddin GR, Sultan F, Zhang K, Khaleeq G. Sulfasalazine induced lung toxicity masquerading as sarcoidosis case report and review of the literature. Sarcoidosis Vasc Diffuse Lung Dis 2013; 30(3): 226-30. [PMID: 24284297]

[17] Ruiz de Angulo D, Ortiz MA, Martínez de Haro LF. Side effects of proton-pump inhibitors: another reason to indicate anti-reflux surgery for Barretts esophagus? Cir Esp 2014; 92(5): 303-4. [http://dx.doi.org/10.1016/j.ciresp.2014.01.009] [PMID: 24625629]

[18] Wilhelm SM, Rjater RG, Kale-Pradhan PB. Perils and pitfalls of long-term effects of proton pump inhibitors. Expert Rev Clin Pharmacol 2013; 6(4): 443-51. [http://dx.doi.org/10.1586/17512433.2013.811206] [PMID: 23927671]

[19] Mirani G, Williams PL, Chernoff M, *et al.* Changing trends in complications and mortality among US youth and young adults with HIV Infection in the era of combination antiretroviral therapy. Clin Infect Dis 2015; 61(12): 1850-61. [http://dx.doi.org/10.1093/cid/civ687] [PMID: 26270680]

[20] Jolobe OM. Dual infection with *S. pneumoniae* and *M. tuberculosis* was also a possibility. Int J Cardiol 2015; 201: 184. [http://dx.doi.org/10.1016/j.ijcard.2015.08.016] [PMID: 26298375]

[21] Minet C, Potton L, Bonadona A, *et al.* Venous thromboembolism in the ICU: main characteristics, diagnosis and thromboprophylaxis. Crit Care 2015; 19: 287. [http://dx.doi.org/10.1186/s13054-015-1003-9] [PMID: 26283414]

[22] Hoskote SS, Devarapally SR, Dasgupta R, Pang Y, Shapiro JM. Fatal pulmonary embolism complicating a postoperative chylothorax despite adequate thromboprophylaxis. Blood Coagul

Fibrinolysis 2013; 24(8): 887-9.
[http://dx.doi.org/10.1097/MBC.0b013e3283626266] [PMID: 23751608]

[23] Zhang Y, Wang R, Mu L. [Two cases of acute pulmonary embolism in head and neck tumor surgery]. Lin Chung Er Bi Yan Hou Tou Jing Wai Ke Za Zhi 2015; 29(2): 177-8.
[PMID: 25989673]

[24] Fernández-Torre JL, Burgueño P, Ballesteros MA, Hernández-Hernández MA, Villagrá-Terán N, de Lucas EM. Super-refractory nonconvulsive status epilepticus secondary to fat embolism: a clinical, electrophysiological, and pathological study. Epilepsy Behav 2015; 49: 184-8.
[http://dx.doi.org/10.1016/j.yebeh.2015.04.045] [PMID: 25986321]

[25] Selvi SK, Kar R, Vadivelan M, Subrahmanyam DK. A fatal case of bone marrow embolism of unknown cause masquerading clinically as dengue shock syndrome. Indian J Pathol Microbiol 2012; 55(4): 572-3.
[http://dx.doi.org/10.4103/0377-4929.107827] [PMID: 23455811]

[26] Gurzu S, Jung I. Basic Concepts of Pathology. University Press. Tîrgu-Mureş: 2011.

[27] Cárdenas-Camarena L, Bayter JE, Aguirre-Serrano H, Cuenca-Pardo J. Deaths Caused by Gluteal Lipoinjection: What Are We Doing Wrong? Plast Reconstr Surg 2015; 136(1): 58-66.
[http://dx.doi.org/10.1097/PRS.0000000000001364] [PMID: 26111314]

[28] Matsumoto K, Yamamoto W, Ohgusa E, *et al.* Disseminated *Cunninghamella bertholletiae* infection with septic pulmonary embolism after allogeneic bone marrow transplantation. Transpl Infect Dis 2014; 16(2): 304-6.
[http://dx.doi.org/10.1111/tid.12190] [PMID: 24593246]

[29] Oh JK, Park JH, Kim SS, *et al.* Thread-like bone cement in the right-side heart and pulmonary arteries causing diffuse pulmonary embolism as a late complication. Heart Lung Circ 2015; 24(7): e104-7.
[http://dx.doi.org/10.1016/j.hlc.2015.02.017] [PMID: 25797324]

[30] Huh S, Lee H. Pulmonary bone cement embolism: CT angiographic evaluation with material decomposition using gemstone spectral imaging. Korean J Radiol 2014; 15(4): 443-7.
[http://dx.doi.org/10.3348/kjr.2014.15.4.443] [PMID: 25053903]

[31] Bhagat R, Forteza RM, Calcote CB, Williams WT, Bigler SA, Dwyer TM. Pulmonary emboli from therapeutic sodium hyaluronate. Respir Care 2012; 57(10): 1670-3.
[http://dx.doi.org/10.4187/respcare.01666] [PMID: 22417476]

[32] Kim HJ, Son JD, Kwak KH. Unexpected and severe postintubation croup after a very short day surgery in a pediatric patient: a case report. Korean J Anesthesiol 2014; 67(4): 287-9.
[http://dx.doi.org/10.4097/kjae.2014.67.4.287] [PMID: 25368790]

[33] Kamachi M, Yoshioka M, Akamatsu Y, Honma K, Yamaguchi K. [Two cases of postintubation granuloma of the larynx]. Masui 2009; 58(10): 1282-5.
[PMID: 19860234]

[34] Cirilla DJ 2nd, Ngo J, Vaisman V, *et al.* Does the incidence of sore throat postoperatively increase with the use of a traditional intubation blade or the GlideScope? J Clin Anesth 2015; 26(8): 646-51.
[http://dx.doi.org/10.1016/j.jclinane.2015.06.005] [PMID: 26277231]

[35] Aydemir B, Celik S, Uncu O, Tanrikulu H, Okay T. Iatrogenic tracheal ruptures: review of the literature and personal experience of 11 cases. Open J Thor Surg 2013; 3: 130-4.
[http://dx.doi.org/10.4236/ojts.2013.34027]

[36] Bakhshaee M, Bameshki AR, Foroughipour M, Zaringhalam MA. Unilateral recurrent laryngeal and hypoglossal nerve paralysis following rhinoplasty: a case report and review of the literature. Iran J Otorhinolaryngol 2014; 26(74): 47-50.
[PMID: 24505575]

[37] Desmots F, Allali L, Radulesco T, Geffroy Y. Serious complication of postextubation laryngeal oedema treated by corticosteroids: septic cricoid chondronecrosis. Eur Ann Otorhinolaryngol Head

Neck Dis 2014; 131(5): 323-4.
[http://dx.doi.org/10.1016/j.anorl.2014.02.005] [PMID: 25027300]

[38] Kar A, Dharmic S, Suryanarayana V, Harish M. A case of mediastinitis secondary to retropharyngeal abscess. J Pharm Bioallied Sci 2015; 7 (Suppl. 1): S63-4.
[http://dx.doi.org/10.4103/0975-7406.155805] [PMID: 26015751]

[39] Atiyeh K, Chitkara A, Achlatis S, Branski RC, Amin MR. Allergic reaction to ortho-phthalaldehyde following flexible laryngoscopy. Laryngoscope 2015; 125(10): 2349-52.
[http://dx.doi.org/10.1002/lary.25421] [PMID: 26199135]

[40] Magzoub TA, Al Ghamdi SA, Dagriri K, Al Fagih A. A delayed spontaneous expulsion of a three teeth bridge after 6 months period of aspiration in the right lung following cardiac surgery. Saudi J Anaesth 2015; 9(3): 330-1.
[http://dx.doi.org/10.4103/1658-354X.154742] [PMID: 26240558]

[41] Obiagwu C, Paul V, Chadha S, Hollander G, Shani J. Acute pulmonary edema secondary to hyperbaric oxygen therapy. Oxf Med Case Reports 2015; 2015(2): 183-4.
[http://dx.doi.org/10.1093/omcr/omv002] [PMID: 25988073]

[42] Cakmak T, Battal B, Kara K, *et al.* A case of tension pneumothorax during hyperbaric oxygen therapy in an earthquake survivor with crush injury complicated by ARDS (adult respiratory distress syndrome). Undersea Hyperb Med 2015; 42(1): 9-13.
[PMID: 26094299]

[43] Ali S, Waheed K, Iqbal ZH. Microbiological pattern of ventilator associated pneumonia. J Ayub Med Coll Abbottabad 2015; 27(1): 117-9.
[PMID: 26182754]

[44] Castro Codesal ML, Featherstone R, Martinez Carrasco C, *et al.* Long-term non-invasive ventilation therapies in children: a scoping review protocol. BMJ Open 2015; 5(8): e008697.
[http://dx.doi.org/10.1136/bmjopen-2015-008697] [PMID: 26270951]

[45] Mc Queen M, Rojas J, Sun SC, *et al.* Safety and Long Term Outcomes with High Flow Nasal Cannula Therapy in Neonatology: A Large Retrospective Cohort Study. J Pulm Resp Med 2014; 4:pii216.

[46] Hoepker A, Seear M, Petrocheilou A, *et al.* Wilson-Mikity syndrome: updated diagnostic criteria based on nine cases and a review of the literature. Pediatr Pulmonol 2008; 43(10): 1004-12.
[http://dx.doi.org/10.1002/ppul.20900] [PMID: 18781642]

[47] Lee YM, Kim CS, Jo K, Sohn EJ, Kim JS, Kim J. Inhibitory effect of Samul-tang on retinal neovascularization in oxygen-induced retinopathy. BMC Complement Altern Med 2015; 15: 271.
[http://dx.doi.org/10.1186/s12906-015-0800-7] [PMID: 26264147]

[48] Carrasco Loza R, Villamizar Rodríguez G, Medel Fernández N. Ventilator-Induced Lung Injury (VILI) in Acute Respiratory Distress Syndrome (ARDS): Volutrauma and Molecular Effects. Open Respir Med J 2015; 9: 112-9.
[http://dx.doi.org/10.2174/1874306401509010112] [PMID: 26312103]

[49] Gurzu S, Jung I, Azamfirei L, *et al.* Vascular endothelial growth factor bioactivity and its receptors in patients with acute respiratory distress syndrome. Korean J Pathol 2011; 45: 139-45.
[http://dx.doi.org/10.4132/KoreanJPathol.2011.45.2.139]

[50] Azamfirei L, Gurzu S, Solomon R, *et al.* Vascular endothelial growth factor: a possible mediator of endothelial activation in acute respiratory distress syndrome. Minerva Anestesiol 2010; 76(8): 609-16.
[PMID: 20661201]

[51] Oliveira GP, Silva JD, Marques PS, *et al.* The effects of Dasatinib in experimental acute respiratory distress syndrome depend on dose and etiology. Cell Physiol Biochem 2015; 36(4): 1644-58.
[http://dx.doi.org/10.1159/000430325] [PMID: 26160269]

[52] Richardson CM, Pointon KS, Manhire AR, Macfarlane JT. Percutaneous lung biopsies: a survey of

UK practice based on 5444 biopsies. Br J Radiol 2002; 75(897): 731-5.
[http://dx.doi.org/10.1259/bjr.75.897.750731] [PMID: 12200241]

[53] Lorenz J, Blum M. Complications of percutaneous chest biopsy. Semin Intervent Radiol 2006; 23(2): 188-93.
[http://dx.doi.org/10.1055/s-2006-941449] [PMID: 21326762]

[54] Olgun DC, Samanci C, Ergin AS, Akman C. Life-threatening complication of percutaneous transthoracic fine-needle aspiration biopsy: systemic arterial air embolism. Eurasian J Med 2015; 47(1): 72-4.
[http://dx.doi.org/10.5152/eajm.2014.51] [PMID: 25745350]

[55] Rapicetta C, Lococo F, Levrini G, Ricchetti T, Sgarbi G, Paci M. Asymptomatic air-embolism following percutaneous radiofrequency ablation of lung tumor: rare or underestimated complication? Thorac Cancer 2015; 6(2): 227-9.
[http://dx.doi.org/10.1111/1759-7714.12180] [PMID: 26273364]

[56] Zhang L, Yang Y, Zhang J, Zhou X, Dong H, Zhou Y. Barium sulfate aspiration: Severe chemical pneumonia induced by a massive reflux of contrast medium during small bowel barium enema. Forensic Sci Int 2015; 253: e16-9.
[http://dx.doi.org/10.1016/j.forsciint.2015.05.016] [PMID: 26077941]

[57] Vicente DA, Solomon NP, Avital I, *et al.* Voice outcomes after total thyroidectomy, partial thyroidectomy, or non-neck surgery using a prospective multifactorial assessment. J Am Coll Surg 2014; 219(1): 152-63.
[http://dx.doi.org/10.1016/j.jamcollsurg.2014.03.019] [PMID: 24745621]

[58] Simon D, Boucher M, Schmidt-Wilcke P. [Intraoperative avoidance and recognition of recurrent laryngeal nerve palsy in thyroid surgery]. Chirurg 2015; 86(1): 6-12.
[http://dx.doi.org/10.1007/s00104-014-2816-9] [PMID: 25502321]

[59] Koelmel JC, Sittel C. [Quality of voice and life after injectionlaryngoplasty using VOX Implants(®) (polydimethylsiloxane)]. Laryngorhinootologie 2014; 93(5): 316-20.
[PMID: 24519317]

[60] Tesei F, Poveda LM, Strali W, Tosi L, Magnani G, Farneti G. Unilateral laryngeal and hypoglossal paralysis (Tapias syndrome) following rhinoplasty in general anaesthesia: case report and review of the literature. Acta Otorhinolaryngol Ital 2006; 26(4): 219-21.
[PMID: 18236639]

[61] Mukherjee R, Müller M, Amstad H, *et al.* [Dysphonia and dysphagia after anterior cervical spine surgery]. HNO 2014; 62(8): 575-81.
[http://dx.doi.org/10.1007/s00106-014-2877-6] [PMID: 24906340]

[62] Goz V, Qureshi S, Hecht AC. Arytenoid dislocation as a cause of prolonged hoarseness after cervical discectomy and fusion. Global Spine J 2013; 3(1): 47-50.
[http://dx.doi.org/10.1055/s-0032-1329890] [PMID: 24436851]

[63] Emohare O, Peterson E, Slinkard N, Janus S, Morgan R. Occam paradox? A variation of tapia syndrome and an unreported complication of guidewire-assisted pedicle screw insertion. Evid Based Spine Care J 2013; 4(2): 132-6.
[http://dx.doi.org/10.1055/s-0033-1357355] [PMID: 24436711]

[64] Bao M, Zhou Y, Jiang G, Chen C. Pulmonary artery pseudoaneurysm after a left upper sleeve lobectomy. World J Surg Oncol 2013; 11: 272-4.
[http://dx.doi.org/10.1186/1477-7819-11-272] [PMID: 24119497]

CHAPTER 6

Iatrogenic Pathology of Gastrointestinal Tract

Simona Gurzu*, **Tivadar Bara** and **Ioan Jung**

Department of Pathology, University of Medicine and Pharmacy, Tirgu-Mures, Romania

Abstract: This chapter includes a synthesis of data regarding iatrogenic injuries of the gastrointestinal tract. In the first section, medical drug-induced lesions are analyzed, while the following sections refer to the diagnostic and/or therapeutic interventions that involve the gastrointestinal segments. ADRs come in a wide spectrum of manifestations, from mucosal inflammation to severe lesions, such as Stevens-Johnson syndrome. The most common agents involved in severe reactions are non-steroidal anti-inflammatory drugs (NSAIDs). Proton pump inhibitors (PPIs) are responsible for the occurrence of cystic polyposis of the stomach. Intestinal iatrogenic disorders primarily involve enterocolitis, but strange complications, such as bezoar formation or intestinal rupture, are also reported. Complications relating to endoscopic examinations, laparotomy and laparoscopy are also presented in detail.

Keywords: Adverse drug reaction, Aspiration, Bezoar, Cystic polyposis, Endoscopy, Enterocolitis, Gingival hyperplasia, Hemorrhage, Laparoscopy, Laparotomy, Malabsorption, Polyp, Proton pump inhibitors, Stevens-Johnson syndrome, Teeth discoloration.

DRUG-INDUCED LESIONS

ADRs of the GI tract (Table **6-1**) can be induced *via* the following mechanisms: dose-dependent direct toxicity (*e.g.,* PPIs), immune hypersensitivity reactions, idiosyncrasy and mixed mechanisms (*e.g.,* NSAIDs) [1].

Lesions of the Oral Cavity, Pharynx And Esophagus

- ***Mucosal Inflammation***

Antibiotics, conventional chemotherapeutics, immunosuppressive drugs and targeted cancer therapeutics (*e.g.,* mTOR and tyrosine kinase inhibitors, antiangiogenic drugs) can cause stomatitis, pharyngitis, esophagitis and angina. These types of mucositis can be ulcerative, mycotic (*e.g.,* candidiasis) or

* **Corresponding author Simona Gurzu:** Department of Pathology, University of Medicine and Pharmacy, Tirgu-Mures, Romania; Tel: 0040-745-673550; Fax: 0040-372-653250; E-mail: simonagurzu@yahoo.com

Simona Gurzu & Ioan Jung (Eds.)

gangrenous [1 - 3].

- ***Other Lesions of the Oral Mucosa***

These are presented in detail in Table **6-1**. For example, *gingival hyperplasia* can be induced by anticonvulsants or contraceptives. In psychiatric patients receiving antipsychotics, *Stevens-Johnson syndrome* has been reported; skin lesions (described in Chapter 13) are associated with edema and ulcers of the oral and ocular mucosa [4].

Tetracyclines can produce *discoloration of the teeth* and can also, during the childhood period, induce hyperplasia or deformities of the teeth enamel. Although iron supplementation confers protection against enamel demineralization, it can also induce black teeth discoloration in children, especially in hypomineralized and decalcified areas. Because staining intensity is directly correlated with the supplements' contact with teeth, and the duration of that contact, simultaneous consumption with liquids or dripping directly to the posterior parts of the mouth is suggested [1, 5].

- ***Other Lesions of the Esophagus***

Doxycycline may induce hemolysis and epithelial injury with subsequent esophageal *erosion*. Polymedication can result in *dysphagia*. Chemotherapeutics can produce taste disorders (*dysgeusia/ageusia*) and esophageal *strictures* [3, 6 - 9].

Table 6-1. ADRs of the salivary glands, oral cavity and esophagus. Data from references [1 - 9].

ADR type	**Drugs**
Acute sialorrhea/hypersalivation	Ketamine (intravenous anesthetic drug)
Hyposalivation/xerostomia	Antihistaminic drugs, atropine, belladonna neuroleptics (promethazine)
Dysphagia, dysgeusia	Chemotherapeutics (vismodegib)
Parotitis	Morphine
Increased appetite	Corticosteroids
Yellow, brown or black teeth (teeth discoloration)	Tetracyclines, iron supplements, augmentin (amoxicillin with clavulanate)
Erythema multiforme of the mouth	Aspirin, barbiturates, bromide, hydantoin, iodine, antibiotics (penicillin, streptomycin), sulfonamides, thiouracil
Mouth ulcerations	Antipsychotics (carbamazepine, phenytoin, clozapine), mTOR inhibitors, chemotherapeutics

(Table 6-1) contd.....

ADR type	Drugs
Gingival hyperplasia	Antiepileptic drugs (hydantoin), contraceptive pills, cyclosporine, atropine, belladonna
Esophageal erosions	Antibiotics (*e.g.,* doxycycline), NSAIDs, potassium chloride, chemotherapeutics (*e.g.,* carboplatin and paclitaxel)
Necrotizing inflammations	Cytotoxic drugs (*e.g.,* cyclophosphamide), immunosuppressives
Esophageal strictures	Chemotherapeutics (vinblastine, doxorubicin, 5-FU, rituximab, methotrexate, *etc.*)
Mycotic infections	Antibiotics, immunosuppressive drugs
Mucosal hyperpigmentation	Cyclophosphamide, doxorubicin, busulfan, augmentin

Gastric Disorders

- ***Acute/Chronic Gastritis with Associated Erosions or Peptic Ulcers***

Gastric mucosal lesions (Table **6-2**) can be induced by several drugs, including antibiotics, sulfonamides, corticosteroids, chemotherapeutics, rauwolfia-based drugs, *etc.* [10, 11]. Ulcerations are present in about 20% of long-term users of NSAIDs [12]. Aspirin is the cause of 50% of gastric erosion. The pathomechanism involves direct injuries to the gastric mucosa-defending barriers. This is followed by increasing ion permeability and back diffusion of hydrogen ions across the gastric mucosa, with further mastocyte degranulation and histamine release. This, in turn, leads to chloride acid hypersecretion and subsequent mucosal erosions, superficial necroses and bleeding [13]. Acute gastritis is common in patients hospitalized in ICUs (Fig. **6-1**).

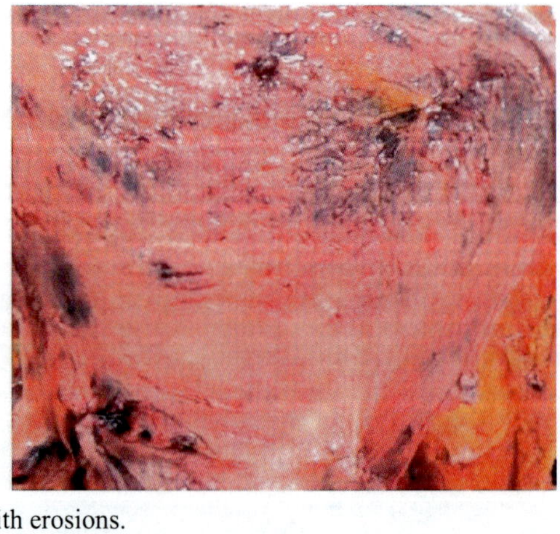

Fig. (6-1). Acute gastritis with erosions.

- ***Dyspepsia and Chronic Peptic Ulcer Complications***

The side effects of NSAIDs include a large spectrum of lesions, from asymptomatic gastric mucosa lesions and submucosal hemorrhages to dyspepsia and ulcer complications, such as perforation and bleeding [10, 11]. Simultaneous intake of NSAIDs, anticoagulants and corticosteroids increases the risk of upper GI bleeding [14].

- ***Fundic Gland Polyps (Cystic Polyposis of the Stomach)***

In patients taking PPIs for at least 12 months, the occurrence of gastric fundic polyps is reported in 23.1% of cases, with this proportion further increasing in elderly patients [15]. In drug-associated polyposis, the number of polyps gradually increases, and a feature that can help to distinguish them is hereditary gastric proximal polyposis of the stomach (GAPPS syndrome). This is an autosomal syndrome produced by mutations of the familial adenomatous polyposis (FAP) gene and is characterized by several polyps of the proximal stomach, without related intestinal or colorectal polyps [16].

Disorders of the Small Intestine and Colorectal Segments

- ***Pseudomembranous/Hemorrhagic Enterocolitis***

This condition is commonly induced by the use of oral antibiotics (Table **6-2**). The lesion is also common in medical oncology units and can be fatal in elderly and immunosuppressed patients (Fig. **6-2**). The pathomechanism involves the destruction of the normal bacterial flora of the intestine, causing the overgrowth of pro-inflammatory bacteria (*e.g., Clostridium difficile, Staphylococcus aureus, Proteus, Enterococcus*). The clinical symptoms are abdominal pain and diarrhea (as this condition can be of the hemorrhagic type). Concomitant administration of probiotics, prebiotics and high volumes of liquids (to prevent long-term contact with mucosa) are mandatory for the prevention of this complication [1, 17]. Immunosuppressive drug-related enterocolitis predominantly affects the ileum and proximal colon [1]. *Clostridium-related enterocolitis* can also be caused by PPIs in a dose-dependent manner [17 - 19]. In surgery departments, an increasing number of cases involving Clostridium infections is the result of extensive use of broad-spectrum antibiotics. This is a pseudomembranous or hemorrhagic inflammation with a high risk of intestinal perforation and death (Fig. **6-3**).

- ***Non-Specific Enterocolitis with Intestinal Ulcerations***

Intestinal ulcers, sometimes large, can be induced by NSAIDs, but also by the long-term use of steroids or contraceptives (*e.g.,* norgestrel, ethinylestradiol). Immunosuppressive drugs can cause cytomegalovirus (CMV)-related colitis [1]. Conventional chemotherapeutics, such as capecitabine, can also induce chronic enterocolitis (Fig. **6-4**) [20].

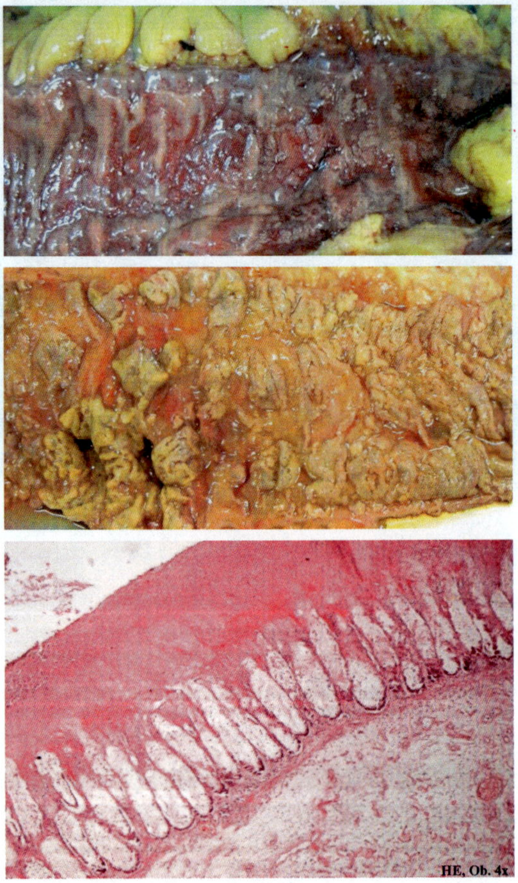

Fig. (6-2). Antibiotic-induced pseudomembranous colitis.

In one of our cases, a 63-year-old female who had undergone hip prosthesis six months previously, presented with acute abdominal ulceration and emergency laparotomy was necessary. Intraoperative examination revealed several perforations of the colorectal segments with associated peritonitis, and a total colectomy was performed. Macroscopic examination also revealed diffuse mucosal atrophy from the cecum to the rectum (Fig. **6-5**). Under the microscope, mucosal atrophy with several fistulae was observed. The patient died one week after surgery due to septicemia. Upon examining the patient's medical history, we found that she had been taking more than 20 drugs in the previous two months, including analgesics, NSAIDs, antihypertensive drugs (five types), oral antidiabetics, sedatives, PPIs, liver protectors and vitamin supplements, such as milgamma (vitamins B1 and B6).

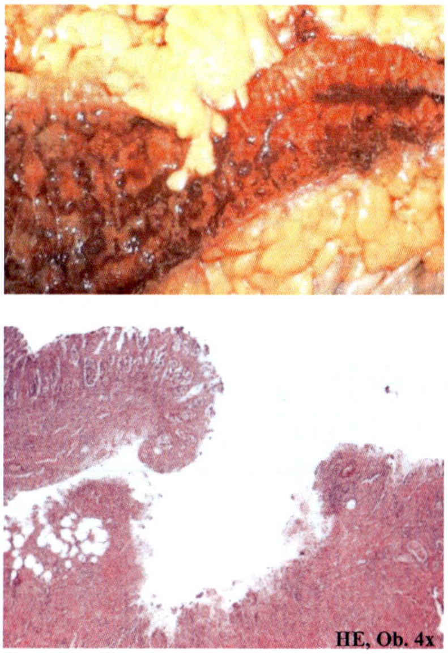

Fig. (6-3). Clostridium-related hemorrhagic colitis.

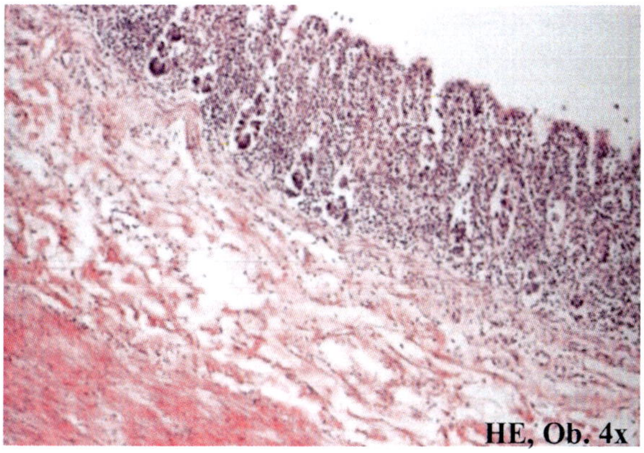

Fig. (6-4). Capecitabine-related non-specific colitis with submucosal fibrosis.

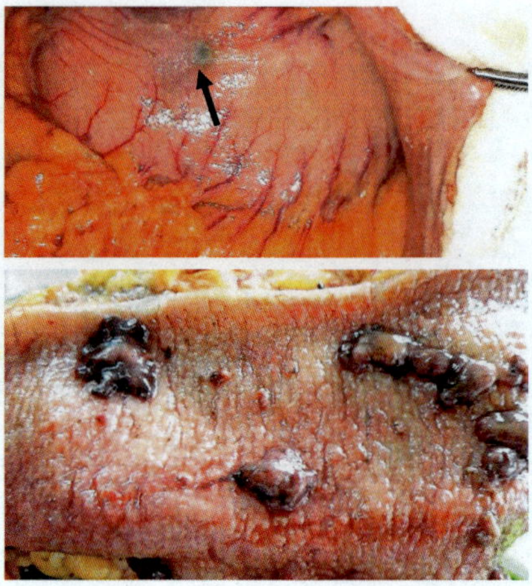

Fig. (6-5). Drug-related ulcers and perforations of the colon (top) and atrophy of the mucosa with inflammatory polyps (bottom).

- ***Anaphylaxis-Related Intestinal Lesions***

Shirai *et al.*, (2006) report a number of cases of intestinal ulcerations that occurred in patients with anaphylaxis. Drugs such as diclofenac, acetaminophen and pranoprofen can be involved in such cases [21].

- ***Intestinal Hemorrhages***

These hemorrhages can be related to anticoagulant therapy, but other substances, such as NSAIDs and sodium fluoride, can also induce intramural hemorrhages [22]. Moreover, PPIs and histamine-H2 receptor antagonists induce dysbiosis that can exacerbate NSAIDs-related intestinal injuries [17, 23].

- ***Malabsorption Syndrome***

This is a common drug-related syndrome that can occur following polymedication (Table **6-2**). PPIs can induce magnesium absorption disorders or iron and vitamin B12 deficiency, in a dose-dependent manner [18].

- ***Targeted Therapy-Related Gastrointestinal Mucositis***

Some of the agents used for the individualized treatment of cancer (Table **6-2**) increase the risk of developing diarrhea, becoming twice to eight times as likely as compared to controls. The highest risk (eight times higher than the baseline) was recently reported for patients treated with lapatinib [3].

Table 6-2. ADRs of the stomach, small intestine and colorectal segments. Data from references [10 - 23].

ADR type	Drugs
Acute/chronic gastritis	Aspirin, antibiotics, corticosteroids, NSAIDs, phenylbutazone, histamine, sulfonamides, cytotoxic drugs (taxanes: docetaxel, paclitaxel), bromocriptine (anti-prolactin drug), iron compounds, bisphosphonates
Acute peptic ulcers/erosions	Aspirin, corticosteroids, NSAIDs, anticoagulants, digitalis, 5-FU, phenylbutazone, histamine, insulin, steroids
GI hemorrhages	Anticoagulants, cytotoxic drugs, sodium fluoride, PPIs
IBD-like enterocolitis (diarrhea, constipation, bloating and eosinophils in the bioptic specimen)	Immunosuppressive drugs (mycophenolate mofetil used in renal transplantation recipients), 5-FU, NSAIDs, gold compounds, alpha-methyldopa, salicylates, sulfasalazine, ipilimumab (an anti-cytotoxic Tlymphocyte human monoclonal antibody used to treat melanoma, lung and prostate cancer)
Fungal inflammations	Antibiotics, corticosteroids, immunosuppressive agents
Non-traumatic rupture of the GI tract	Corticosteroids
Pseudomembranous/hemorrhagic enterocolitis	Antibiotics (*e.g.*, augmentin or amoxicillin with clavulanate), cytotoxic drugs, PPIs
Ulcerative colitis	Phenylbutazone, oral contraceptives, antifungal flucytosine, potassium chloride, NSAIDs, immunosuppressive drugs
Colitis, constipation, GI bezoars (with crystals)	Kayexalate® (sodium polystyrene sulfonate) – used to treat chronic renal failure Calcium and vitamin D
Nausea, loss of appetite, diarrhea	Augmentin (amoxicillin with clavulanate), chemotherapeutics (5-FU, capecitabine, irinotecan, tegafur, *etc.*), targeted cancer drugs (lapatinib, erlotinib, gefitinib, sorafenib, sunitinib, anti-EGFR agents), thyreostatic drugs, lithium topiramate (anticonvulsant)
Intestinal infarction	Digitalis toxicity
Malabsorption syndrome	Cytotoxic drugs, neomycin, colchicine, phenolphthalein, PPIs
Vasculitis	Serum sickness

IATROGENIC LESIONS DURING DIAGNOSTIC AND THERAPEUTIC PROCEDURES

Endoscopic Examinations

Perforation of the *esophagus* is reported in fewer than 0.1% of patients who undergo upper GI endoscopic examination. The risk of rupture is higher for the upper esophagus at the level of the cricopharyngeal muscle. The distal esophagus can be perforated in patients with chronic inflammations, previous stenosis and hiatal hernia. Perforation can lead to mediastinitis, peritonitis, septic shock, hemorrhagic shock, pneumoperitoneum (10 cases reported in 2012), *etc.* [1, 24].

Gastric perforation is extremely rare, but has been reported in patients with chronic atrophic gastritis or gastric cancer. Gastroscopy-related splenic rupture, as a result of excessive stretching of the splenogastric and splenodiaphragmatic ligaments, can also occur [25].

Perforation of the *colorectal segments,* both with and without subsequent peritonitis, occur in 0.05-0.6% of patients who undergo colonoscopy [26, 27]. Hemorrhages are seen in 0.28% of patients [27, 28].

In patients with coagulation disorders (such as hemophilia A), pericolic hematoma, splenic rupture and hemoperitoneum can emerge immediately or up to two weeks after intervention [27]. The risk of splenic rupture should also be taken into account in patients with difficult intubation, traction of the splenocolic ligament, looping of the colonoscope, adhesions between the spleen and colon, and presence of a large mass or polyp at the splenic flexure [27]. Other rare complications of colonoscopy are pneumothorax, pneumoperitoneum, interstitial emphysema, pulmonary emboli, congestive heart failure and sepsis. The colonoscopy-related mortality rate is approximately 0.4% (0.2% for diagnostic procedures and 1.2% for therapeutic procedures) [28].

Endoscopic Mucosal Resection and Submucosal Dissection for Early Gastric Cancer

Delayed bleeding is the most common complication occurring after mucosal resection of gastric tumors. Perforation of the stomach and/or bleeding can occur in 2-3% of cases [29]. Following endoscopic submucosal dissection, perforation occurs in 1-4% of cases. This risk exceeds 10% for fundic tumors, which can be repaired with hemoclips. The rate of periprocedural bleeding is 1.7-16% [30, 31]. A rare complication is tension pneumoperitoneum [32].

Laparotomy

Most laparotomy-related lesions are induced by surgical excision, but other lesions occur as a result of uncertain mechanisms. These lesions are presented in detail in Chapter 17.

Acute Gastric Dilatation

This is a multifactorial event induced by transient postoperative gastric wall atony. It occurs in almost all patients who undergo an abdominal intervention, presenting a spontaneous resolution. In rare cases, the fluid accumulated in the dilated stomach can induce mesenteric traction and subsequent intestinal compression. Patients can present vomiting, abdominal pain, gastric distension, tachycardia, oliguria and even abdominal compartment syndrome. The latter complication can be avoided through permanent aspiration of the gastric fluid. The most severe complications are gastric necrosis with perforation, sepsis and prolonged gastroparetic state. Patients with diabetes or preexisting dysmotility disorders present a higher risk of postoperative complications [1, 33].

Ogilvie's Syndrome (pseudomegacolon)

This syndrome represents a postoperative acute paralytic dilatation of the cecum and ascending colon. It is primarily a complication of abdominal surgery and cesarean section, but can also emerge after coronary bypass grafting (0.046%), spinal surgery and joints arthroplasty (0.29-1.3%). Intestinal rupture is observed in 13-15% of cases, especially in patients with cecum dilatation greater than 12 cm. The risk of intestinal gangrene is relatively high for elderly patients with associated comorbidities (cardiovascular, neurological, infectious, inflammatory, metabolic, *etc.*). In refractory cases, in addition to gastric and intestinal decompression, fluid and electrolyte balance correction should be accompanied by administration of neostigmine [1, 34, 35].

Lesions of the Gastric Stump

Functional Disorders are the most common postoperative complications. These include GI dysmotility and biliary dyskinesia. Bloating, nausea, vomiting and malnutrition are the main symptoms [1].

Decrease of Immune Mechanisms has been recorded in several studies. The incidence of pulmonary tuberculosis is three times higher in patients who have undergone a gastric resection as compared to the control group. Due to the low acidity that emerges in 90% of cases (pH between four and eight, as compared to a normal pH between one and two), multiplication of bacteria and fungi, especially Candida albicans, is also noted [1].

Morphological Disorders of Remnant Gastric Mucosa are chronic gastritis and intestinal metaplasia that occur as a result of biliary and duodenal reflux. Gastric foveolar polypous hyperplasia (50% of patients) and cystic glandular dilatation (60%) can also be seen [1].

Gastric Stump Carcinoma can occur as a result of postoperatively emerging chronic gastritis, bloating of the anastomotic area with bile acids and an increasing number of bacteria, including those with the capacity to transform nitrates into nitrosamines [1, 36].

Gastric stump carcinoma usually occurs within 30-32 years of gastrectomy performed for benign diseases. The time interval is shorter in patients who presented a primary malignant lesion (10-18 years). Regarding surgical technique, the time interval is longer following Billroth-II than it is following Billroth-I reconstruction (30-32 years *vs*. 12-20 years). This carcinoma is usually located near the suture line and remnant gastric wall, in the case of Billroth-I, and at the anastomotic area, in the case of Billroth-II procedures [36 - 38].

Delayed Consequences at the Incision Line of the Abdominal Wall

Acute lesions are presented in Chapter 17. In this section, we present consequences related to delayed laparotomy.

Foreign Body Granuloma can be formed surrounding the suture material, extensive inflammatory infiltrate, talc or other foreign bodies.

Localized Myositis Ossificans is a rapidly growing, well-circumscribed metaplastic bone formation that can occur as a nodule on the incision line between weeks and years following surgery, usually without clinical consequences [39]. Under the microscope, bone lamellae lined by osteoblasts are seen (Fig. **6-6**).

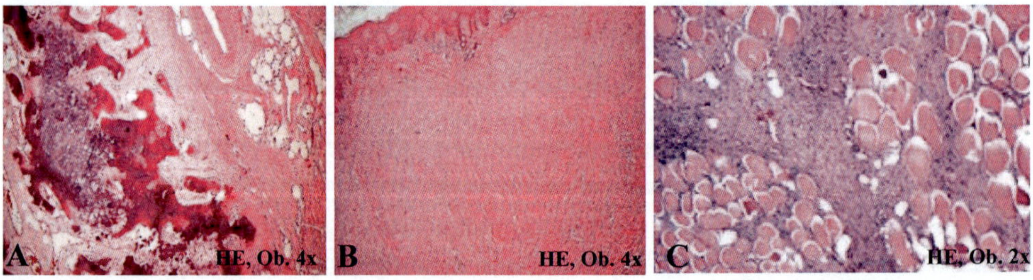

Fig. (6-6). Post-laparoscopy delayed injuries of the abdominal wall. **A** – Localized myositis ossificans with bone lamellae and cartilage. **B** – Cheloid scar shown as subepithelial hyalinized connective tissue. **C** – Desmoid tumor indicated by proliferation of connective cells among the skeletal muscle fibers. This lesion occurred in a 25-year-old female, two years after laparoscopy. Due to the infiltrating aspect, removal of the rectus abdominis muscle was necessary.

Cheloid Scars (Fig **6-6**) are primarily reported in females. *Scar endometriosis* is rare and especially reported following appendectomy and in the laparoscopic trocar, usually with spontaneous regression [40].

Desmoid Tumors are slow-growing pseudotumoral lesions produced by mutations of the *CTNNB1* gene that encodes β-catenin. They occur more frequently in females, within one to two years of laparotomy, in most cases being reported following cesarean section of the abdominal muscle. In patients with desmoid tumors, the risk of occurrence of FAP is 1000 times greater than in the general population [41]. In one of our cases, the pseudotumor occurred in a 25-year-old female, two years after a previous laparotomy performed for a hepatectomy after a motorcycle accident (Fig. **6-6**).

Postoperative Parotitis

Although rare (<0.3% of cases) postoperative parotitis can occur after abdominal surgery. It has been hypothesized that allergic mechanisms, postoperative dehydration or glandular autodigestion by substances released during surgery are responsible for its pathogenesis. It can be associated with other complications, such as abscesses, direct spread along the facial nerve and thrombophlebitis of the jugular vein [42].

Other Therapeutic Procedures

Surgical Interventions

Laparoscopy – air embolism and bowel injury are the most common consequences [43]. Carbon dioxide (CO_2) embolism can also occur during laparoscopic surgery, which usually requires pneumoperitoneum by insufflating CO_2 into the peritoneal cavity. It can be a consequence of vascular injuries (*e.g.,* to the middle hepatic vein during laparoscopic cholecystectomy). Clinical indications include significantly decreased arterial blood pressure, arrhythmia and pulmonary hypertension [43]. Massive dilatation of the stomach, or gas-bloat syndrome, which can be associated with delayed gastric necrosis, is known to be a relatively common consequence (1-85%) of laparoscopic Nissen fundoplication. This intervention is performed in patients with PPIs, refractory gastroesophageal reflux disease (GERD) and in patients with hiatal hernia [44]. Details regarding the potential complications of laparoscopy are presented in Chapter 17.

Surgery for Head and Neck Tumors can induce functional disorders of the GI tract, such as dysphagia [7].

Cervical Spine Surgery especially *anterior cervical discectomy,* can be followed by soft tissue injuries and esophageal perforation (0.25-1.49%). The most common late postoperative complication is dysphagia, which occurs as a result of plate migration and esophageal erosion through the posterior pharyngeal wall. It is more common in females over the age of 60 and is directly correlated with the length of the surgical intervention [45 - 47]. About 98% of cases present spontaneous regression within two years of surgery. Recurrent pneumonias, cervical abscesses, sepsis, mediastinitis, meningitis and unexplained fever can be associated [47]. Tapia's syndrome (hoarse voice, impaired breathing and tongue paresis) have also been reported following spinal surgery [48].

Endoscopic Interventions

Sclerotherapy for Esophageal Varices can be followed by esophageal ulcerations and hemorrhages [49]. Rebleeding is reported in 2.2% of patients in the first two weeks following the obliteration, 3.9% of patients within four weeks, 18.9% of patients within six months and 27.6% of patients within 12 months [50]. The risk of squamous cell carcinoma of the esophagus is observed to increase within about 20 months of sclerotherapy [51].

Augmentation of the Lower Esophageal Sphincter can be performed in patients with severe GERD using magnetic devices approved by the FDA in 2012. These are considered to be safe devices, without significant side effects. The most common complications are moderate to severe regurgitation (57% in the first months and only 1.2% after five years), gas-bloat syndrome (52% at baseline and 8.3% at five years) and dysphagia (5%) [52].

Parenteral Nutrition

This can lead to intestinal atrophy (due to lack of use) or cholecystitis (due to prolonged biliary stasis and absence of cholecystokinin that is synthesized into the small intestine). Postprocedural pneumonia, sepsis and metabolic and electrolyte imbalances can be associated [53].

Enteral Nutrition

This can induce gastroesophageal reflux, pulmonary aspiration of gastric content, gastrohepatic fistulae and sepsis [53, 54]. Long-term enteral nutrition can lead to esophageal ulcerations and plasma deficiency of iron, zinc, phosphorus, calcium and vitamin D (micronutrient deficiency), especially in children. Diarrhea, vomiting, necrotizing enterocolitis, malabsorption and metabolic disorders (hypo-/hypernatremia, hypokalemia and hyperglycemia) can also occur [55]. In patients with severe acute pancreatitis, enteral feeding increases the severity of chylous ascites [56].

Hemodialysis-Related Gastric Lesions

Hyperplasia of the Gastric Mucosa can be caused by hypergastrinemia, hyperchlorhydria or uremia. It involves hyperplasia of gastric parietal cells, antral G-cells and Brunner's duodenal glands [1, 57].

Gastric Angiodysplasia refers to gastric antral vascular ectasia (GAVE), which is also known as watermelon stomach. It can be a consequence of continuous peritoneal dialysis and can induce anemia and hematemesis [58].

Other Colorectal Lesions

Radiotherapy-Related Lesions are usually without significant clinical consequences and present as actinic proctitis and rectal stenosis [59].

Post-Transplant Injuries of the GI Tract are relatively common. Following kidney transplantation, uremia-related pseudomembranous colitis (Fig. **6-7**) can be complicated by colorectal ulcerations and/or perforations. The immunosuppressive drug mycophenolate mofetil induces colitis and diarrhea (Table **6-2**) in 45% of patients [60].

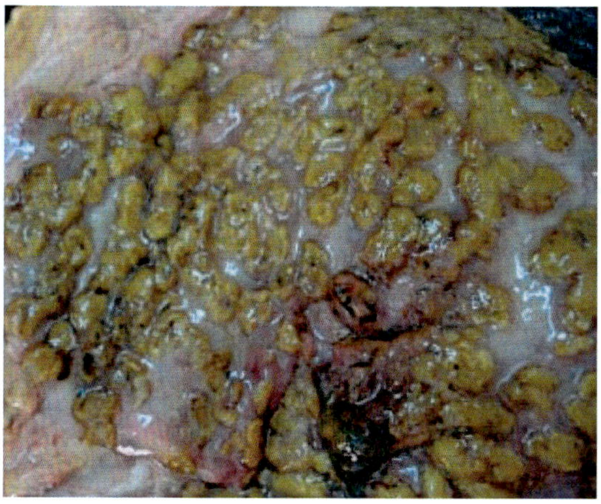

Fig. (6-7). Uremia-induced pseudomembranous proctitis.

Foreign Body Granulomas can be formed surrounding vegetable fibers or suture material (Fig. **6-8**), but an excessive amount of inflammatory infiltrate can also induce their genesis. In some cases, they can mimic a tumor relapse. *Talc powder proctitis* is the result of accumulation of starch granules or talc crystals from surgical gloves. It is an immune-induced granulomatous inflammation that can lead to rectal wall fibrosis and stenosis. Barium passage can be followed by the formation of intramural *barium granulomas*, while the treatment of hemorrhoids using oil-based substances can be followed by the occurrence of *oleogranulomas* [1].

Other Postoperative Colorectal Lesions include surgical dehiscence (with accompanying risk of sepsis) and hemorrhages (with accompanying risk of hemoperitoneum or hemorrhagic shock). In one of our cases, two weeks after a colectomy was performed to treat a colonic tumor, the patient was hospitalized with mechanical ileus. At this point, a partial colectomy was performed. In the surgical specimen, on the cut section, a total luminal obstruction produced by forgotten surgical meshes, surrounded by a rich granulation tissue was found (Fig. **6-9**).

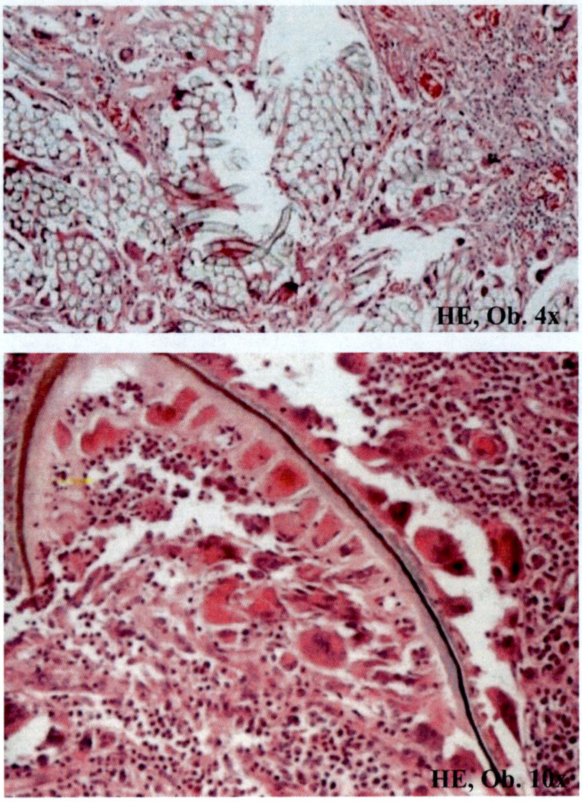

Fig. (6-8). Foreign body granulomas surrounding suture material (top) and vegetable tissue (bottom).

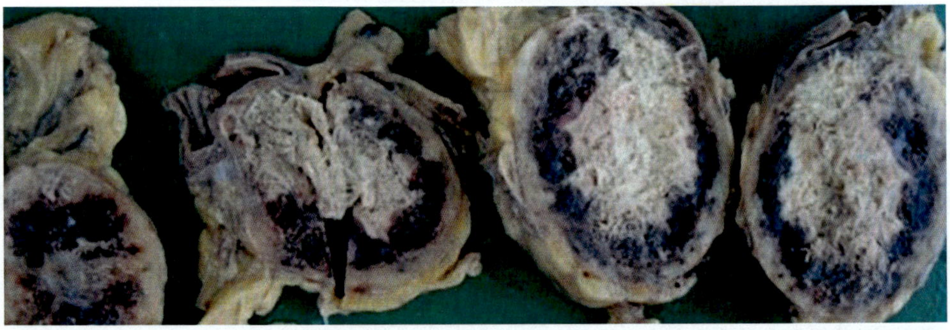

Fig. (6-9). Postoperative intestinal obstruction with surgical meshes.

CONFLICT OF INTEREST

The authors confirm that this chapter content has no conflict of interest.

ACKNOWLEDGEMENTS

Declared none.

REFERENCES

[1] Jung J, Ed. Patologie iatrogenă. Tîrgu-Mureş, Romania: University Press 2006.

[2] Carenco C, Faure S, Ursic-Bedoya J, Herrero A, Pageaux GP. Solid, non-skin, post-liver transplant tumors: Key role of lifestyle and immunosuppression management. World J Gastroenterol 2016; 22(1): 427-34.
[http://dx.doi.org/10.3748/wjg.v22.i1.427] [PMID: 26755888]

[3] Peterson DE, Boers-Doets CB, Bensadoun RJ, Herrstedt J. Management of oral and gastrointestinal mucosal injury: ESMO Clinical Practice Guidelines for diagnosis, treatment, and follow-up. Ann Oncol 2015; 26 (Suppl. 5): v139-51.
[http://dx.doi.org/10.1093/annonc/mdv202] [PMID: 26142468]

[4] Wu MK, Chung W, Wu CK, Tseng PT. The severe complication of Stevens-Johnson syndrome induced by long-term clozapine treatment in a male schizophrenia patient: a case report. Neuropsychiatr Dis Treat 2015; 11: 1039-41.
[PMID: 25914536]

[5] Talebi M, Parisay I, Mokhtari N. The parents knowledge and behavior towards the effects of using iron supplements on tooth staining and dental caries in Mashhad, Iran. Dent Res J (Isfahan) 2012; 9(6): 715-8.
[PMID: 23559947]

[6] Tutuian R. Adverse effects of drugs on the esophagus. Best Pract Res Clin Gastroenterol 2010; 24(2): 91-7.
[http://dx.doi.org/10.1016/j.bpg.2010.02.005] [PMID: 20227023]

[7] Schwemmle C, Jungheim M, Miller S, Kühn D, Ptok M. [Medication-induced dysphagia : A review]. HNO 2015; 63(7): 504-10.
[http://dx.doi.org/10.1007/s00106-015-0015-8] [PMID: 26148562]

[8] Benatta MA, Loumi A. Oesophagogastric junction stricture: a rare complication of chemotherapy for malignant lymphoma. Hepatobiliary Surg Nutr 2015; 4(4): 295-6.
[PMID: 26312247]

[9] Reyes-Habito CM, Roh EK. Cutaneous reactions to chemotherapeutic drugs and targeted therapy for cancer: Part II. Targeted therapy. J Am Acad Dermatol 2014; 71(2): 217.e1-217.e11.
[http://dx.doi.org/10.1016/j.jaad.2014.04.013] [PMID: 25037801]

[10] Thiéfin G. [Epidemiology and treatment of gastroduodenal lesions caused by non-steroidal anti-inflammatory agents]. Rev Med Interne 1991; 12(3): 227-36.
[PMID: 1896717]

[11] Roĭtberg GE, Polunina TE. [Drug lesions of the gastroduodenal zone]. Eksp Klin Gastroenterol 2002; 117(3): 9-15, 117.
[PMID: 12353401]

[12] Aabakkeri L. Clinical symptoms, endoscopic findings and histological features of gastroduodenal NSAIDs lesions. Ital J Gastroenterol Hepatol 1999; 31: 19-22.
[PMID: 10091099]

[13] Ivey KJ, Clifton JA. Back diffusion of hydrogen ions across gastric mucosa of patients with gastric ulcer and rheumatoid arthritis. BMJ 1974; 1(5896): 16-9.
[http://dx.doi.org/10.1136/bmj.1.5896.16] [PMID: 4808814]

[14] Aalykke C, Lauritsen K. Epidemiology of NSAID-related gastroduodenal mucosal injury. Best Pract Res Clin Gastroenterol 2001; 15(5): 705-22.
[http://dx.doi.org/10.1053/bega.2001.0230] [PMID: 11566036]

[15] Huang CZ, Lai RX, Mai L, Zhou HL, Chen HJ, Guo HX. Relative risk factors associated with the development of fundic gland polyps. Eur J Gastroenterol Hepatol 2014; 26(11): 1217-21.
[http://dx.doi.org/10.1097/MEG.0000000000000199] [PMID: 25187299]

[16] Worthley DL, Phillips KD, Wayte N, *et al.* Gastric adenocarcinoma and proximal polyposis of the stomach (GAPPS): a new autosomal dominant syndrome. Gut 2012; 61(5): 774-9.
[http://dx.doi.org/10.1136/gutjnl-2011-300348] [PMID: 21813476]

[17] Fujimori S. What are the effects of proton pump inhibitors on the small intestine? World J Gastroenterol 2015; 21(22): 6817-9.
[PMID: 26078557]

[18] Ruiz de Angulo D, Ortiz MA, Martínez de Haro LF. Side effects of proton-pump inhibitors: another reason to indicate anti-reflux surgery for Barretts esophagus? Cir Esp 2014; 92(5): 303-4.
[http://dx.doi.org/10.1016/j.ciresp.2014.01.009] [PMID: 24625629]

[19] Wilhelm SM, Rjater RG, Kale-Pradhan PB. Perils and pitfalls of long-term effects of proton pump inhibitors. Expert Rev Clin Pharmacol 2013; 6(4): 443-51.
[http://dx.doi.org/10.1586/17512433.2013.811206] [PMID: 23927671]

[20] Gurzu S, Jung I, Comsulea M, Kadar Z, Azamfirei L, Molnar C. Lethal cardiotoxicity, steatohepatitis, chronic pancreatitis, and acute enteritis induced by capecitabine and oxaliplatin in a 36-year-old woman. Diagn Pathol 2013; 8: 150.
[http://dx.doi.org/10.1186/1746-1596-8-150] [PMID: 24041405]

[21] Shirai T, Mori M, Uotani T, Chida K. Gastrointestinal disorders in anaphylaxis. Intern Med 2007; 46(6): 315-6.
[http://dx.doi.org/10.2169/internalmedicine.46.6126]

[22] Müller P, Schmid K, Warnecke G, Setnikar I, Simon B. Sodium fluoride-induced gastric mucosal lesions: comparison with sodium monofluorophosphate. Z Gastroenterol 1992; 30(4): 252-4.
[PMID: 1604908]

[23] Wallace JL, de Nucci G, Sulaieva O. Toward More GI-Friendly Anti-Inflammatory Medications. Curr Treat Options Gastroenterol 2015; 13(4): 377-85.
[http://dx.doi.org/10.1007/s11938-015-0064-9] [PMID: 26303996]

[24] Symeonidis N, Ballas K, Pavlidis E, Psarras K, Pavlidis T, Sakantamis A. Tension pneumoperitoneum: a rare complication of upper gastrointestinal endoscopy. JSLS 2012; 16(3): 495-7.
[http://dx.doi.org/10.4293/108680812X13462882736655] [PMID: 23318083]

[25] Estevez-Boullosa P, Alonso-Aguirre PA, Couto-Worner I, Blanco-Rodriguez M, de Llano-Monelos P, Sanchez-Gonzalez F. Splenic rupture following a diagnostic upper endoscopy. World J Gastrointest Endosc 2010; 2(6): 235-6.
[http://dx.doi.org/10.4253/wjge.v2.i6.235] [PMID: 21160940]

[26] Doran H, Marin IT, Iaciu M, Pătraşcu T. Iatrogenic perforations during colonoscopy. Chirurgia (Bucur) 2014; 109(4): 523-6.
[PMID: 25149617]

[27] Mazulis A, Lakha A, Qazi B, Shapiro A. Delayed presentation of splenic rupture after endoscopy in a patient with hemophilia A: case report and review of the literature. ACG Case Rep J 2014; 1(4): 175-7.
[PMID: 26157867]

[28] Pourmand A, Shokoohi H. Tension pneumothorax, pneumoperitoneum, and cervical emphysema following a diagnostic colonoscopy. Case Rep Emerg Med 2013; 2013: 583287. [http://dx.doi.org/10.1155/2013/583287] [PMID: 23819071]

[29] Jeon SW, Jung MK, Kim SK, *et al.* Clinical outcomes for perforations during endoscopic submucosal dissection in patients with gastric lesions. Surg Endosc 2010; 24(4): 911-6. [http://dx.doi.org/10.1007/s00464-009-0693-y] [PMID: 19789921]

[30] Lee JS, Kim GH, Park DY, *et al.* Endoscopic Submucosal Dissection for Gastric Subepithelial Tumors: A Single-Center Experience. Gastroenterol Res Pract 2015; 2015: 425469. [http://dx.doi.org/10.1007/s00464-009-0693-y] [PMID: 19789921]

[31] Chung IK, Lee JH, Lee SH, *et al.* Therapeutic outcomes in 1000 cases of endoscopic submucosal dissection for early gastric neoplasms: Korean ESD Study Group multicenter study. Gastrointest Endosc 2009; 69(7): 1228-35. [http://dx.doi.org/10.1016/j.gie.2008.09.027] [PMID: 19249769]

[32] Siboni S, Bona D, Abate E, Bonavina L. Tension pneumoperitoneum following endoscopic submucosal dissection of leiomyoma of the cardia. Endoscopy 2010; 42 (Suppl. 2): E152. [http://dx.doi.org/10.1055/s-0029-1244048] [PMID: 20556708]

[33] Gauci JL, Stoven S, Szarka L, Papadakis KA. Prolonged idiopathic gastric dilatation following revascularization for chronic mesenteric ischemia. Ann Gastroenterol 2014; 27(3): 273-5. [PMID: 24975870]

[34] Valle RG, Godoy FL. Neostigmine for acute colonic pseudo-obstruction: A meta-analysis. Ann Med Surg (Lond) 2014; 3(3): 60-4. [http://dx.doi.org/10.1016/j.amsu.2014.04.002] [PMID: 25568788]

[35] Latunde-Dada AO, Alleemudder DI, Webster DP. Ogilvies syndrome following caesarean section. BMJ Case Rep 2013; 2013: bcr2013010013. [http://dx.doi.org/10.1136/bcr-2013-010013] [PMID: 23784768]

[36] Gurzu S, Copotoiu C, Azamfirei L, Jung I. Caliber persistent artery (Dieulafoys lesion) which is associated with an early-stage gastric stump cancer following distal gastrectomy. J Clin Diagn Res 2013; 7(8): 1717-9. [PMID: 24086889]

[37] Komatsu S, Ichikawa D, Okamoto K, *et al.* Progression of remnant gastric cancer is associated with duration of follow-up following distal gastrectomy. World J Gastroenterol 2012; 18(22): 2832-6. [http://dx.doi.org/10.3748/wjg.v18.i22.2832] [PMID: 22719193]

[38] Tanigawa N, Nomura E, Lee SW, *et al.* Current state of gastric stump carcinoma in Japan: based on the results of a nationwide survey. World J Surg 2010; 34(7): 1540-7. [http://dx.doi.org/10.1007/s00268-010-0505-5] [PMID: 20182716]

[39] Gurzu S, Bara T, Bara T Jr, Jung I. Metaplastic bone formation in the abdominal wall an incidental finding in a patient with gastric cancer. Case report and hypothesis about its histogenesis. Am J Dermatopathol 2013; 35(8): 844-6. [http://dx.doi.org/10.1097/DAD.0b013e318285db5c] [PMID: 24257191]

[40] Vural B, Vural F, Müezzinoglu B. An abdominal wall desmoid tumour mimicking cesarean scar endometriomas: a case report and review of the literature. J Clin Diagn Res 2015; 9(9): QD14-6. [PMID: 26500967]

[41] Jung I, Gurzu S, Turdean GS. Current status of familial gastrointestinal polyposis syndromes. World J Gastrointest Oncol 2015; 7(11): 347-55. [http://dx.doi.org/10.4251/wjgo.v7.i11.347] [PMID: 26600934]

[42] Sermoneta D, Lodoli C, Di Mugno M, De Cosmo G, Gui D. An unusual case of acute unilateral parotitis following abdominal surgery. Report of a case and review of the literature. Ann Ital Chir 2009; 80(3): 221-3.

[PMID: 20131541]

[43] Shin HY, Kim DW, Kim JD, *et al.* Paradoxical carbon dioxide embolism during laparoscopic cholecystectomy as a cause of cardiac arrest and neurologic sequelae: a case report. Korean J Anesthesiol 2014; 67(6): 425-8.
[http://dx.doi.org/10.4097/kjae.2014.67.6.425] [PMID: 25558345]

[44] Salinas J, Georgiev T, González-Sánchez JA, López-Ruiz E, Rodríguez-Montes JA. Gastric necrosis: A late complication of nissen fundoplication. World J Gastrointest Surg 2014; 6(9): 183-6.
[http://dx.doi.org/10.4240/wjgs.v6.i9.183] [PMID: 25276288]

[45] Mukherjee R, Müller M, Amstad H, *et al.* [Dysphonia and dysphagia after anterior cervical spine surgery]. HNO 2014; 62(8): 575-81.
[http://dx.doi.org/10.1007/s00106-014-2877-6] [PMID: 24906340]

[46] Anderson KK, Arnold PM. Oropharyngeal Dysphagia after anterior cervical spine surgery: a review. Global Spine J 2013; 3(4): 273-86.
[http://dx.doi.org/10.1055/s-0033-1354253] [PMID: 24436882]

[47] Nathani A, Weber AE, Wahlquist TC, Graziano GP, Park P, Patel RD. Delayed presentation of pharyngeal erosion after anterior cervical discectomy and fusion. Case Rep Orthop 2015; 2015: 173687.
[http://dx.doi.org/10.1155/2015/173687] [PMID: 25699193]

[48] Emohare O, Peterson E, Slinkard N, Janus S, Morgan R. Occam paradox? A variation of tapia syndrome and an unreported complication of guidewire-assisted pedicle screw insertion. Evid Based Spine Care J 2013; 4(2): 132-6.
[http://dx.doi.org/10.1055/s-0033-1357355] [PMID: 24436711]

[49] Wienbeck M, Berges W, Lübke HJ. Drug-induced oesophageal lesions. Baillieres Clin Gastroenterol 1988; 2(2): 263-74.
[http://dx.doi.org/10.1016/0950-3528(88)90003-6] [PMID: 3044462]

[50] Kim KR, Jun CH, Cho KM, *et al.* Can proton pump inhibitors reduce rebleeding following Histoacryl sclerotherapy for gastric variceal hemorrhage? Korean J Intern Med 2015; 30(5): 593-601.
[http://dx.doi.org/10.3904/kjim.2015.30.5.593] [PMID: 26354053]

[51] Kokudo N, Sanjo K, Umekita N, Harihara Y, Tada Y, Idezuki Y. Squamous cell carcinoma after endoscopic injection sclerotherapy for esophageal varices. Am J Gastroenterol 1990; 85(7): 861-4.
[PMID: 2196786]

[52] Ganz RA, Edmundowicz SA, Taiganides PA, *et al.* Long-Term Outcomes of Patients Receiving a Magnetic Sphincter Augmentation Device for Gastroesophageal Reflux. Clin Gastroenterol Hepatol 2016; 14(5): 671-7.
[http://dx.doi.org/10.1016/j.cgh.2015.05.028] [PMID: 26044316]

[53] Tamiya H, Yasunaga H, Matusi H, Fushimi K, Akishita M, Ogawa S. Comparison of short-term mortality and morbidity between parenteral and enteral nutrition for adults without cancer: a propensity-matched analysis using a national inpatient database. Am J Clin Nutr 2015; 102(5): 1222-8.
[http://dx.doi.org/10.3945/ajcn.115.111831] [PMID: 26447149]

[54] Rafiq A, Abbas N, Tariq H, Nayudu SK. Gastro-hepatic fistula with liver abscess: a rare complication of a common procedure. Am J Case Rep 2015; 16: 652-7.
[http://dx.doi.org/10.12659/AJCR.895098] [PMID: 26402902]

[55] Davidson P, Kwiatkowski CA, Wien M. Management of hyperglycemia and enteral nutrition in the hospitalized patient. Nutr Clin Pract 2015; 30(5): 652-9.
[http://dx.doi.org/10.1177/0884533615591057] [PMID: 26084507]

[56] Zhang SY, Liang ZY, Yu WQ, Wang ZE, Chen ZB, Zhang Y. Early enteral nutrition with polymeric feeds was associated with chylous ascites in patients with severe acute pancreatitis. Pancreas 2014; 43(4): 553-8.

[http://dx.doi.org/10.1097/MPA.0000000000000067] [PMID: 24632544]

[57] Carlei F, Caruso U, Lezoche E, *et al.* Hyperplasia of antral G cells in uraemic patients. Digestion 1984; 29(1): 26-30.
[http://dx.doi.org/10.1159/000199004] [PMID: 6724166]

[58] Tomori K, Nakamoto H, Kotaki S, *et al.* Gastric angiodysplasia in patients undergoing maintenance dialysis. Adv Perit Dial 2003; 19: 136-42.
[PMID: 14763050]

[59] Karamanolis G, Psatha P, Triantafyllou K. Endoscopic treatments for chronic radiation proctitis. World J Gastrointest Endosc 2013; 5(7): 308-12.
[http://dx.doi.org/10.4253/wjge.v5.i7.308] [PMID: 23858374]

[60] Calmet FH, Yarur AJ, Pukazhendhi G, Ahmad J, Bhamidimarri KR. Endoscopic and histological features of mycophenolate mofetil colitis in patients after solid organ transplantation. Ann Gastroenterol 2015; 28(3): 366-73.
[PMID: 26126799]

CHAPTER 7

Iatrogenic Pathology of the Peritoneum and Retroperitoneum

Ioan Jung, Vlad Butiurca and **Simona Gurzu***

Department of Pathology, University of Medicine and Pharmacy, Tirgu-Mures, Romania

Abstract: This chapter presents a synthesis of data regarding the iatrogenic injuries of the peritoneum and retroperitoneum. Similar to the previous chapters, medical drug-induced lesions and the consequences of diagnostic and/or therapeutic interventions are presented in detail. Iatrogenic retroperitoneal fibrosis can emerge following radiotherapy or as a consequence of long-term use of drugs such as beta blockers or antiepileptic substances. Pneumoperitoneum is usually a postoperative transient lesion, but it can also be a severe consequence of barotrauma or mechanical ventilation. The causes and consequences of iatrogenic peritonitis and ascites are also analyzed.

Keywords: Adverse drug reaction, Ascites, Barotrauma, Beta blockers, Hematoma, Hemoperitoneum, Hydralazine, Iatrogenic, Peritoneum, Peritonitis, Pneumoperitoneum, Retroperitoneal emphysema, Retroperitoneal fibrosis, Retroperitoneum.

DRUG-INDUCED LESIONS

Hemoperitoneum can occur in patients taking anticoagulants as a spontaneous lesion or secondary to drug-induced spleen rupture [1, 2].

Retroperitoneal Fibrosis is, in 85% of cases, an idiopathic primary lesion known as Ormond's disease. Secondary fibrosis can be induced by drugs (Table **7-1**), radiotherapy performed for abdominal tumors or surgical intervention. It is accompanied by a high risk of developing progressive renal failure; uretero-hydronephrosis is associated in 63% of patients. The treatment comprises steroids and immunosuppressive drugs, but azathioprine, methotrexate and cyclosporine are sometimes necessary [3, 4].

Sclerosing Peritonitis involves extensive fibrosis of the wall of the small intestine and mesenterium followed by intestinal stenosis or obstruction. The

* **Corresponding author Simona Gurzu:** Department of Pathology, University of Medicine and Pharmacy, Tirgu-Mures, Romania; Tel: 0040-745-673550; Fax: 0040-372-653250; E-mail: simonagurzu@yahoo.com

Simona Gurzu & Ioan Jung (Eds.)

idiopathic type was first reported by Owtschinnikow in 1907, whereas the secondary type was only identified in 1978, occurring after prolonged peritoneal dialysis. It can also be induced by drugs (*e.g.*, beta blockers, antiepileptics) or as a complication of intestinal transplantation [4 - 6].

Table 7-1. Drug-related peritoneal lesions. Data from references [1 - 4].

LESION	Drugs
Hemorrhages	Anticoagulants, antiplatelet drugs, cytotoxic drugs
Fibrosis	Hydralazine, beta blockers (*e.g.*, propranolol), methyldopa, LSD analogs (dose-dependent effect), nicotinic acid, procaine-polyvinylpyrrolidone, ergotamine, belladonna, analgesics, methysergide, antiepileptic drugs

IATROGENIC LESIONS DURING DIAGNOSTIC AND THERAPEUTIC PROCEDURES

Pneumoperitoneum and Retroperitoneal Emphysema

Transient ***pneumoperitoneum*** without associated bowel perforations occurs in 60-80% of abdominal surgical interventions and is usually without clinical impact. About 500-1000 ml of air is accumulated in the peritoneal cavity and is spontaneously absorbed within 10 days. In most cases, no clinical consequences are reported, but secondary fibrotic adherences or compression of the abdominal organs can occur. Besides abdominal surgery, pneumoperitoneum can also be a consequence of gynecological surgery or GI tract endoscopy as a result of bowel perforation [4, 7, 8]. Endoscopic resection of gastric tumors and endosonography-guided biliary drainage are also reported to induce pneumoperitoneum [9, 10].

Tension Pneumoperitoneum can be a consequence of barotrauma. It produces progressive compression of the abdominal organs and large vessels (abdominal aorta, inferior cava vein) and can induce abdominal compartment syndrome [4, 11]. Tension pneumoperitoneum can also emerge after laparoscopic interventions and can lead to subcutaneous emphysema, tension pneumothorax and pneumomediastinum [12]. In 4% of children undergoing pneumatic reduction of ileal intussusception, tension pneumoperitoneum emerged during air enema reduction. Needle decompression and subsequent laparotomy with bowel resection is the treatment of choice [13].

Retroperitoneal Emphysema can be a consequence of mechanical ventilation. The pathomechanism involves high pressure-induced interstitial emphysema of the lung and mediastinal tissues, with subsequent propagation of the air through the retroperitoneum and peritoneal cavity. The air is either totally absorbed or its accumulation leads to peritoneal adherences and/or emphysema of the abdominal tissues [4, 7].

Retroperitoneal Hematoma and Hemoperitoneum

In patients undergoing cardiac angiography or angioplasty, retroperitoneal hematoma can occur during catheter advancement as a result of dissection and/or rupture of the abdominal aorta [14]. In our experience, this lesion has been identified at autopsy in only one case. This was the case of a 62-year-old male with severe atherosclerosis who presented a periprocedural intramural hematoma as a result of rupture of an atherosclerotic plaque of the abdominal aorta. Within a few hours of intervention, rupture of the hematoma led to fatal retroperitoneal hematoma and hemorrhagic shock.

Retroperitoneal bleeding can also occur during open or laparoscopic abdominal, urological or gynecological surgery as a result of rupture of the major vessels [15, 16]. During spinal surgery, injuries of the lumbar artery can lead to formation of a pseudoaneurysm and delayed retroperitoneal hematoma [17]. Moreover, because the aortic bifurcation is near to the anterior surface of the L4-L5 disc, lumbar discectomy can lead to dilacerations of the aorta and subsequent retroperitoneal hemorrhage [18].

In patients with polycystic kidney, hemodialysis can induce rupture of the cystic structures and retroperitoneal hemorrhage [19]. In children, retroperitoneal hemorrhage can occur after cardiopulmonary resuscitation [20].

Postoperative Peritonitis

Iatrogenic peritonitis can be an infective or non-infective, acute or chronic, localized or diffuse, exudative or granulomatous inflammation.

- ***Diffuse Purulent Peritonitis***

  This is an infective inflammation that can occur after abdominal surgery, including laparoscopy, or as a complication of hemodialysis [21]. Incidental rupture of the intestine can occur in pediatric surgery, but can be intraoperatively handled (Fig. **7-1**).

- ***Bile Peritonitis***

  This is a non-infective peritonitis caused by bile extravasation into the abdominal cavity. The bile can be released following rupture of the bile ducts (during cholecystectomy, endoscopic retrograde cholangiopancreatography or endosonography-guided biliary drainage) or of the liver (during liver biopsy or abdominal surgery). The reported mortality rate is approximately 0-1.8% [4, 10, 22].

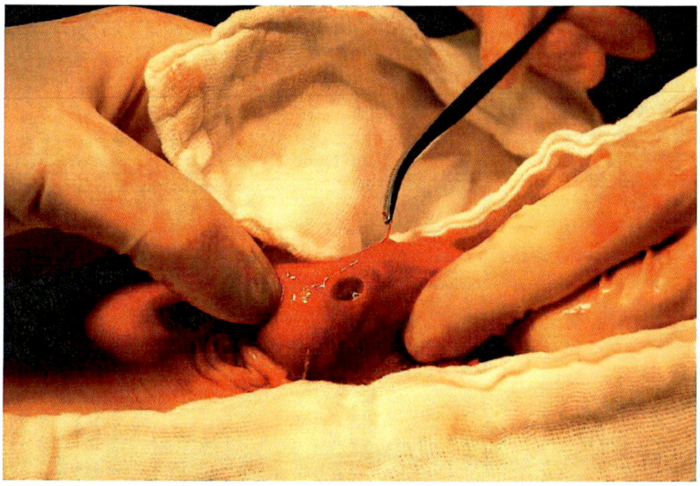

Fig. (7-1). Incidental perforation of the intestine during pediatric abdominal surgery.

- ***Granulomatous Peritonitis***

This is characterized by the formation of foreign body granulomas and can be induced by several substances that can enter the abdominal cavity.

Starch and Talc Granulomatous Peritonitis is the result of accumulation in the peritoneal cavity of granules/crystals released from surgical gloves. Foreign body granulomas forming around talc crystals occur within between 10 days and weeks after surgery, presenting as small white nodules that can mimic peritoneal carcinomatosis or miliary tuberculosis. Superinfection with Staphylococcus can be associated. Under the microscope, the talc crystals present a Maltese cross birefringence [4, 23].

Surgical Materials-Related Peritonitis is a granulomatous inflammation produced by cellulose and cotton fibers derived from disposable surgical gowns, drapes and meshes [21, 24]. Under the microscope, the cellulose fibers are birefringent [4]. An intraperitoneal mesh forgotten in the abdominal cavity can induce a granulomatous-purulent inflammation (Fig. **7-2**).

Barium Peritonitis is rare and can occur following a barium enema and subsequent bowel perforation. The incidence is between two and eight cases per 10,000 examinations. The barium crystals are non-birefringent upon microscopic examination and granulomas are primarily located at the anastomotic site [4, 25].

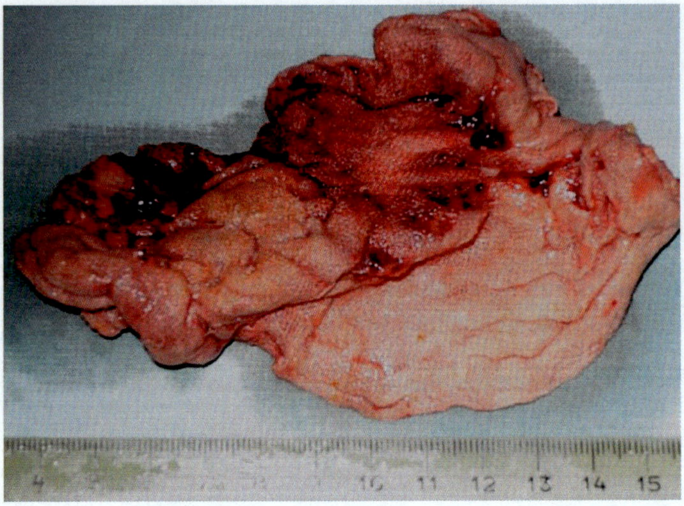

Fig. (7-2). A forgotten mesh that induced a postoperative peritonitis.

IATROGENIC ASCITES

• *Postoperative Chylous Ascites*

Although uncommon, this is reported following pelvic irradiation and abdominal/retroperitoneal surgical interventions, including hepatopancreatobiliary surgery (1%). In patients undergoing pancreatic resection, the risk of developing chylous ascites is about 3.3%, and even higher after distal pancreatectomy. The main risk factors are manipulation of the para-aortic structures, retroperitoneal invasion and early postoperative enteral feeding [26 - 29].

Chylous ascites is also reported within the first weeks following radical surgery for gynecological cancer, including hysterectomy, bilateral adnexectomy and extended lymph node dissection [30, 31]. It can also be a complication of mediastinal surgeries, such as thoracic duct embolization [32].

Its diagnosis is based on the presence of at least 100 ml of milky fluid per day in the abdominal cavity, which is amylase-free and has a triglyceride concentration of at least 110 mg/dl [26]. Chyluria test is positive. Its consequences are hypoproteinemia, electrolyte imbalance, malnutrition, immunodeficiency, fungal infections and even death [26, 30].

• *Eosinophilic Ascites*

This is a rare lesion that can be associated with parasitic infections, eosinophilic gastroenteritis, abdominal lymphomas or rupture of a hydatid cyst. Iatrogenic eosinophilic ascites is also reported in patients undergoing chronic peritoneal dialysis [4, 33].

- ***Urinary Ascites and Peritonitis***

Uroperitoneum and urinary peritonitis occur most particularly in pediatrics departments. Their incidence is about 0.5% of all pediatric abdominal emergencies and 5% of urological emergencies. Bladder rupture is an uncommon lesion that can occur during surgery and can induce sepsis and acute renal failure [34, 35].

CONFLICT OF INTEREST

The authors confirm that this chapter content has no conflict of interest.

ACKNOWLEDGEMENTS

Declared none.

REFERENCES

[1] Hosseini M, Hosseinzadeh A, Raufian K, Hedjazi A. Nontraumatic retroperitoneal hematoma after warfarin administration: fatal case report and review of the literature. Am J Forensic Med Pathol 2015; 36(4): 245-8. [http://dx.doi.org/10.1097/PAF.0000000000000190] [PMID: 26280884]

[2] Gazel E, Açıkgöz G, Kasap Y, Yiğman M, Güneş ZE. Spontaneous splenic rupture due to uremic coagulopathy and mortal sepsis after splenectomy. Int J Crit Illn Inj Sci 2015; 5(2): 119-22. [http://dx.doi.org/10.4103/2229-5151.158419] [PMID: 26157658]

[3] Labidi J, Ariba YB, Chargui S, Bousetta N, Louzir B, Othmani S. Retroperitoneal fibrosis: a retrospective review of clinical presentation, treatment and outcomes. Saudi J Kidney Dis Transpl 2015; 26(4): 816-22. [http://dx.doi.org/10.4103/1319-2442.160226] [PMID: 26178567]

[4] Jung J, Ed. Patologie iatrogenă. Tîrgu-Mureş, Romania: University Press 2006.

[5] Candido PdeC, Werner AdeF, Pereira IM, Matos BA, Pfeilsticker RM, Silva R. Sclerosing encapsulating peritonitis: a case report. Radiol Bras 2015; 48(1): 56-8. [http://dx.doi.org/10.1590/0100-3984.2013.1909] [PMID: 25798009]

[6] Rumbo C, Zambernardi A, Cabanne A, Rumbo M, Gondolesi G. Sclerosing peritonitis, a rare complication after intestinal transplant. Report of one case successfully treated with adjustment of immunosuppression. Pediatr Transplant 2013; 17(5): E125-9. [http://dx.doi.org/10.1111/petr.12110] [PMID: 23902605]

[7] Pourmand A, Shokoohi H. Tension pneumothorax, pneumoperitoneum, and cervical emphysema following a diagnostic colonoscopy. Case Rep Emerg Med 2013; 2013: 583287. [http://dx.doi.org/10.1155/2013/583287]

[8] Symeonidis N, Ballas K, Pavlidis E, Psarras K, Pavlidis T, Sakantamis A. Tension pneumoperitoneum: a rare complication of upper gastrointestinal endoscopy. JSLS 16(3): 495-7. [http://dx.doi.org/10.4293/108680812X13462882736655]

[9] Siboni S, Bona D, Abate E, Bonavina L. Tension pneumoperitoneum following endoscopic submucosal dissection of leiomyoma of the cardia. Endoscopy 2010; 42 (Suppl. 2): E152. [http://dx.doi.org/10.1055/s-0029-1244048] [PMID: 20556708]

[10] Prachayakul V, Aswakul P. Successful endoscopic treatment of iatrogenic biloma as a complication of endosonography-guided hepaticogastrostomy: The first case report. J Interv Gastroenterol 2012; 2(4): 202-4.
[http://dx.doi.org/10.4161/jig.23750] [PMID: 23687611]

[11] Garcia-Santos E, Puerto-Puerto A, Sanchez-Garcia S, Ruescas-Garcia FJ, Alberca-Paramo A, Martin-Fernandez J. Abdominal compartment syndrome by tension pneumoperitoneum secondary to barotrauma. Presentation case Cir Cir 2015; 83(5): 429-32.
[http://dx.doi.org/10.1016/j.circir.2015.05.046] [PMID: 26159366]

[12] Fedun S, Mateu P, Gratiae E, Gelisse E, Just B. [An unusual case of tension pneumoperitoneum causing subcutaneous emphysema, tension pneumothorax and pneumomediastinum after laparoscopic hysterectomy]. Ann Fr Anesth Reanim 2013; 32(9): 628-9.
[http://dx.doi.org/10.1016/j.annfar.2013.07.803] [PMID: 23958177]

[13] Fallon SC, Kim ES, Naik-Mathuria BJ, Nuchtern JG, Cassady CI, Rodriguez JR. Needle decompression to avoid tension pneumoperitoneum and hemodynamic compromise after pneumatic reduction of pediatric intussusception. Pediatr Radiol 2013; 43(6): 662-7.
[http://dx.doi.org/10.1007/s00247-012-2604-y] [PMID: 23283408]

[14] Chan YC, Morales JP, Reidy JF, Taylor PR. Management of spontaneous and iatrogenic retroperitoneal haemorrhage: conservative management, endovascular intervention or open surgery? Int J Clin Pract 2008; 62(10): 1604-13.
[http://dx.doi.org/10.1111/j.1742-1241.2007.01494.x] [PMID: 17949429]

[15] Christensen JG, Achiam MP. [Retroperitoneal haematoma as a complication at the beginning of a laparoscopic operation]. Ugeskr Laeger 2015; 177(2A): 98-9.
[PMID: 25612988]

[16] Vagnoni V, Gaudiano C, Passaretti G, *et al.* Massive hematuria due to ruptured iatrogenic aortic pseudoaneurysm: a case report. Arch Ital Urol Androl 2013; 85(2): 96-8.
[http://dx.doi.org/10.4081/aiua.2013.2.96] [PMID: 23820658]

[17] Oh YM, Choi HY, Eun JP. Delayed retroperitoneal hemorrhage due to lumbar artery pseudoaneurysm after lumbar posterolateral fusion. J Korean Neurosurg Soc 2013; 54(4): 344-6.
[http://dx.doi.org/10.3340/jkns.2013.54.4.344] [PMID: 24294460]

[18] Yip SL, Woo SB, Kwok TK, Mak KH. Nightmare of lumbar diskectomy: aorta laceration. Spine 2011; 36(26): E1758-60.
[http://dx.doi.org/10.1097/BRS.0b013e3182194e1c] [PMID: 22138785]

[19] Biyik Z, Solak Y, Gaipov A, Ozbek O, Esen H, Turk S. Spontaneous retroperitoneal hemorrhage presenting as hemoperitoneum secondary to renal cyst rupture in a peritoneal dialysis patient with acquired cystic kidney disease. Indian J Nephrol 2015; 25(4): 251-4.
[http://dx.doi.org/10.4103/0971-4065.147371] [PMID: 26199480]

[20] Bush CM, Jones JS, Cohle SD, Johnson H. Pediatric injuries from cardiopulmonary resuscitation. Ann Emerg Med 1996; 28(1): 40-4.
[http://dx.doi.org/10.1016/S0196-0644(96)70137-3] [PMID: 8669737]

[21] Strik C, Stommel MW, Ten Broek RP, van Goor H. Adhesiolysis in patients undergoing a repeat median laparotomy. Dis Colon Rectum 2015; 58(8): 792-8.
[http://dx.doi.org/10.1097/DCR.0000000000000405] [PMID: 26163959]

[22] Ahmed M, Diggory RT. Case-based review: bile peritonitis after T-tube removal. Ann R Coll Surg Engl 2013; 95(6): 383-5.
[http://dx.doi.org/10.1308/003588413X13629960048596] [PMID: 24025283]

[23] Juaneda I, Moser F, Eynard H, Diller A, Caeiro E. [Granulomatous peritonitis due to the starch used in surgical gloves]. Medicina (B Aires) 2008; 68(3): 222-4.
[PMID: 18689154]

[24] Tinker MA, Burdman D, Deysine M, Teicher I, Platt N, Aufses AH Jr. Granulomatous peritonitis due to cellulose fibers from disposable surgical fabrics: laboratory investigation and clinical implications. Ann Surg 1974; 180(6): 831-5.
[http://dx.doi.org/10.1097/00000658-197412000-00006] [PMID: 4611359]

[25] Kitajima T, Tomizawa K, Hanaoka Y, *et al.* Anastomotic stenosis of the descending colon caused by barium granuloma formation following barium peritonitis: report of a case. Surg Today 2014; 44(11): 2153-6.
[http://dx.doi.org/10.1007/s00595-013-0696-0] [PMID: 23955478]

[26] Kuboki S, Shimizu H, Yoshidome H, *et al.* Chylous ascites after hepatopancreatobiliary surgery. Br J Surg 2013; 100(4): 522-7.
[http://dx.doi.org/10.1002/bjs.9013] [PMID: 23288577]

[27] Zhang SY, Liang ZY, Yu WQ, Wang ZE, Chen ZB, Zhang Y. Early enteral nutrition with polymeric feeds was associated with chylous ascites in patients with severe acute pancreatitis. Pancreas 2014; 43(4): 553-8.
[http://dx.doi.org/10.1097/MPA.0000000000000067] [PMID: 24632544]

[28] Shah SS, Ahmed K, Smith R, Mallina R, Akhbari P, Khan MS. Chylous ascites following radical nephrectomy: a case report. J Med Case Reports 2008; 2: 3.
[http://dx.doi.org/10.1186/1752-1947-2-3] [PMID: 18190695]

[29] Ouakaa-Kchaou A, Ennaifer R, Elloumi H, *et al.* [Chylous ascites after pelvic irradiation for urologic malignancy]. Presse Med 2008; 37(6 Pt 1): 978-81.
[http://dx.doi.org/10.1016/j.lpm.2007.09.025] [PMID: 18313885]

[30] Qi Z, Zhang Y. Rare case of concurrent severe chylous ascites after radical surgery for cervical cancer. Eur J Gynaecol Oncol 2015; 36(3): 356-8.
[PMID: 26189272]

[31] Janco JM, Gloviczki P, Friese JL, Cliby WA. Lymphatic mapping and ligation for persistent ascites after surgery for gynecologic malignancy. Obstet Gynecol 2015; 125(2): 434-7.
[http://dx.doi.org/10.1097/AOG.0000000000000550] [PMID: 25569016]

[32] Gaba RC, Owens CA, Bui JT, Carrillo TC, Knuttinen MG. Chylous ascites: a rare complication of thoracic duct embolization for chylothorax. Cardiovasc Intervent Radiol 2011; 34 (Suppl. 2): S245-9.
[http://dx.doi.org/10.1007/s00270-010-9900-4] [PMID: 20517611]

[33] Van Laethem JL, Jacobs F, Braude P, Van Gossum A, Deviere J. Toxocara canis infection presenting as eosinophilic ascites and gastroenteritis. Dig Dis Sci 1994; 39(6): 1370-2.
[http://dx.doi.org/10.1007/BF02093807] [PMID: 8200273]

[34] Raherinantenaina F, Rambel AH, Rakotosamimanana J, *et al.* [Urinary ascites, uroperitoneum and urinary peritonitis in children: management of nine case reports in Madagascar]. Prog Urol 2013; 23(12): 1004-11.
[http://dx.doi.org/10.1016/j.purol.2013.04.017] [PMID: 24090786]

[35] Mischianu D, Bratu O, Ilie C, Madan V. Notes concerning the peritonitis of urinary aetiology. J Med Life 2008; 1(1): 66-71.
[PMID: 20108482]

CHAPTER 8

Iatrogenic Pathology of the Liver, Gallbladder and Pancreas

Simona Gurzu* and **Ioan Jung**

Department of Pathology, University of Medicine and Pharmacy, Tirgu-Mures, Romania

Abstract: This chapter presents a synthesis of data regarding iatrogenic injuries of the liver, gallbladder and pancreas. For each of these organs, medical drug-induced lesions are presented. The second part of the chapter includes the consequences of diagnostic and/or therapeutic interventions for the above-mentioned organs. The liver is the second most common organ involved in drug effects, following the skin. Its destruction can be an indication for transplantation. The hepatic disorders include metabolic disturbances, cholestasis, hepatitis, cirrhosis and risk of malignancy. The biliary channels can be injured during open surgical interventions or laparoscopic cholecystectomy, leading to fistulae, peritonitis, bilirrhagia and even death. Endoscopic retrograde cholangiopancreatography (ERCP) can be associated with local complications, such as pancreatitis and cholangitis, but pneumothorax, pneumomediastinum and pneumoretroperitoneum are also encountered in rare cases.

Keywords: Adverse drug reaction, Allergy, Bilirrhagia, Cholangiopancreatography, Cholecystectomy, Cholestasis, Cirrhosis, Gallbladder, Hematoma, Hepatitis, Hepatocellular carcinoma, Hepatoportal sclerosis, Iatrogenic, Liver, Pancreas, Pancreatitis, Peritonitis.

DRUG-INDUCED LESIONS

Besides the skin, the liver is the most common organ that presents drug-induced lesions. Moreover, liver injuries are the most common reason for drug withdrawal from the pharmaceutical market (*e.g.,* troglitazone, bromfenac) and the leading cause for liver transplantation [1]. The worldwide incidence of drug-induced liver injuries is between two and 24 cases per 100,000 people per year [1]. These injuries can include metabolic disorders, acute cholestasis with reversible focal necroses, granulomatous/fulminant hepatitis, chronic liver injury (toxic hepatitis, steatosis, cirrhosis, hepatoportal sclerosis), high serum levels of transaminases,

* **Corresponding author Simona Gurzu:** Department of Pathology, University of Medicine and Pharmacy, Tirgu-Mures, Romania; Tel: 0040-745-673550; Fax: 0040-372-653250; E-mail: simonagurzu@yahoo.com

hepatomegaly and neoplastic lesions (hepatocellular carcinoma, cholangiocarcinoma, angiosarcoma) [2]. In our practice, we have encountered a few cases in which liver transplantation was necessary due to severe liver failure that occurred as a result of consumption of weight-loss pills, in young females, or anabolic substances, in males.

Mechanisms of ADRs

Hepatopancreatic drug-related lesions can be induced through dose-dependent toxicity or through allergic or idiosyncratic mechanisms (dose-independent ADR) [1].

Dose-Dependent Hepatopancreatic Toxicity

The most common dose-dependent *hepatotoxic drugs* are aspirin, salicylates, chemotherapeutics, steroids, methyltestosterone and estrogen (Table **8-1**). Chemotherapeutics, such as capecitabine and oxaliplatin, can induce steatohepatitis (Fig. **8-1**), sinusoidal obstruction syndrome, liver fibrosis and liver failure [3 - 5]. Long-term consumption of androgenic steroids-based contraceptive pills is a risk factor for hepatocellular adenoma (with an annual incidence of between three and four cases per 100,000 females) and even hepatocellular carcinoma [6].

Drug-related *pancreatitis* is reported by the WHO to be induced by more than 500 drugs, but direct toxic effect has been proven for 31 drugs only [7]. These include chemotherapeutics (Fig. **8-1**), paracetamol, steroids, procainamide, *etc.* [8]. Simultaneous administration of capecitabine and oxaliplatin can also induce hypertriglyceridemia [3 - 5].

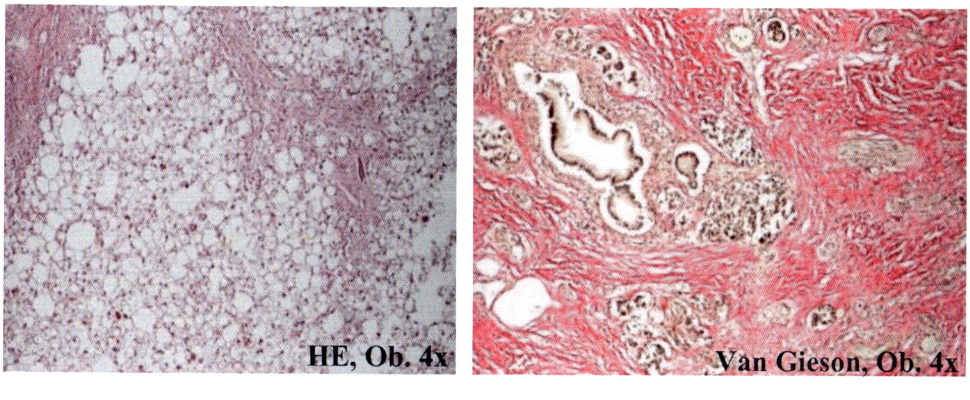

Fig. (8-1). Chemotherapy-associated hepato-pancreatic lesions. Steatohepatitis (left) and chronic pancreatitis (right) induced by capecitabine and oxaliplatin.

Allergic and Idiosyncratic Drug Reactions

These mechanisms are more frequently involved in drug-induced hepatic disorders than dose-dependent lesions. Hepatopancreatic lesions arise within several weeks of the completion of treatment. Systemic reactions, such as fever, rash, arthralgia and eosinophilia, can be associated [1, 2, 9].

Hepatopancreatic Lesions Induced Through Mixed Mechanisms

Halothane-related hepatitis is produced through direct toxicity combined with hypersensitivity and genetic susceptibility [10]. The associated yellowish liver presents large necrotic areas under the microscope (Fig. **8-2**).

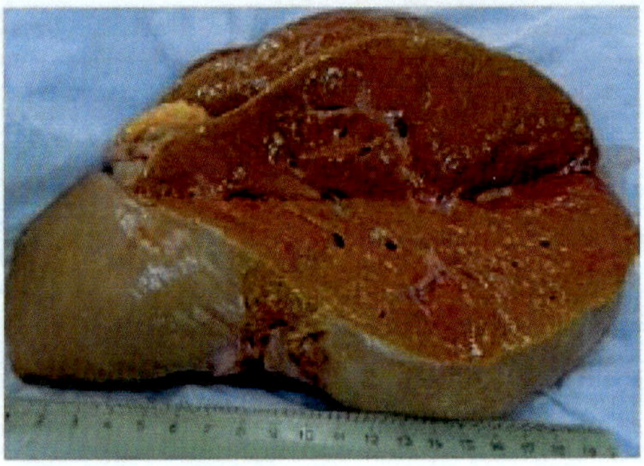

Fig. (8-2). Halothane-induced hepatitis with necrosis.

Drug-Induced Diabetes and Hyperglycemia can be the result of direct toxic effect or alterations in insulin secretion and sensitivity. They can be caused by several drugs, including steroids, nicotinic acid, statins, thiazide diuretics, fluoroquinolones, phenytoin, valproic acid, pentamidine, growth hormones, somatostatin analogs, beta blockers, calcium channel blockers and inhibitors of the renin-angiotensin system (Table **8-1**) [11]. In pediatric departments, medication-induced diabetes is especially reported in children with leukemia treated with L-asparaginase and glucocorticoids [12].

Table 8-1. Drug-induced hepatopancreatic injuries. Data from references [1 - 20].

Lesion	**Drugs**
High level of serum transaminases, jaundice	Augmentin (amoxicillin with clavulanic), neuroleptic/antidepressant drugs (chlorpromazine, lithium, tiotixen, triflupromazine, tranylcypromine)

(Table 8-1) contd.....

Lesion	Drugs
Dose-dependent hepatotoxicity	Aspirin, salicylates, NSAIDs, chemotherapeutics (daunorubicin, methotrexate, antifolates, oxaliplatin, 5-FU, capecitabine), steroids, estrogen, methyltestosterone immunosuppressive drugs (cyclosporine, tacrolimus), thyreostatic drugs, halothane
Cholestasis/cholestatic hepatitis	Methyltestosterone, analgesics, erythromycin, nitrofurantoin, rifampicin, contraceptive pills, busulfan, tamoxifen, carbamazepine, cyclosporine, nifedipine chlorpromazine, phenothiazines, azathioprine, nicotinic acid, ketamine
Fatty liver	Tetracycline, asparaginase, sodium valproate, methotrexate, amiodarone, 5-FU
Perisinusoidal fibrosis	Excess of vitamin A, oxaliplatin
Peliosis	Anabolic steroids, oral contraceptives, azathioprine, corticosteroids, immunoglobulins, tamoxifen, methotrexate, 6-thioguanine, 6-merc--ptopurine
Toxic hepatitis	Chlorpromazine, phenothiazines, halothane
Reactive hepatitis	Sulfonamides, methyldopa, phenylbutazone
Viral-like hepatitis	Antituberculosis agents (isoniazid, rifampicin, 4-aminosalicylic acid), methyldopa, phenytoin, halothane
Autoimmune-like hepatitis	Sofosbuvir, masitinib, nitrofurantoin
Granulomatous hepatitis	Sulfonamides, chlorpromazine, phenylbutazone, allopurinol, carbamazepine
Chronic aggressive hepatitis/ cirrhosis	Isoniazid, methyldopa, methotrexate, phenolisatine-containing laxatives
Risk of tumors (adenoma, HCC)	Anabolic steroids, oral contraceptives
Risk of angiosarcoma	Inhalation of toxins (*e.g.,* chemical plants, arsenic)
Risk of gallstones	Octreotide (anti-growth hormone drug), contraceptive pills
Oddi sphincter spasm (narcotics)	Fentanyl
Iatrogenic diabetes and hyperglycemia	Corticosteroids, growth hormone-releasing drugs (genotropin), somatostatin analogs, nicotinic acid, statins, thiazide, diuretics, fluoroquinolones, phenytoin, valproic acid, pentamidine, beta blockers, calcium channel blockers, inhibitors of the renin-angiotensin system
Acute or chronic pancreatitis, steatonecrosis	Calcium/vitamin D overdose, azathioprine, sulfonamides, L-asparaginase, 6-mercaptopurin, pentamidine, furosemide, estrogens, tetracyclines, piroxicam, acetaminophen (paracetamol), corticosteroids, chemotherapeutics (oxaliplatin, capecitabine, pazopanib, sunitinib, sorafenib, axitinib), antithyroid methimazole

Morphology of Drug-Induced Hepatopancreatic Disorders

Cholestasis occurs as a result of damage to the basal membrane of the biliary channels and can be induced by several drugs, such as anabolic steroids, tranquilizers, antibiotics, *etc.* (Table **8-1**) [13].

Hepatitis can be similar to acute viral hepatitis, associated with focal eosinophilic necroses, or can display other morphological features (Table **8-1**). Tuberculostatic drugs can cause the occurrence of bridging necrosis. *Cholestatic hepatitis* comprises the association of cholestasis with periportal inflammatory infiltrate rich in eosinophils. This can be a side effect of drugs used for patients with psychiatric disorders (*e.g.,* phenothiazines). Azathioprine (imuran), which is used in patients with Crohn's disease, nicotinic acid (vitamin B3 or niacin) and the antithyroid drug methimazole can also be responsible for the occurrence of cholestatic hepatitis [2, 7, 9, 14]. *Reactive hepatitis* is characterized by the presence of periportal inflammatory infiltrate rich in eosinophils and Kupffer cells hyperplasia. It can occur following consumption of sulfonamides, methyldopa or phenylbutazone. *Autoimmune-like hepatitis* can be diagnosed based on elevated titers of antinuclear and anti-smooth muscle antibodies, along with elevated IgG, transaminases and gamma globulin serum levels. Microscopically, large areas of necrosis with fibrous septa and distorted architecture can be seen. This hepatitis can be induced by the immunomodulator drug masitinib, which is used in patients with amyotrophic lateral sclerosis [15], but also by nitrofurantoin [16] and by drugs used to treat patients with chronic viral hepatitis such as sofosbuvir [17]. *Chronic aggressive hepatitis* can be caused by long-term consumption of methyldopa, tuberculostatic drugs, cytotoxic agents or laxatives [18]. *Granulomatous hepatitis* is microscopically characterized by granulomatous proliferation of Kupffer cells and inflammatory cells. It can be induced by allopurinol, sulfonamides, *etc.* [2].

Perisinusoidal Fibrosis can be the result of vitamin A overdose and involves proliferation of Ito cells.

Hepatic Peliosis is characterized by proliferation of blood-filled spaces and can occur following long-term consumption of oral contraceptives or androgens [6].

Fatty Liver can be seen in long-term users of antibiotics, methotrexate, *etc.*

Pancreatitis can be induced by several drugs (Table **8-1**), including antiangiogenic agents (*e.g.,* pazopanib, axitinib) and kinase inhibitors (*e.g.,* sunitinib, sorafenib) [7]. After excluding other potential causes, the diagnosis of drug-induced pancreatitis is based on its occurrence during drug administration, resolution after drug cessation and reoccurrence after re-administration of the specific drug [7]. In drug-induced acute pancreatitis, the blood lipase levels usually decrease after drug cessation [2, 19, 20].

IATROGENIC LESIONS DURING DIAGNOSTIC AND THERAPEUTIC PROCEDURES

Surgery-Related Injuries of the Biliary Channels

The first iatrogenic bile duct injury was reported by Sprengel in 1891 following a classic cholecystectomy. The laparoscopic cholecystectomy was firstly performed in 1985 by the German surgeon Erich Müche, and the rate of complications has progressively decreased since then. However, the biliary channels can be injured in 0.2-9% of patients undergoing laparoscopic cholecystectomy, especially in cases of gangrenous or sclerosing cholecystitis. These channels can be crushed, sectioned or tied. The early consequences are biliary fistulae, biliary peritonitis and bilirrhagia. Postoperative jaundice and pancreatitis can occur as a consequence of incidental suture of biliary channels or lesions of the Oddi sphincter. The mortality rate related to laparoscopic cholecystectomy is approximately 1%. This rate increases to 4% in octogenarians, due to associated comorbidities (ischemic heart disease, diabetes, chronic renal failure, *etc.*), the higher incidence of gangrenous cholecystitis and bile duct stones in this group, and greater conversion from laparoscopic to open surgery as compared to younger patients. Consequences that emerge later include excessive scarring with further biliary stenosis, biliary cirrhosis and hepatic failure [21 - 24].

Endoscopic Retrograde Cholangiopancreatography (ERCP)

ERCP and endoscopic papillotomy are associated with a rate of complications of 5-6.9%, mainly involving pancreatitis and cholangitis [25]. Lesions of the papilla of Vater can induce periampular hemorrhages. In 10% of cases, delayed ampullary strictures are reported [26]. Perforation of the ampulla of Vater can be a life-threatening complication. The ERCP-related mortality rate is 0.33% [25].

Pneumothorax, pneumomediastinum and pneumoretroperitoneum are rare complications of ERCP that primarily occur following sphincterotomy and in patients with juxtapapillary diverticula. The mechanism involves interruption of the duodenal barrier due to a deep sphincterotomy. As a result, air enters the peritoneum, retroperitoneum and mediastinum [25].

Endoscopic ultrasound-guided biliary drainage, which is performed in patients with biliary obstruction, can be followed by bile leakage, biloma formation, pneumoperitoneum, peritonitis, stent malposition and stent migration [27].

Liver Biopsy

Liver biopsy can be followed by biliary peritonitis, especially in patients with mechanical jaundice. Accidental bioptic incision of a hydatid cyst can produce anaphylactic shock. Other rare complications are hemorrhages, perforation of the surrounding organs, subcutaneous or mediastinal emphysema and air embolism. Barium intravasation into the portal vein can lead to pylephlebitis and subsequent liver abscesses. The mortality rate is 0.03% [2, 28].

Liver Resection

Post-hepatectomy liver failure is the most severe associated complication, with an incidence of 5-10%. This risk is directly correlated with the size of the resected specimen but is also patient-related. Hepatocellular failure and postoperative ascites are more common in patients with a remnant liver volume of <1% of body weight or 50% of initial total liver volume [29]. Portal vein ligation is usually used to rapidly induce liver regeneration. It is associated with a mortality rate of 12-20%. Other post-vein ligation complications are complete ischemia of the deportalized liver, biliary fistulae and ascites. An improper suture of the hepatic artery can produce necroses of liver parenchyma [30].

In patients with hepatic tumors treated with transcatheter chemoembolization, expanded necrosis of the hepatic parenchyma surrounded by gas collection, as a result of nitrogen release, can be observed upon CT examination [2, 28].

Iatrogenically induced lesions of the liver should be differentiated from inflammatory disorders and benign tumors or pseudotumors, such as adenoma, hemangioma, cysts, focal nodular hyperplasia, biliary hamartoma, *etc.* [2, 28, 31].

Surgery-Related Injuries of the Liver Parenchyma

Focal Necroses are primarily related to the intrahepatic circulatory disorders that can be caused by abdominal surgery. *Diffuse necroses* can occur following ligation of the hepatic artery. *Steatohepatitis, hepatic cirrhosis and increased risk of hepatocellular carcinoma* are reported following jejuno-ileal bypass surgery performed for morbid obesity [2].

Percutaneous endoscopic gastrostomy is a safety procedure that is commonly used for enteral nutrition. In rare cases, life-threatening complications, such as dislodging of the tube with further gastrohepatic fistulae and formation of liver abscesses, have been reported [32].

Surgery-Related Pancreatic Lesions

Independently of the type of surgery, postoperative shock can be associated with acute pancreatitis, which is, in some cases, a life-threatening complication.

In patients with pancreatitis who undergo pancreatectomy, damage to the portal vein or mesenteric/splenic artery with subsequent hemorrhage is reported [2].

CONFLICT OF INTEREST

The authors confirm that this chapter content has no conflict of interest.

ACKNOWLEDGEMENTS

Declared none.

REFERENCES

[1] Khoury T, Rmeileh AA, Yosha L, Benson AA, Daher S, Mizrahi M. Drug induced liver injury: review with a focus on genetic factors, tissue diagnosis, and treatment options. J Clin Transl Hepatol 2015; 3(2): 99-108.
[http://dx.doi.org/10.14218/JCTH.2015.00007] [PMID: 26356634]

[2] Jung J, Ed. Patologie iatrogenă. Tîrgu-Mureş, Romania: University Press 2006.

[3] Gurzu S, Jung I, Comsulea M, Kadar Z, Azamfirei L, Molnar C. Lethal cardiotoxicity, steatohepatitis, chronic pancreatitis, and acute enteritis induced by capecitabine and oxaliplatin in a 36-year-old woman. Diagn Pathol 2013; 8: 150.
[http://dx.doi.org/10.1186/1746-1596-8-150] [PMID: 24041405]

[4] Chan HY, Ng CM, Tiu SC, Chan AO, Shek CC. Hypertriglyceridaemia-induced pancreatitis: a contributory role of capecitabine? Hong Kong Med J 2012; 18(6): 526-9.
[PMID: 23223655]

[5] Pessaux P. [Chemotherapys hepatotoxicity: what is the impact on surgery?]. J Chir (Paris) 2010; 147 (Suppl. 1): S7-S11.
[PMID: 20172202]

[6] Gurzu S, Jung I, Contac AO, *et al.* Atypical hepatocellular neoplasm with peliosis in cirrhotic liver *versus* hepatocellular carcinoma: A diagnostic trap. Medicine (Baltimore) 2015; 94(29): e1189.
[http://dx.doi.org/10.1097/MD.0000000000001189] [PMID: 26200629]

[7] Agito K, Manni A. Acute pancreatitis induced by methimazole in a patient with subclinical hyperthyroidism. J Investig Med High Impact Case Rep 2015; 3(2): 2324709615592229.
[http://dx.doi.org/10.1177/2324709615592229] [PMID: 26425645]

[8] Feyles F, Mussa A, Peiretti V, *et al.* Iatrogenic acute pancreatitis due to hypercalcemia in a child with pseudohypoparathyroidism. J Pediatr Endocrinol Metab 2013; 10: 1-4.
[PMID: 23934639]

[9] Zou H, Jin L, Wang LR, Braddock M, Cai WW, Zheng MH. Methimazole-induced cholestatic hepatitis: two cases report and literature review. Oncotarget 2016; 7(4): 5088-91.
[http://dx.doi.org/10.18632/oncotarget.6144] [PMID: 26498145]

[10] Kurth MJ, Yokoi T, Gershwin ME. Halothane-induced hepatitis: paradigm or paradox for drug-induced liver injury. Hepatology 2014; 60(5): 1473-5.
[http://dx.doi.org/10.1002/hep.27253] [PMID: 24913773]

[11] Fathallah N, Slim R, Larif S, Hmouda H, Ben Salem C. Drug-induced hyperglycaemia and diabetes. Drug Saf 2015; 38(12): 1153-68. In press
[http://dx.doi.org/10.1007/s40264-015-0339-z] [PMID: 26370106]

[12] Yeshayahu Y, Koltin D, Hamilton J, Nathan PC, Urbach S. Medication-induced diabetes during induction treatment for ALL, an early marker for future metabolic risk? Pediatr Diabetes 2015; 16(2):

104-8.
[http://dx.doi.org/10.1111/pedi.12138] [PMID: 24673941]

[13] Zhou J, Shaw SG, Gilleece Y. Dilated common bile duct and deranged liver function tests associated with ketamine use in two HIV-positive MSM. Int J STD AIDS 2013; 24(8): 667-9.
[http://dx.doi.org/10.1177/0956462413479894] [PMID: 23970577]

[14] de Jong DJ, Goullet M, Naber TH. Side effects of azathioprine in patients with Crohns disease. Eur J Gastroenterol Hepatol 2004; 16(2): 207-12.
[http://dx.doi.org/10.1097/00042737-200402000-00014] [PMID: 15075996]

[15] Salvado M, Vargas V, Vidal M, Simon-Talero M, Camacho J, Gamez J. Autoimmune-like hepatitis during masitinib therapy in an amyotrophic lateral sclerosis patient. World J Gastroenterol 2015; 21(36): 10475-9.
[http://dx.doi.org/10.3748/wjg.v21.i36.10475] [PMID: 26420975]

[16] Sorin B, Pineton de Chambrun M, Haroche J, *et al.* Autoimmune hepatitis triggered by nitrofurantoin: A rare drug-induced toxicity. Rev Med Interne 2016; 37(2): 131-4.
[http://dx.doi.org/10.1016/j.revmed.2015.07.003] [PMID: 26404522]

[17] Gupta N, Bodin R, Sule S. Autoimmune hepatitis in association with sofosbuvir. Am J Ther 2015. In press
[http://dx.doi.org/10.1097/MJT.0000000000000233] [PMID: 26448334]

[18] Tomich LG, Núñez M, Mendes-Correa MC. Drug-induced liver injury in hospitalized HIV patients: high incidence and association with drugs for tuberculosis. Ann Hepatol 2015; 14(6): 888-94.
[http://dx.doi.org/10.5604/16652681.1171778] [PMID: 26436361]

[19] Kawakubo K, Hata H, Kawakami H, *et al.* Pazopanib-induced severe acute pancreatitis. Case Rep Oncol 2015; 8(2): 356-8.
[http://dx.doi.org/10.1159/000439124] [PMID: 26464570]

[20] Péron J, Khenifer S, Potier V, *et al.* Axitinib-induced acute pancreatitis: a case report. Anticancer Drugs 2014; 25(4): 478-9.
[http://dx.doi.org/10.1097/CAD.0000000000000076] [PMID: 24398664]

[21] Jabłońska B, Lampe P. Iatrogenic bile duct injuries: etiology, diagnosis and management. World J Gastroenterol 2009; 15(33): 4097-104.
[http://dx.doi.org/10.3748/wjg.15.4097] [PMID: 19725140]

[22] Archer SB, Brown DW, Smith CD, Branum GD, Hunter JG. Bile duct injury during laparoscopic cholecystectomy: results of a national survey. Ann Surg 2001; 234(4): 549-58.
[http://dx.doi.org/10.1097/00000658-200110000-00014] [PMID: 11573048]

[23] Negi SS, Sakhuja P, Malhotra V, Chaudhary A. Factors predicting advanced hepatic fibrosis in patients with postcholecystectomy bile duct strictures. Arch Surg 2004; 139(3): 299-303.
[http://dx.doi.org/10.1001/archsurg.139.3.299] [PMID: 15006888]

[24] Nikfarjam M, Yeo D, Perini M, *et al.* Outcomes of cholecystectomy for treatment of acute cholecystitis in octogenarians. ANZ J Surg 2014; 84(12): 943-8.
[http://dx.doi.org/10.1111/ans.12313] [PMID: 23910372]

[25] Noeofytou K, Petrou A, Savva C, *et al.* Pneumothorax following ERCP: report of two cases with different pathophysiology. Case Rep Med 2013; 2013: 206564.
[http://dx.doi.org/10.1155/2013/206564]

[26] Malas A, Roberts KE. Endoscopic Retrograde Cholangiopancreatography 2015. Available at: http://emedicine.medscape.com/article/1829797-overview

[27] Prachayakul V, Aswakul P. Successful endoscopic treatment of iatrogenic biloma as a complication of endosonography-guided hepaticogastrostomy: The first case report. J Interv Gastroenterol 2012; 2(4): 202-4.
[http://dx.doi.org/10.4161/jig.23750] [PMID: 23687611]

[28] Guerra JA, Trippia M, Pissaia A, Teixeira BC, Ivantes CA. Acoustic radiation force impulse is equivalent to liver biopsy to evaluate liver fibrosis in patients with chronic hepatitis c and nonalcoholic fatty liver disease. Arq Gastroenterol 2015; 52(3): 234-8.
[http://dx.doi.org/10.1590/S0004-28032015000300015] [PMID: 26486293]

[29] Lhuaire M, Piardi T, Bruno O, Sibert A, Kianmanesh R, Sommacale D. Post-hepatectomy liver failure: Should we consider venous outflow? Int J Surg Case Rep 2015; 16: 154-6.
[http://dx.doi.org/10.1016/j.ijscr.2015.10.001] [PMID: 26476052]

[30] Sanjeevi S, Sparrelid E, Gilg S, Jonas E, Isaksson B. Arterial ischemia in the deportalized liver following associating liver partition and portal vein ligation for staged hepatectomy. World J Hepatol 2015; 7(23): 2492-6.
[http://dx.doi.org/10.4254/wjh.v7.i23.2492] [PMID: 26483871]

[31] Anderson SW, Kruskal JB, Kane RA. Benign hepatic tumors and iatrogenic pseudotumors. Radiographics 2009; 29(1): 211-29.
[http://dx.doi.org/10.1148/rg.291085099] [PMID: 19168846]

[32] Rafiq A, Abbas N, Tariq H, Nayudu SK. Gastro-hepatic fistula with liver abscess: a rare complication of a common procedure. Am J Case Rep 2015; 16: 652-7.
[http://dx.doi.org/10.12659/AJCR.895098] [PMID: 26402902]

CHAPTER 9

Iatrogenic Pathology of the Kidney and Urinary System

Ioan Jung and **Simona Gurzu***

Department of Pathology, University of Medicine and Pharmacy, Tirgu-Mures, Romania

Abstract: This chapter presents a synthesis of data regárding acute and chronic drug-related lesions of the kidneys and urinary tract, as well as the urologic injuries that can result from diagnostic and/or therapeutic interventions. Reversible or irreversible renal injuries can be caused by prerenal, intrarenal or postrenal damage. Identification of the pathomechanism is mandatory for proper treatment of the side effects. Those drugs that are excreted through the kidneys can induce ischemic or obstructive lesions and can predispose the patient to stone formation. Analgesic nephropathy is a particular type of nephritis that can be reversible after drug cessation. Glomerulonephritis can be caused by several drugs, including vaccines, anti-inflammatory agents and beta blockers. Regarding surgical interventions, upper urinary tract deterioration can occur following direct injuries or as a consequence of iatrogenic lumbosacral spinal cord lesions. Complications relating to peritoneal dialysis are also presented in detail.

Keywords: Adverse drug reaction, Analgesic nephropathy, Azotemia, Cystitis, dialysis, Glomerulopathy, Hemolysis, Iatrogenic, Kidney, Lithiasis, Nephritis, Papillary necrosis, Percutaneous intervention, Urinary tract, Vasculitis.

DRUG-INDUCED LESIONS

Drug-induced renal injuries can be reversible or irreversible, acute or chronic processes (Table **9-1** and Table **9-2**). The mechanism involves damage at one of the following three levels: prerenal (volume depletion and electrolytes disturbances), intrarenal (direct toxicity, pro-inflammatory effect or drug-induced obstructive or ischemic lesions) and postrenal (promoters of stone formation) [1].

Acute kidney injuries are identified based on albuminuria and elevated levels of serum creatinine and blood urea nitrogen. Other recently proposed serum biomarkers are kidney injury molecule-1, neutrophil gelatinase-associated lipocalin and N-acetyl-β-d-glucosaminidase [2].

* **Corresponding author Simona Gurzu:** Department of Pathology, University of Medicine and Pharmacy, Tirgu-Mures, Romania; Tel: 0040-745-673550; Fax: 0040-372-653250; E-mail: simonagurzu@yahoo.com

Prerenal Azotemia can be caused by mannitol, diuretics and antihypertensive drugs that act as vasodilators and induce hypovolemia [1].

Intrarenal Injuries primarily refer to tubular lesions, but secondary parenchymatous damage is associated. Glomerulonephritis and interstitial nephritis are generated through immune complex hypersensitivity (type III) reaction. Acute interstitial nephritis can be a dose-dependent lesion in long-term users of proton pump inhibitors (PPIs). Vascular lesions can also occur. Due to the inhibition of prostaglandin synthesis, NSAIDs produce impaired perfusion with subsequent acute allergic interstitial nephritis and/or acute toxic tubular necrosis [1, 3].

Postrenal Injuries are primarily dose-dependent lesions and include urethral obstruction and risk of stone formation [4].

Analgesic Nephropathy

This is a particular type of *drug-induced chronic nondestructive interstitial nephritis* that is characterized by interstitial fibrosis and tubular atrophy. In severe forms, papillary necrosis can occur (Fig. **9-1**). Sclerosis of the medullary capillaries and fibrosis of the mucosa lining calices, pelvis and ureters can be associated [5, 6]. Chronic renal failure is reported in one third of patients. This type of nephritis is caused by the chronic use of analgesics (phenacetin, acetaminophen, saridon, *etc.*) or NSAIDs [4, 7].

The treatment involves drug cessation. Due to progressive renal failure, the clinical symptoms are polyuria, polydipsia and hypertension. This lesion predisposes the patient to urothelial carcinoma, the incidence of which is 13 times higher than in the control group. The risk of urothelial carcinoma of the renal pelvis, furthermore, is 75 times higher than in the control group [4, 7].

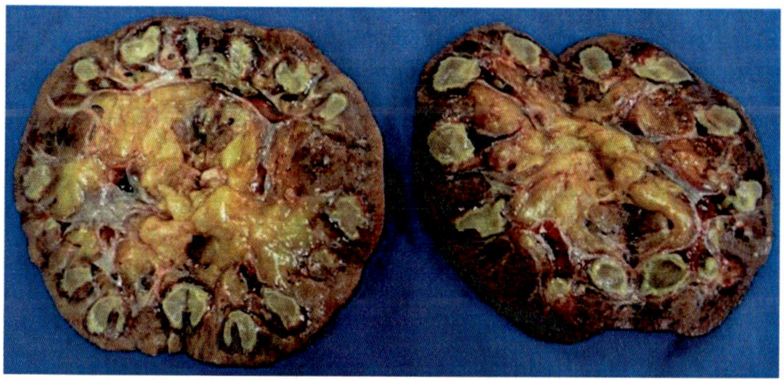

Fig. (9-1). Bilateral papillary necrosis in a patient with chronic interstitial nephritis.

Other Drug-Induced Renal Injuries

These lesions are presented in Table **9-1** and Table **9-2**. The most common specific drug-related effects are the following [4, 8 - 10]:

Contrast Agents (*e.g.*, iodine-based substances) can produce tubular lesions which induce acute/chronic renal failure, acute/chronic nephrotic syndrome, fluid and electrolyte imbalance, acid-base disorders, *etc.*

Antibiotics (*e.g.*, gentamicin, tobramycin, cephalosporin) present a dose-dependent tubular toxicity. The tetracyclines present an anabolic effect and can induce tubulonephrosis. Amphotericin produces vasoconstriction of the small arteries and arterioles.

Diethylenetriamine (DETA) is an organic compound used in patients with lead or other metal intoxications, which can induce tubulonecrosis of the proximal tubes.

Cyclosporine and Rapamycin induce functional disorders due to their inhibition of calcineurin.

Serum Immunization and Vaccination can cause an immune-mediated crescentic or membranous glomerulonephritis.

Lithium Nephropathy can occur in patients with mood or bipolar disorders, or other psychiatric illnesses, who take lithium compounds for more than one or two years. It is characterized by a wide range of spectrum injuries, from a minimal decrease of the glomerular filtration rate to tubulointerstitial nephropathy and renal failure. The consequences are more severe in young females.

Table 9-1. Drug-induced tubular lesions and functional disorders. Data from references [1 - 10].

ADR type	**Drugs**
Tubular toxicity	Cisplatin, nedaplatin, amphotericin B, tacrolimus, carbamazepine, aminoglycosides, quinolones, ifosfamide, radiocontrast substances, mannitol, dextran, mithramycin, pentamidine, methoxyflurane, tetracycline, cephaloridine, streptozotocin, foscarnet, zoledronate, cidofovir, adefovir, tenofovir, hydroxyethyl starch, intravenous gamma globulin
Acute tubulonecrosis	NSAIDs, aminoglycosides, amphotericin, cyclosporine, sulfonamides, cephalosporins, tetracycline, rifampicin, cytotoxic drugs (cisplatin, methotrexate, mithramycin, nitrosourea)
Rhabdomyolysis (obstructive tubulopathy)	Lovastatin, ethanol, barbiturates, diazepam, codeine

(Table 9-1) contd.....

ADR type	Drugs
Severe hemolysis (obstructive tubulopathy)	Quinine, quinidine, nitrofurantoin, hydralazine, sulfonamides, triamterene
Crystalluria/lithiasis (obstructive tubulopathy)	Methotrexate, acyclovir, ganciclovir, indinavir, sulfanilamide
Ureteral obstruction secondary to retroperitoneal fibrosis	Ergotamine, dihydroergotamine, hydralazine, methyldopa, methysergide, pindolol
Risk of stone formation	Simultaneous administration of topiramate (anticonvulsant) and acetazolamide (carbonic anhydrase inhibitor)
Phospholipoidosis mimicking Fabry disease	Chloroquine (antimalarial and antirheumatic effect, antiretroviral in patients with HIV infection)
Polyuria	Neuroleptic/antidepressant drugs (chlorpromazine, lithium)
Oliguria	Neuroleptic/antidepressant drugs (haloperidol, fluphenazine), cyclosporine
Prerenal azotemia (functional renal failure)	Diuretics, NSAIDs, cyclosporine, ACE inhibitors, hydralazine, calcium blockers, radiocontrast agents, sulfonamides, interleukin-2, amphotericin B, rapamycin, influenza immunization
Pseudo-elevation of serum levels of urea and creatinine	Trimethoprim, cimetidine, diuretics (spironolactone, amiloride), probenecid, triamterene

Table 9-2. Drug-induced glomerular, interstitial and vascular disorders. Data from references [1 - 10].

ADR type	Drugs
Glomerular lesions (glomerulopathy)	Captopril, NSAIDs, penicillamine, lithium, mefenamate, interferon-alpha, gold salts, captopril, NSAIDs, fenoprofen, mercury compounds, pamidronate, fenclofenac, tolmetin, foscarnet
Minimal change glomerulonephritis	NSAIDs
Crescentic glomerulonephritis	Infliximab, influenza vaccine
Lupus-like (membranous) glomerulonephritis	Procainamide, hydralazine, isoniazid, penicillamine, gold salts, serum sickness, mercury compounds, trimethadione, probenecid (used for patients with gout)
Focal and segmental glomerulosclerosis	Pamidronate, cyclosporine, tacrolimus
Nephritic syndrome or isolated proteinuria	NSAIDs, captopril, interferon-alpha, D-penicillamine
Nephrotic syndrome	Thyreostatic drugs (perchlorate)
Acute interstitial nephritis	NSAIDs, allopurinol, thiazides, sulfonamides, cephalosporins, penicillin, methicillin, cyclosporine, proton pump inhibitors (PPIs)
Chronic interstitial nephritis, with/without papillary necroses	Phenacetin, NSAIDs (ibuprofen, phenylbutazone), acetaminophen, aspirin, acyclovir, indinavir, lithium

(Table 9-2) contd.....

ADR type	Drugs
Immune-mediated interstitial nephritis	Ampicillin, methicillin, penicillin, rifampicin, sulfonamides, phenytoin, allopurinol, furosemide, pantoprazole, cephalosporins, ciprofloxacin, thiazides, NSAIDs, cytosine arabinoside, cimetidine
Chronic tubulointerstitial nephritis/nephrocalcinosis	NSAIDs, thiazides, lithium, germanium, oral sodium phosphate purgative, cephalosporins, tetracyclines, augmentin (amoxicillin with clavulanate), sulfonamides analgesics
Endothelial lesions, thrombotic microangiopathy, thrombotic thrombocytopenic purpura – hemolytic uremic syndrome	Antiangiogenic drugs (*e.g.*, bevacizumab), antiplatelets (ticlopidine, clopidogrel, quinine), immunosuppressive drugs (cyclosporine, tacrolimus [calcineurin inhibitor], muromonab-CD3), antivirals (interferon, valacyclovir), chemotherapeutics (mitomycin C, gemcitabine)
Vasculitis	Antibiotics (penicillin), sulfonamides, aspirin, phenylbutazone, cytotoxic/immunosuppressive drugs, serum sickness
Obliterative arteriopathy	Cyclosporine, tacrolimus

Drug-Induced Lesions of the Bladder

Eosinophilic Cystitis is a drug-induced allergic reaction. It is associated with unspecific symptoms, such as gross hematuria, lumbar pain and lower abdominal pain. In some cases, it can mimic a bladder cancer. Disseminated intravascular coagulation syndrome can also be associated [11].

Hemorrhagic Cystitis can be induced by cytotoxic drugs, such as cyclophosphamide, or by chemotherapeutics, such as cabazitaxel, used in patients with metastatic castration-resistant prostate cancer. The primary clinical symptom is gross hematuria with negative urine cytology and culture. The differential diagnosis includes tuberculosis and bladder tumors [12, 13].

Intravesical Immunotherapy with Bacillus Calmette-Guerin (BCG) for Treating Bladder Cancer can induce storage symptoms such as dysuria, pollakiuria and hematuria. These usually emerge after the third BCG administration. Cystitis is a common local complication caused by *Mycobacterium bovis*. Bladder contracture is a rare but severe consequence that occurs in 0.05-1% of patients. Cystoprostatectomy with orthotopic ileal neobladder reconstruction is sometimes necessary in these patients [14]. Other severe complications include ureteral obstruction, periurethral diverticulum, orchiepididymitis, multiorgan granulomata (prostate, kidney, lung, liver), life-threatening sepsis with disseminated mycobacterial infection, reactive arthritis and hypersensitivity reactions [15].

IATROGENIC LESIONS DURING DIAGNOSTIC AND THERAPEUTIC PROCEDURES

Disorders of the Urinary Tract

Surgery-Related Complications

The bladder, ureters and urethra can be injured during various types of surgery, primarily those involving the retroperitoneum, pelvis and abdominal cavity. During gynecological, intestinal and vascular surgeries, ureteral sections or clamping and ureterovaginal or uretero-uterine fistulae can occur. The terminal ureter is the most commonly damaged [16]. During *hysterectomy*, bladder injuries are reported in 0.3-6% of cases and urethral lesions in 0.2-7.3%. *Caesarean sections* are associated with bladder lesions in fewer than 0.3% of cases [17].

Iatrogenic lumbosacral spinal cord lesions are followed by upper urinary tract deterioration in more than 65% of cases [18]. Later complications include risk of bladder stone formation and bladder cancer [19]. In one of our cases, involving a diabetic male, a spinal injury induced paralysis and urinary retention. He survived for 15 years following the injury. At his autopsy, necrosis of the penis and huge bladder stones were found.

Postoperative rhabdomyolysis with *myoglobinuria and obstructive tubulopathy* has been reported following urological, bariatric and orthopedic interventions [20 - 22], and as a consequence of thoraco-abdominal aortic repair [23].

Suture of the ureters can be accompanied by *vascular damage*. For example, in one case, a pelvic surgery complicated by an accidental injury of the right ureter sutured with an end-to-end anastomosis was followed by massive hematuria two months after surgery. This was caused by the rupture of a pseudoaneurysm of the abdominal aorta that was periprocedurally formed below the renal vessels [24].

General/rachidian anesthesia can induce hypovolemia and oliguria (<0.5 ml urine/kg/hour).

Endoscopic Examination of the Urinary Tract

This is a safety procedure that can be followed by mucosal damage, hemorrhages and perforations of the urinary tract. These consequences can lead to the formation of periurethral phlegmon/abscess, ureterovaginal or uretero-uterine fistulae and peritonitis. The risk of infections is higher for diabetics and patients with low immunity. In diabetics with associated Klebsiella infection, an emphysematous periurethral abscess can emerge [25].

Urethral Catheter-Related Lesions

Indwelling urethral and suprapubic catheterization can induce upper urinary tract injuries with hematuria, urinary tract infections and catheter obstruction [18]. Misplacement of the catheter can lead to bleeding at the urethral meatus, high-riding (nonpalpable) prostate, perineal hematoma, perforation of the small bowel and enterocutaneous fistulae. Intestinal resection is necessary in such cases [26]. Bladder perforation is the most severe complication of catheterization, is more common in infants and can lead to deadly peritonitis [27]. Later complications are more common in older and male patients, and can include iatrogenic hypospadias, chronic infections, urethral diverticulum, bladder stone formation and risk of bladder cancer [19, 28, 29].

Transurethral Resection (TUR)

Resection of a bladder tumor can be followed by bladder perforation with further urinary ascites and pseudo-renal failure with elevated creatinine [30]. Following tumor resection, intravesical therapy with BCG can induce renal tuberculosis [31].

In patients with prostatic hyperplasia, the most common post-TUR complications are urinary infections, urethral stricture and TUR syndrome (transient hypotension, hyponatremia and anuria). Urinary incontinence and bladder neck contracture can also occur [32, 33].

Renal Biopsy and Nephrectomy

Ultrasonographic-guided Percutaneous Renal Biopsy is followed by vascular injuries with macroscopic hematuria in 3.5% of patients. The renal artery and, more rarely, the aorta, lumbar artery, superior mesenteric artery and left colic artery can be injured. However, most lesions do not have clinical implications. Transfusion is necessary in 0.9% of patients with vascular injuries and reinterventions are required in just 0.6% of cases. The main complications are arteriovenous fistulae and pseudoaneurysms of the injured arteries (1-2%). Perirenal or retroperitoneal hematomas are seen in 17% of cases. The risk of bleeding is higher for patients with acute kidney injury and high creatinine serum levels, as well as in cases of large bore needle use [34].

Radical Nephrectomy can be followed by chylous ascites, with about 35 cases having been reported by 2008 [35]. This lesion can also be a consequence of pelvic irradiation for tumors [36].

Sclerotherapy of Simple Renal Cysts is not associated with significant complications. Although uncommon, sclerotherapy-induced renal cell carcinoma has been reported [37].

Complications of Hemodialysis And Peritoneal Dialysis

Catheter-Related Complications

The most common complications are infections, catheter dysfunctions (thrombosis, malposition or kinking, and fibrin shell formation), vascular access disorders and central vein stenosis. According to Wang *et al.*, the risk of infection is directly correlated with increased age, diabetes, low serum albumin and high ferritin levels [38]. In children, peritoneal dialysis is usually preferred, and catheter-related complications include catheter loss with further intra-abdominal injuries, mechanical flow dysfunction (blockage/kinking of the tube or tip migration), infections (peritonitis, sepsis), bleeding and hernia of the abdominal wall [39].

Complications in End-Stage Renal Disease

In patients with chronic dialysis and persistent renal failure, the consequences are uremia-related. In one of our cases, a 27-year-old male with rejection of the transplanted kidney, who underwent hemodialysis for three years, was hospitalized with high serum levels of urea and severe cardiorespiratory failure. At autopsy, uremia-induced fibrinous pericarditis and bilateral pleuritis were found (Fig. **9-2**). Renal failure-induced secondary hyperparathyroidism has been reported in patients undergoing hemodialysis with a median duration of 122 months. In drug-resistant cases, subtotal parathyroidectomy is indicated [40].

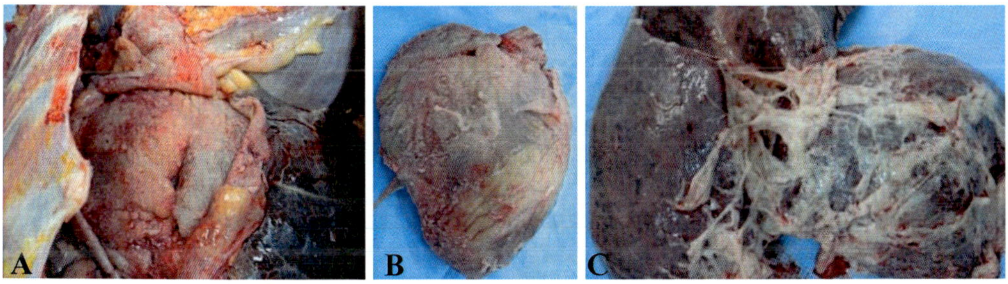

Fig. (9-2). The features of fibrinous pericarditis (A, B) and pleuritis (C) in a patient with chronic renal failure. He underwent hemodialysis for three years.

Peritonitis

This is an uncommon lesion in patients undergoing chronic peritoneal dialysis. It is more commonly reported in children and can present in several forms [39, 41,

42]:

Infective Peritonitis is a lesion induced by *Staphylococcus aureus* and can be catheter-related. In 10-20% of patients, relapsing peritonitis has been noted at four weeks after completion of antibiotherapy, especially in cases of chronic use of systemic antibiotics.

Eosinophilic Peritonitis is characterized by the presence of more than 100 white cells/mL with ≥10% eosinophils in the peritoneal fluid. It can be a spontaneously reversed or chronic lesion.

Sclerosing Peritonitis with subsequent ileal obstruction occurs in 0.9-7.3% of patients. The main risk factors are the duration of hemodialysis and recurrent peritonitis.

Culture-Negative or Aseptic Peritonitis accounts for 5-20% of hemodialysis-related peritonitis. It can be caused by fungi, mycobacteria or non-infective factors, such as drugs or tumors.

Lesions of the Gastric Mucosa

Mucosal hyperplasia (gastric parietal, G-cells and Brunner's duodenal glands) is induced by hemodialysis-related hypergastrinemia and hyperchlorhydria [4, 43]. Hemodialysis-induced GAVE syndrome can lead to upper GI bleeding [44].

Splenic Rupture

Splenic rupture is reported in patients using heparin during hemodialysis and in patients with uremic coagulopathy (hyperuricemia increases platelet adhesion), infections and secondary amyloidosis. The occurrence of hemoperitoneum calls for emergency splenectomy [45].

Spontaneous Retroperitoneal Hemorrhage

This is an exceedingly rare but life-threatening complication of peritoneal dialysis that can emerge in patients with polycystic kidneys as a result of rupture of a renal cyst [45, 46].

Systemic Amyloidosis

This condition is primarily reported in patients undergoing long-term dialysis. Renal failure, hematuria and carpal tunnel syndrome (compression of the median nerve) are the most common complications, affecting 1-2% of patients [47, 48].

Renal Malignancy

In patients with polycystic kidneys and undergoing long-term dialysis, malignant transformation has been infrequently reported [46].

CONFLICT OF INTEREST

The authors confirm that this chapter content has no conflict of interest.

ACKNOWLEDGEMENTS

Declared none.

REFERENCES

[1] Choudhury D, Ahmed Z. Drug-associated renal dysfunction and injury. Nat Clin Pract Nephrol 2006; 2(2): 80-91.
[http://dx.doi.org/10.1038/ncpneph0076] [PMID: 16932399]

[2] Gobe GC, Coombes JS, Fassett RG, Endre ZH. Biomarkers of drug-induced acute kidney injury in the adult. Expert Opin Drug Metab Toxicol 2015; 11(11): 1683-94.
[http://dx.doi.org/10.1517/17425255.2015.1083011] [PMID: 26548752]

[3] Wilhelm SM, Rjater RG, Kale-Pradhan PB. Perils and pitfalls of long-term effects of proton pump inhibitors. Expert Rev Clin Pharmacol 2013; 6(4): 443-51.
[http://dx.doi.org/10.1586/17512433.2013.811206] [PMID: 23927671]

[4] Jung J, Ed. Patologie iatrogenă. Tîrgu-Mureş, Romania: University Press 2006.

[5] Available at: www.rhombnet.com

[6] Thurner J. Iatrogene Pathologie. München, Berlin, Wien: Urban&Schwarzenberg 1970.

[7] Jochum E, Janssen U. [Chronic interstitial nephritis in an 18-year-old due to intake of a compound analgesic]. Med Klin (Munich) 2006; 101(10): 830-4.
[http://dx.doi.org/10.1007/s00063-006-1111-z] [PMID: 17039326]

[8] Shine B, McKnight RF, Leaver L, Geddes JR. Long-term effects of lithium on renal, thyroid, and parathyroid function: a retrospective analysis of laboratory data. Lancet 2015; 386(9992): 461-8.
[http://dx.doi.org/10.1016/S0140-6736(14)61842-0] [PMID: 26003379]

[9] Duggal T, Segal P, Shah M, Carter-Monroe N, Manoharan P, Geetha D. Antineutrophil cytoplasmic antibody vasculitis associated with influenza vaccination. Am J Nephrol 2013; 38(2): 174-8.
[http://dx.doi.org/10.1159/000354084] [PMID: 23941822]

[10] Solez K, Racusen LC, Mihatsch M. Nephrotoxicity of cyclosporine and newer immunosuppressive agents. Handout XXII International Congress of the International Academy of Pathology. 20-44.

[11] Okazaki S, Hori J, Kita M, Yamaguchi S, Kawakami N, Kakizaki H. [A case of eosinophilic cystitis mimicking an invasive bladder cancer]. Hinyokika Kiyo 2014; 60(12): 635-9.
[PMID: 25602481]

[12] Kosaka T, Oya M. Hemorrhagic cystitis in a patient without a past history of radiation therapy who was treated with cabazitaxel for CRPC. Ann Oncol 2015; 26(11): 2355-6.
[http://dx.doi.org/10.1093/annonc/mdv362] [PMID: 26347111]

[13] Webb H, Jaureguiberry G, Dufek S, Tullus K, Bockenhauer D. Cyclophosphamide and rituximab in frequently relapsing/steroid-dependent nephrotic syndrome. Pediatr Nephrol 2016; 31(4): 589-94.
[http://dx.doi.org/10.1007/s00467-015-3245-9] [PMID: 26525199]

[14] Vetorazzo Filho JE, Bahia LA, Vedovato BC, *et al.* Cystectomy with orthotopic ileal neobladder reconstruction for treatment of bladder contracture after intravesical bacillus Calmette-Guerin therapy. Einstein (Sao Paulo) 2014; 12(4): 502-4. [Sao Paolo].
[http://dx.doi.org/10.1590/S1679-45082014RC2794] [PMID: 25628205]

[15] Macleod LC, Ngo TC, Gonzalgo ML. Complications of intravesical bacillus calmette-guérin. Can Urol Assoc J 2014; 8(7-8): E540-4.
[http://dx.doi.org/10.5489/cuaj.1411] [PMID: 25210559]

[16] Fernández Gómez JM, Sahagun JL, Regadera FJ, *et al.* [Iatrogenic lesions of the urinary tract. II. Bladder and urethra]. Actas Urol Esp 1994; 18(3): 190-9.
[PMID: 8036945]

[17] Jasonni VM, Matonti G. [Management of iatrogenic gynecologic injuries with urologic relevance. Causes and prevention of complications: the gynecologists opinion]. Urologia 2013; 80 (Suppl. 22): 24-7.
[http://dx.doi.org/10.5301/RU.2013.10619] [PMID: 23341201]

[18] Zhang Z, Liao L. Risk factors predicting upper urinary tract deterioration in patients with spinal cord injury: a prospective study. Spinal Cord 2014; 52(6): 468-71.
[http://dx.doi.org/10.1038/sc.2014.63] [PMID: 24777160]

[19] Ho CH, Sung KC, Lim SW, *et al.* Chronic indwelling urinary catheter increase the risk of bladder cancer, even in patients without spinal cord injury. Medicine (Baltimore) 2015; 94: e1736.
[http://dx.doi.org/10.1097/MD.0000000000001736]

[20] Collier B, Goreja MA, Duke BE III. Postoperative rhabdomyolysis with bariatric surgery. Obes Surg 2003; 13(6): 941-3.
[http://dx.doi.org/10.1381/096089203322618821] [PMID: 14738687]

[21] Hiratsuka Y, Ishii T, Takeuchi F, Okadome A, Taira H. Risk of elevated creatine kinase and myoglobulinemia due to incised muscles in patients who underwent urological surgery. J Urol 2003; 170(1): 119-21.
[http://dx.doi.org/10.1097/01.ju.0000070660.41083.a3] [PMID: 12796661]

[22] Sudarsanan S, Omar AS, Pattath RA, Al Mulla A. Acute kidney injury associated with rhabdomyolysis after coronary artery bypass graft: a case report and review of the literatures. BMC Res Notes 2014; 7: 152-7.
[http://dx.doi.org/10.1186/1756-0500-7-152] [PMID: 24636137]

[23] Miller CC, Villa MA. Sutton mJ, Keyhani LD, Estera Al, Safi HJ. Serum myoglobin and renal morbidity and mortality following thoracic and thoraco-abdominal aortic repair: does rhabdomyolysis play a role? Eur J Vasc Endovasc Surg 2009; 37: 388-94.
[http://dx.doi.org/10.1016/j.ejvs.2008.12.020] [PMID: 19232502]

[24] Vagnoni V, Gaudiano C, Passaretti G, *et al.* Massive hematuria due to ruptured iatrogenic aortic pseudoaneurysm: a case report. Arch Ital Urol Androl 2013; 85(2): 96-8.
[http://dx.doi.org/10.4081/aiua.2013.2.96] [PMID: 23820658]

[25] Lee CY, Tsai HC, Lee SS, Chen YS. Concomitant emphysematous prostatic and periurethral abscesses due to *Klebsiella pneumoniae*: a case report and review of the literature. Southeast Asian J Trop Med Public Health 2014; 45(5): 1099-106.
[PMID: 25417511]

[26] Barai KP, Islam S. Suprapubic catheterization complicated by an iatrogenic enterocutaneous fistula: a case report. Cases J 2009; 2: 9311.
[http://dx.doi.org/10.1186/1757-1626-2-9311] [PMID: 20062634]

[27] Samiee-Zafarghandy S, Guerra L, Koujok K, Rebollo-Polo M, Daboval T. Urethral catheter-related bladder wall lesions simulating inflammatory pseudotumor in a neonate. Am J Case Rep 2015; 16: 268-71.

[http://dx.doi.org/10.12659/AJCR.891097] [PMID: 25937365]

[28] Ogawa S, Date T, Muraki O. Intraperitoneal urinary bladder perforation observed in a patient with an indwelling urethral catheter. Case Rep Urol 2013; 2013: 765704.
[http://dx.doi.org/10.1155/2013/765704]

[29] Kaur G, Jain S, Sharma A, Suneja A, Guleria K. Urethral diverticulum masquerading as anterior vaginal wall cyst: A diagnostic dilemma. J Clin Diagn Res 2015; 9(10): QD08-9.
[PMID: 26557574]

[30] Matsumura M, Ando N, Kumabe A, Dhaliwal G. Pseudo-renal failure: bladder rupture with urinary ascites. BMJ Case Rep 2015; 2015: bcr2015212671.
[http://dx.doi.org/10.1136/bcr-2015-212671] [PMID: 26590189]

[31] Higashioka K, Miyake N, Nishida R, Chong Y, Shimoda S, Shimono N. Bilateral granulomatous renal masses after intravesical BCG therapy for non-muscle-invasive bladder cancer and carcinoma *in situ* of the upper urinary tract: A case study. Kansenshogaku Zasshi 2015; 89(4): 481-4.
[PMID: 26554225]

[32] Sivarajan G, Borofsky MS, Shah O, Lingeman JE, Lepor H. The role of minimally invasive surgical techniques in the management of large-gland benign prostatic hypertrophy. Rev Urol 2015; 17(3): 140-9.
[PMID: 26543428]

[33] Parker DC, Simhan J. Management of complications after surgical outlet reduction for benign prostatic obstruction. Can J Urol 2015; 22 (Suppl. 1): 88-92.
[PMID: 26497349]

[34] Madhusudhan KS, Gamanagatti S, Gupta AK. Endovascular embolization of pseudoaneurysm of left colic artery developing after renal biopsy. Indian J Nephrol 2015; 25(4): 242-5.
[http://dx.doi.org/10.4103/0971-4065.146029] [PMID: 26199477]

[35] Shah SS, Ahmed K, Smith R, Mallina R, Akhbari P, Khan MS. Chylous ascites following radical nephrectomy: a case report. J Med Case Reports 2008; 2: 3.
[http://dx.doi.org/10.1186/1752-1947-2-3] [PMID: 18190695]

[36] Ouakaa-Kchaou A, Ennaifer R, Elloumi H, *et al.* [Chylous ascites after pelvic irradiation for urologic malignancy]. Presse Med 2008; 37(6 Pt 1): 978-81.
[http://dx.doi.org/10.1016/j.lpm.2007.09.025] [PMID: 18313885]

[37] Hashimoto Y, Imai A, Tokui N, *et al.* Unexpected outcome after sclerotherapy of simple renal cyst. BMC Nephrol 2012; 13: 63.
[http://dx.doi.org/10.1186/1471-2369-13-63] [PMID: 22827879]

[38] Wang K, Wang P, Liang X, Lu X, Liu Z. Epidemiology of haemodialysis catheter complications: a survey of 865 dialysis patients from 14 haemodialysis centres in Henan province in China. BMJ Open 2015; 5(11): e007136.
[http://dx.doi.org/10.1136/bmjopen-2014-007136] [PMID: 26589425]

[39] Fraser N, Hussain FK, Connell R, Shenoy MU. Chronic peritoneal dialysis in children. Int J Nephrol Renovasc Dis 2015; 8: 125-37.
[http://dx.doi.org/10.2147/IJNRD.S82419] [PMID: 26504404]

[40] Skalli Z, Elouazzani H, Alhamany Z, *et al.* Kinetics of parathyroid hormone after parathyroidectomy in chronic hemodialysis patients. Saudi J Kidney Dis Transpl 2015; 26(6): 1199-204.
[http://dx.doi.org/10.4103/1319-2442.168622] [PMID: 26586059]

[41] Candido PdeC, Werner AdeF, Pereira IM, Matos BA, Pfeilsticker RM, Silva R. Sclerosing encapsulating peritonitis: a case report. Radiol Bras 2015; 48(1): 56-8.
[http://dx.doi.org/10.1590/0100-3984.2013.1909] [PMID: 25798009]

[42] Johnson DW, Gray N, Snelling P. A peritoneal dialysis patient with fatal culture-negative peritonitis. Nephrology (Carlton) 2003; 8(1): 49-55.

[http://dx.doi.org/10.1046/j.1440-1797.2003.00119.x] [PMID: 15012750]

[43] Carlei F, Caruso U, Lezoche E, *et al.* Hyperplasia of antral G cells in uraemic patients. Digestion 1984; 29(1): 26-30.
[http://dx.doi.org/10.1159/000199004] [PMID: 6724166]

[44] Tomori K, Nakamoto H, Kotaki S, *et al.* Gastric angiodysplasia in patients undergoing maintenance dialysis. Adv Perit Dial 2003; 19: 136-42.
[PMID: 14763050]

[45] Gazel E, Açıkgöz G, Kasap Y, Yiğman M, Güneş ZE. Spontaneous splenic rupture due to uremic coagulopathy and mortal sepsis after splenectomy. Int J Crit Illn Inj Sci 2015; 5(2): 119-22.
[http://dx.doi.org/10.4103/2229-5151.158419] [PMID: 26157658]

[46] Biyik Z, Solak Y, Gaipov A, Ozbek O, Esen H, Turk S. Spontaneous retroperitoneal hemorrhage presenting as hemoperitoneum secondary to renal cyst rupture in a peritoneal dialysis patient with acquired cystic kidney disease. Indian J Nephrol 2015; 25(4): 251-4.
[http://dx.doi.org/10.4103/0971-4065.147371] [PMID: 26199480]

[47] Hsiao PJ, Chiang WF, Chao TK, Lin SH. Life-threatening hematuria in a hemodialysis patient with systemic light-chain amyloidosis. Clin Chim Acta 2015; 451: 180-2.
[http://dx.doi.org/10.1016/j.cca.2015.09.027] [PMID: 26434538]

[48] Hoshino J, Yamagata K, Nishi S, *et al.* Significance of the decreased risk of dialysis-related amyloidosis now proven by results from Japanese nationwide surveys in 1998 and 2010. Nephrol Dial Transplant 2016; 31(4): 595-602.
[http://dx.doi.org/10.1093/ndt/gfv276] [PMID: 26206763]

CHAPTER 10

Iatrogenic Pathology of the Female Genital System and Breast

Ioan Jung, Simona Gurzu* and **Sabin Turdean**

Department of Pathology, University of Medicine and Pharmacy, Tirgu-Mures, Romania

Abstract: The female genital system and breast can be injured by drugs or during diagnostic and/or therapeutic interventions. Drug-induced lesions of the female genitalia primarily involve contact dermatitis and fixed drug eruptions. Galactorrhea can be caused by several drugs, including neuroleptics and antihypertensive agents. In females with breast cancer, tamoxifen can induce endometrial hyperplasia and transformation into carcinoma. Diagnostic and therapeutic procedures rarely lead to severe complications, but such complications are specific and require knowledge for clinicians. The final section of this chapter is reserved for specific lesions related to pregnancy and the effects of the intrauterine environment on newborns.

Keywords: Adverse drug reaction, Allergy, Breast, Dermatitis, Endocervical hyperplasia, Endometrial atrophy, Endometrial hyperplasia, Female genitalia, Fixed drug eruption, Galactorrhea, Genital system, Iatrogenic, Newborn, Pregnancy, Urticaria.

DRUG-INDUCED LESIONS

Lesions of the Female Genitalia

These lesions are local injuries produced by gels, creams and topical antiseptics, as well as lesions secondary to the systemic administration of drugs.

Iatrogenic Contact Dermatitis And/Or Urticaria is the most common local injury of the female genitalia and is produced through type IV hypersensitivity reaction. It can be induced by topical agents, a patient's latex allergy, methylisothiazolinone, *etc.* [1].

Genital Fixed Drug Eruptions represent recurrent, well-defined lesions appearing on the external genital organs each time the responsible drug is taken.

* **Corresponding author Simona Gurzu:** Department of Pathology, University of Medicine and Pharmacy, Tirgu-Mures, Romania; Tel. 0040-745-673550; Fax 0040-372-653250; E-mail: simonagurzu@yahoo.com

They may be related to oral or systemic administration of several drugs (Table **10-1**). Genital ulcers can be associated [1 - 5].

Gonadotropin-Releasing Hormone (GnRH) Agonists are used to preoperatively shrink leiomyomas, to control bleeding and for patients with contraindications for myomectomy. These drugs induce several side effects, including the climacteric effect. To avoid these effects, other combinations are introduced in daily practice. Administration of combined oral contraceptives, progestins- or levonorgestrel-releasing intrauterine devices (IUDs) have proven to be appropriate for bleeding control but not for quick and significant fibroids shrinkage. A new selective progesterone receptor modulator is ulipristal acetate (UPA), which induces amenorrhea and seems to cause long-term shrinkage of leiomyomas [6].

Other female genitalia-related ADRs are presented in Chapter 18.

Table 10-1. Female genitalia-related ADRs. Data from references [1-6].

ADR type	Drugs
Genital fixed drug eruptions	Antifungals (ketoconazole), antiparasitic agents (metronidazole, miconazole) quinine, antibacterial sulfonamides, NSAIDs (ibuprofen), antimalarial drugs, antibiotics (amoxicillin), antihistamines, steroids, *etc.*
Genital ulcers	NSAIDs, antimalarials, ACE inhibitors, beta blockers, lithium, salicylates, corticosteroids, tyrosine kinase inhibitors (*e.g.,* sunitinib)
Hypermenorrhea	Neuroleptics/antidepressant drugs (reserpine)
Amenorrhea, low prolactin levels	Antiemetics, neuroleptics/tricyclic antidepressants (haloperidol, chlorpromazine, sulpiride), cytotoxic drugs (cyclophosphamide)
Time-dependent amenorrhea (more than three months of daily use)	Ulipristal acetate (UPA, a progesterone receptor modulator used to preoperatively shrink symptomatic leiomyomas)
Fungal infections (vulvovaginitis)	Immunosuppressive drugs, corticosteroids, antibiotics
Endocervical hyperplasia, endometrial atrophy, uterine hemorrhages, anovulatory infertility and virilization	Contraceptive pills, progesterone (gestagens)
Endometrial hyperplasia/adenocarcinoma, anovulatory infertility, increased risk of thrombosis and breast cancer	Estrogens, tamoxifen
Ovarian hyperstimulation syndrome, multiple gestation, ectopic pregnancy, adnexal torsion, hemoperitoneum	Gonadotropin

Lesions of the Breast

The most common drug-induced lesions of the breast are galactorrhea, lactation abnormalities and necroses (Table **10-2**).

Table 10-2. Drug-induced lesions of the breast. Data from references [1-6].

ADR type	Drugs
Galactorrhea	Neuroleptic drugs, contraceptive pills, antihypertensive agents, antiemetics
Lactation abnormalities	Antiemetics, antipsychotics, tricyclic antidepressants
Breast hemorrhagic necrosis	Anticoagulants
Breast tenderness	Gonadotropin

IATROGENIC LESIONS DURING DIAGNOSTIC AND THERAPEUTIC PROCEDURES

Non-Surgical or Minimally Invasive Procedures

Endoscopic Examinations can be followed, though rarely, by local hemorrhages and/or ascending infections [7].

Hysterosalpingography can be associated with contrast agent-related complications. Such substances can initiate an allergy or can induce granulomatous salpingitis or peritonitis [8].

Contraceptive IUDs can induce several complications, such as acute/chronic endometritis, cervicitis, vaginitis, tubo-ovarian abscess with subsequent ectopic pregnancy, pelvic actinomycosis, endometrial atrophy/fibrosis, endometrial carcinoma, *etc.* [7].

Curettage of the Intrauterine Cavity (after delivery, abortion or tumor removal) can be followed by infections (endomyometritis), Asherman's syndrome (trauma-related endometrial atrophy, hypo-/amenorrhea, sterility), *etc.* [9].

Uterine Artery Embolization is performed in patients with leiomyomas and can be complicated by Asherman's syndrome. It can also be followed by formation of intrauterine fibrous membranes; the outcome of hysteroscopic adhesiolysis is worse in females with Asherman's syndrome [9]. Other complications are infections, necrosis, ovarian insufficiency and premature menopause (amenorrhea, high follicle stimulating hormone [FSH] levels) [10].

Lesions of the Breast – Excisional Biopsy can be associated with hemorrhages, necroses and formation of lipogranulomas [8].

Surgical Interventions

Hysterectomy can be accompanied by injuries of the bladder, ureters (especially the terminal ureter) and/or urethra. Vesico-vaginal/ureterovaginal fistulae, hematuria, nosocomial infections and surgical wound dehiscence with presence of urine in the wound can also occur. Other possible consequences are scar endometriosis (1.08-2% of cases) and unusual formation of bladder stones incorporating surgical threads. Other organs, such as the intestine and peripheral nerves, can also be damaged [11 - 15]. Radical surgery for uterine or ovarian tumors that involve hysterectomy and extended lymph node dissection can induce chylous ascites [16, 17].

Myomectomy can be followed by hemorrhages that are more common in females with huge or multiple leiomyomas. Periprocedural formation of uterine diverticulum can induce abnormal uterine bleeding, pelvic pain, dysmenorrhea and adverse obstetric events [18].

Breast Reconstruction With Silicone Implants can be complicated by pain, hypo-/hypersensitivity of the breast/nipple, purulent/granulomatous inflammations, infections (Staphylococcus aureus, Candida albicans, Curvularia species, Aspergillus niger, mycobacteria, Clostridium perfringens, *etc*.), hemorrhages, formation of peri-implant seroma, implant displacement, asymmetry, wrinkling, rupture, capsular contracture, difficulty in breastfeeding and malignant transformation (T-cell lymphoma). In June 2013, the FDA approved implants for breast reconstruction in women of any age, but their use for breast augmentation was approved only for women at least 18 years of age (for saline implants) or 22 (for silicone gel-filled implants) [19, 20]. This intervention can be followed by migration of the silicone particles into the lymph nodes, inducing foreign body granuloma formation (siliconoma) [21]. Silicone implants-related hypersensitivity reactions can induce, rarely, a systemic disorder similar to Sjogren's syndrome or scleroderma [22, 23].

IATROGENIC LESIONS DURING PREGNANCY

Lesions in Mothers

Cesarean Sections can be complicated by bladder lesions (0.3%), obstetric fistulae (2%), scar endometriosis (0.03-0.4%), venous air or amniotic fluid embolism, acute pulmonary edema (0.08%), nosocomial infections, aspiration pneumonia, *etc*. Scar endometriosis is presented as a nodular lesion within or underneath the scar and should be differentiated from desmoid tumors. Endometriotic nodules (endometriomas) can be painful during menstruation and can present malignant transformation in an endometrial carcinoma or clear cell ovarian-type carcinoma. The incidence of labor-related air embolism is higher following use of self-collapsible polyvinyl chloride or a polypropylene-based intravenous fluid bag. Other risk factors for air embolism are placenta previa, previous uterine surgery, hypovolemia, maternal positioning, prolonged labor, manual extraction of the placenta, *etc*. In most cases, the air is absorbed into the tissues, without clinical consequences, but rapid entry of 200-300 ml of air or 3-5 ml/kg can result in significant morbidity and mortality. The main risk factors of postpartum pulmonary edema are the administration of tocolytic agents, underlying cardiac disease, iatrogenic fluid overload and preeclampsia. Amniotic embolism is rare but represents the second most common cause of maternal death. It can lead to pulmonary amniotic embolism or induce the onset of DIC [13 - 15, 24 - 28].

Episiotomy/Symphysiotomy can be followed by rupture of the vaginal wall, anal canal injury, risk of postoperative fistulae, opportunistic infections (*e.g.*, pyoderma gangrenosum), delayed scarring, scar endometriosis, *etc*. Epidermoid cysts can occur as a result of migration of epithelial fragments into connective tissue [8, 15, 24, 29, 30].

Iatrogenic Spontaneous Abortion or Preterm Delivery can be induced by inhalational anesthetics, such as nitrous oxide or halothane. Progesterone increases the risk of delivery <14 days and preterm birth <37 weeks [31].

Lesions in Newborns

Intrauterine Environmental Factors such as medical/toxic substances ingested by the mother and viral infections, can lead to hepatic lesions in the newborn (Table **10-3**).

Radiotherapy performed on the mother during pregnancy can lead to embryo-/fetopathy. The potential consequences range from malformations to mental retardation and embryonic death [32]. Details regarding fetal-related radiotherapy were presented in Chapter 2.

Fetoscopic Laser Ablative Surgery performed to treat twin-to-twin transfusion syndrome, induces iatrogenic premature rupture of membranes in 18.5% of cases [33].

Table 10-3. Effects of intrauterine environments upon newborns. Data from references [31-33].

Newborn's disorder	Intrauterine environmental factor
Fetal alcohol syndrome	Alcohol consumption of mother
Veno-occlusive disease	Alkaloids
Risk of hepatoblastoma	Alcohol consumption of mother, or occupational exposure of mother or father to metals, petroleum products, paints or pigments
Neonatal hepatitis, biliary atresia	Rubella, cytomegalovirus (CMV), herpes simplex
Congenital syphilis, neonatal listeriosis, neonatal toxoplasmosis	Treponema pallidum, listeria monocytogenes, Toxoplasma gondii
Disorders of osteogenesis	Tetracycline

CONFLICT OF INTEREST

The authors confirm that this chapter content has no conflict of interest.

ACKNOWLEDGEMENTS

Declared none.

REFERENCES

[1] Eubel J, Diepgen TL, Weisshaar E. Allergic diseases in the genital area. Hautarzt 2015; 66(1): 45-52. [http://dx.doi.org/10.1007/s00105-014-3561-1] [PMID: 25532902]

[2] Kastalli S, El Aïdli S, Lakhoua G, Daghfous R. Genital fixed drug eruption induced by miconazole with positive provocation test. Tunis Med 2014; 92(11): 703. [PMID: 25867162]

[3] Lonsdale-Eccles E, Wallett A, Ward AM. A case of fixed drug eruption secondary to quinine in tonic water presenting to a sexual health clinic. Sex Transm Infect 2014; 90(5): 356-7. [http://dx.doi.org/10.1136/sextrans-2013-051458] [PMID: 24583965]

[4] Saka B, Kombaté K, Médougou BH, *et al.* Fixed drug eruption in dermatology setting in Lomé (Togo): a retrospective study of 321 cases. Bull Soc Pathol Exot 2012; 105(5): 384-7. [http://dx.doi.org/10.1007/s13149-012-0237-x] [PMID: 22669581]

[5] Roett MA, Mayor MT, Uduhiri KA. Diagnosis and management of genital ulcers. Am Fam Physician 2012; 85(3): 254-62. [PMID: 22335265]

[6] Hoellen F, Griesinger G, Bohlmann MK. Therapeutic drugs in the treatment of symptomatic uterine fibroids. Expert Opin Pharmacother 2013; 14(15): 2079-85. [http://dx.doi.org/10.1517/14656566.2013.825607] [PMID: 23914973]

[7] Kurman RJ. Blaustein's Pathology of the Female Genital Tract. New York, Berlin, Heidelberg, London, Paris, Tokyo: Springer Verlag 1989.

[8] Jung J, Ed. Patologie iatrogenă. Tîrgu-Mureş, Romania: University Press 2006.

[9] Song D, Liu Y, Xiao Y, Li TC, Zhou F, Xia E. A matched cohort study comparing the outcome of intrauterine adhesiolysis for Ashermans syndrome after uterine artery embolization or surgical trauma.

J Minim Invasive Gynecol 2014; 21(6): 1022-8.
[http://dx.doi.org/10.1016/j.jmig.2014.04.015] [PMID: 24842805]

[10] Woźniakowska E, Milart P, Paszkowski T, *et al.* Uterine artery embolization clinical problems. Ginekol Pol 2013; 84(12): 1051-4.
[PMID: 24505954]

[11] Hampel C, Neisius A, Thomas C, Thüroff JW, Roos F. Vesicovaginal fistula. Incidence, etiology and phenomenology in Germany Urologe A 2015; 54: 349-58.
[http://dx.doi.org/10.1007/s00120-014-3679-x] [PMID: 25784445]

[12] Fernández Gómez JM, Sahagun JL, Regadera FJ, *et al.* Iatrogenic lesions of the urinary tract. II. Bladder and urethra. Actas Urol Esp 1994; 18(3): 190-9.
[PMID: 8036945]

[13] Jasonni VM, Matonti G. Management of iatrogenic gynecologic injuries with urologic relevance. Causes and prevention of complications: the gynecologists opinion. Urologia 2013; 80 (Suppl. 22): 24-7.
[http://dx.doi.org/10.5301/RU.2013.10619] [PMID: 23341201]

[14] Gregor M, Paterová P, Buchta V, Ketřánek J, Špaček J. Healthcare-associated infections in gynecology and obstetrics at a university hospital in the Czech Republic. Int J Gynaecol Obstet 2014; 126(3): 240-3.
[http://dx.doi.org/10.1016/j.ijgo.2014.04.001] [PMID: 24890744]

[15] Vural B, Vural F, Müezzinoglu B. An abdominal wall desmoid tumour mimicking cesarean scar endometriomas: a case report and review of the literature. J Clin Diagn Res 2015; 9(9): QD14-6.
[PMID: 26500967]

[16] Janco JM, Gloviczki P, Friese JL, Cliby WA. Lymphatic mapping and ligation for persistent ascites after surgery for gynecologic malignancy. Obstet Gynecol 2015; 125(2): 434-7.
[http://dx.doi.org/10.1097/AOG.0000000000000550] [PMID: 25569016]

[17] Qi Z, Zhang Y. Rare case of concurrent severe chylous ascites after radical surgery for cervical cancer. Eur J Gynaecol Oncol 2015; 36(3): 356-8.
[PMID: 26189272]

[18] DeStephano CC, Jernigan AM, Szymanski LM. Iatrogenic uterine diverticulum in pregnancy after robotic-assisted myomectomy. J Minim Invasive Gynecol 2015; 22(5): 902-5.
[http://dx.doi.org/10.1016/j.jmig.2015.03.016] [PMID: 25827328]

[19] US Food and Drug Administration. FDA approves a new silicone gel-filled breast implant. 2013 [August 18, 2013]; Available at: www.fda.gov/NewsEvents/Newsroom/PressAnnouncements/ucm356990.htm

[20] Brooks M. FDA approves new silicone breast implant. 2013 [August 18, 2013]; Available at: www.medscape.com/viewarticle/806432

[21] Vaamonde R, Cabrera JM, Vaamonde-Martín RJ, Jimena I, Marcos Martín J. Silicone granulomatous lymphadenopathy and siliconomas of the breast. Histol Histopathol 1997; 12(4): 1003-11.
[PMID: 9302562]

[22] Lappe MA. Silicone-reactive disorder: a new autoimmune disease caused by immunostimulation and superantigens. Med Hypotheses 1993; 41(4): 348-52.
[http://dx.doi.org/10.1016/0306-9877(93)90081-Z] [PMID: 8289701]

[23] Cohen Tervaert JW, Kappel RM. Silicone implant incompatibility syndrome (SIIS): a frequent cause of ASIA (Shoenfelds syndrome). Immunol Res 2013; 56(2-3): 293-8.
[http://dx.doi.org/10.1007/s12026-013-8401-3] [PMID: 23576058]

[24] Barageine JK, Tumwesigye NM, Byamugisha JK, Almroth L, Faxelid E. Risk factors for obstetric fistula in Western Uganda: a case control study. PLoS One 2014; 9(11): e112299.
[http://dx.doi.org/10.1371/journal.pone.0112299] [PMID: 25401756]

[25] Dobrosz Z, Paleń P, Stojko R, Właszczuk P, Niesłuchowska-Hoxha A, Piechuta-Kośmider I. Clear cell carcinoma derived from an endometriosis focus in a scar after a caesarean section a case report and literature review. Ginekol Pol 2014; 85(10): 792-5. [PMID: 25546933]

[26] Bakan M, Topuz U, Esen A, Basaranoglu G, Ozturk E. Inadvertent venous air embolism during cesarean section: Collapsible intravenous fluid bags without self-sealing outlet have risks. Case report. Braz J Anesthesiol 2013; 63: 362-5. [http://dx.doi.org/10.1016/j.bjane.2012.09.001]

[27] Dunne C, Meriano A. Acute postpartum pulmonary edema in a 23-year-old woman 5 days after cesarean delivery. CJEM 2009; 11(2): 178-81. [http://dx.doi.org/10.1017/S1481803500011179] [PMID: 19272222]

[28] Falzone E, Ricard JD, Pachy F, Mandelbrot L, Keïta H. [Amniotic fluid embolism: report of the successful outcome of a case with inaugural cardiac arrest and early DIVC complicated by hemoperitoneum of iatrogen origin and bleeding of an hepatic adenoma]. Ann Fr Anesth Reanim 2012; 31(10): 802-5. [http://dx.doi.org/10.1016/j.annfar.2012.07.004] [PMID: 22925937]

[29] Alani A, Sadlier M, Ramsay B, Ahmad K. Pyoderma gangrenosum induced by episiotomy. BMJ Case Rep 2016; 2016: bcr2015213574. [http://dx.doi.org/10.1136/bcr-2015-213574] [PMID: 26786531]

[30] Menard S, Poupon C, Bourguignon J, Theau A, Goffinet F, Le Ray C. Predictive factors of 2-month postpartum anal incontinence among patients with an obstetrical anal sphincter injury. J Gynecol Obstet Biol Reprod (Paris) 2016; 45(8): 900-7. [http://dx.doi.org/10.1016/j.jgyn.2015.12.008] [PMID: 26780843]

[31] Hermans FJ, Karolinski A, Othenin-Girard V, *et al.* Population differences and the effect of vaginal progesterone on preterm birth in women with threatened preterm labor. J Matern Fetal Neonatal Med 2015; 23: 1-6. [http://dx.doi.org/10.3109/14767058.2015.1121476] [PMID: 26586448]

[32] Geng C, Moteabbed M, Seco J, *et al.* Dose assessment for the fetus considering scattered and secondary radiation from photon and proton therapy when treating a brain tumor of the mother. Phys Med Biol 2016; 61(2): 683-95. [http://dx.doi.org/10.1088/0031-9155/61/2/683] [PMID: 26716718]

[33] Maggio L, Carr SR, Watson-Smith D, *et al.* Iatrogenic preterm premature rupture of membranes after fetoscopic laser ablative surgery. Fetal Diagn Ther 2015; 38(1): 29-34. [http://dx.doi.org/10.1159/000369250] [PMID: 25427832]

CHAPTER 11

Iatrogenic Pathology of the Male Genital System

Ioan Jung, Simona Gurzu* and **Sabin Turdean**

Department of Pathology, University of Medicine and Pharmacy, Tirgu-Mures, Romania

Abstract: Similar to the female genital system, the male genitalia can be injured by drugs or during diagnostic and/or therapeutic interventions. The drug-induced lesions of the male genitalia that are analyzed in this chapter include contact dermatitis, fixed drug eruptions, scrotal blisters and other specific lesions, such as red scrotum syndrome and scrotum hemangioma. Iatrogenic functional disorders are also presented in detail. The final section of this chapter is dedicated to surgical-related lesions of the male genitalia.

Keywords: Adverse drug reaction, Allergy, Circumcision, Dermatitis, Fixed drug eruption, Genital system, Gynecomastia, Hemangioma, Hyperplasia, Iatrogenic, Male genitalia, Prostate, Red scrotum syndrome, Urticaria.

DRUG-INDUCED LESIONS

Lesions of the External Genitalia

Local Irritation or Contact Dermatitis may be the result of local application of topical agents, such as miconazole [1].

Genital Fixed Drug Eruptions with/without genital ulcerations or necroses may occur following oral or systemic administration of several drugs (Table **11-1**). For example, in a 55-year-old man, a scrotal erythematous patch with pruritus was reported a few days after receiving miconazole and sulpiride for buccal mycosis. Three months later, the patient self-medicated with miconazole gel and the lesion reoccurred accompanied by a penile rash. This disappeared after drug cessation [1 - 6].

Scrotal Blisters can be seen in patients with chemotherapy-related hand-foot syndrome. Tyrosine kinase inhibitors, such as sorafenib, can be involved in their occurrence [7].

* **Corresponding author Simona Gurzu:** Department of Pathology, University of Medicine and Pharmacy, Tirgu-Mures, Romania; Tel: 0040-745-673550; Fax: 0040-372-653250; E-mail: simonagurzu@yahoo.com

Red Scrotum Syndrome is characterized by a burning or itching painful erythema of the scrotum and can be a side effect of topical steroids. Under the microscope, erythematotelangiectatic rosacea-like lesions can be seen [8].

Vitiligo of the penis and scrotum has been reported in males using imiquimod 5% cream for HPV-related condylomata accuminata, Bowen's disease, warts or superficial carcinoma [9].

Scrotum Hemangioma can develop in patients receiving the multi-targeted tyrosine kinase receptor inhibitor sunitinib. This progressively increasing lesion occurs approximately 20 days after the third cycle of targeted therapy. Ulceration can be associated [10].

Isolated Genital Edema is an angioneurotic edema that can occur in patients taking ACE inhibitors or other drugs [11]. Iatrogenic scrotal edema is especially frequently reported in children as a result of perfusion-related hyperhydration (Fig. **11-1**) or in patients with poorly controlled diabetes following administration of insulin [12].

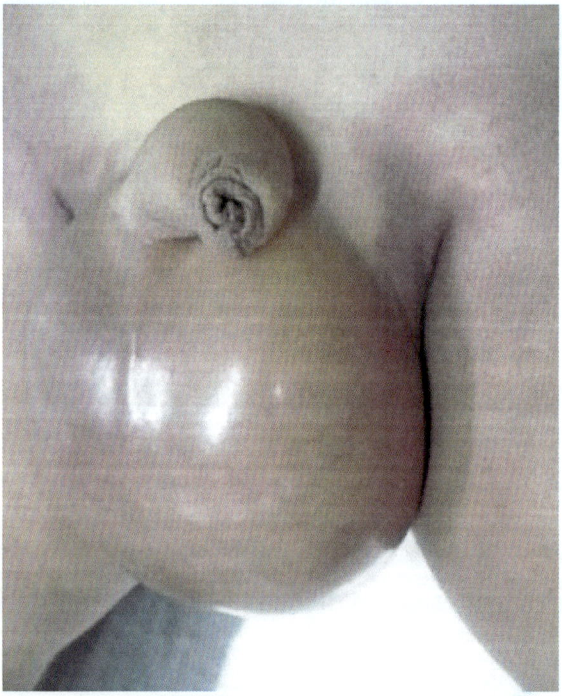

Fig. (11-1). Hyperhydration-related scrotal edema.

Functional Disorders and Hormone-Induced Lesions

Hypogonadism with Aspermia and Sterility can be produced by several drugs (Table **11-1**) and is difficult to differentiate from primary hypogonadism [13].

Sexual Dysfunctions can occur in patients taking antihypertensive drugs (*e.g.*, guanethidine) or psychotropics. These dysfunctions include diminished libido, delayed orgasm, ejaculatory disturbances (especially in the case of antipsychotics), gynecomastia, impotence (especially when taking antihypertensivcs) and priapism (Table **11-1**). Guanethidine inhibits prostate sperm production [14, 15]. Male infertility/germ cells apoptosis can also be caused, in a dose-dependent manner, by cytotoxic agents such as cyclophosphamide [16].

Estrogen-Induced Disorders relate to inhibition of gonadotropin release from the hypothalamus. This can lead to testicular atrophy, decreased libido and gynecomastia. Under the microscope, progressive disappearance of spermatogonia and Leydig cells is characteristic. This is a reversible lesion (following drug cessation) but fibrosis of the seminiferous tubules can emerge [13].

Antiandrogens-Induced Disorders also relate to impairment of the hypothalamic-pituitary-testicular axis. Transient sexual dysfunctions are common, but testicular atrophy, gynecomastia and cardiovascular lesions are more rare than following estrogen use [13, 17]. Details regarding these drugs are presented in Chapter 15.

Gynecomastia can be induced by more than 55 drugs/drug groups (Table **11-1**) and 10-20% of all cases are drug-induced [18 - 21].

Table 11-1. Drug-induced lesions of the male genitalia and breast. Data from references [1 - 25].

ADR type	Drugs
Genital fixed drug eruptions	Antifungals (ketoconazole), antiparasitic agents (metronidazole, miconazole) quinine, sulfonamides, NSAIDs (ibuprofen), antimalarials, antibiotics (amoxicillin), antihistamines, steroids
Genital ulcers/necroses	NSAIDs, antimalarials, ACE inhibitors, beta blockers, lithium, salicylates, steroids, trans-retinoic acid, vasoconstrictors (terlipressin), tyrosine kinase inhibitors (*e.g.*, sunitinib), mTOR inhibitors
Isolated genital edema	ACE inhibitors
Suppression of testicular function (aspermia, hypogonadism, ejaculatory dysfunctions)	Antiandrogens, estrogens, cimetidine, cytotoxic drugs (cyclophosphamide), beta blockers, antiarrhythmic drugs, digitalis, spironolactone (aldactone), phenothiazine, salazosulfapyridine, reserpine, guanethidine, psychotropics, steroids, isoniazid

(Table 11-1) contd.....

ADR type	Drugs
Impotence	Antihypertensives (methyldopa, guanethidine, clonidine, propranolol)
Hyperprolactinemia with decreased libido and erectile dysfunction	Neuroleptics, antihypertensives, antiemetics, estrogens, antiandrogens
Prostate hyperplasia	Estrogens, antiandrogens, anabolic androgenic steroids
Gynecomastia	ACE inhibitors (captopril, enalapril), amiodarone, calcium channel blockers (amlodipine), anabolic steroids (*e.g.,* fluoxymesterone), androgen hormone inhibitors (finasteride, cyproterone acetate), atorvastatin, benserazide, beta blockers (nebivolol), cimetidine, cladribine, cytotoxic drugs, cyclosporine, dasatinib, diazepam, didanosine, diethylpropion, digoxin, diltiazem, domperidone, D-penicillamine, estrogens, etretinate, efavirenz (HIV), fenofibrate, finasteride, fluorenone, fluoxetine, gabapentin, H1-antihistamines (ebastine), highly active retroviral therapy, imatinib, indinavir, isoniazid, ketoconazole, Marinol, methotrexate, metronidazole, nettle, nifedipine, omeprazole, paroxetine, phenytoin, pregabalin, ranitidine, reserpine, rosuvastatin, saquinavir, spironolactone, stavudine, sulindac, sulpiride, sunitinib, tandospirone, thalidomide, theophylline, tricyclic antidepressants, tuberculostatics (ethionamide), venlafaxine, verapamil, vincristine

Drug Effects on Spermatogenesis and Sperm Function

Many drugs can directly inhibit sperm or testicular function or indirectly affect spermatogenesis and sperm function by inhibiting the hypothalamic-testicular axis [17]. For sperm donation, it is necessary to be able to identify the drugs released through semen. For example, vismodegib, which is used for metastatic basal cell carcinoma and other solid malignancies, are detectable in blood and semen and patients cannot donate semen during treatment or within three months following the final dose of treatment [22].

Semen quality can also be impacted by several drugs, including antiepileptics. Of this group, carbamazepine and valproate affect sperm function, while lamotrigine does not. Sperm concentration, viability, motility and morphology are especially affected by valproate. Carbamazepine does not modify quantity, but concentration, progressive motility, motile/functional sperm count and morphology are impacted [23, 24].

The histamine-2 receptor antagonists, especially cimetidine, have also been proven to influence semen quality. Ranitidine and nizatidine rarely affect sperm function, while famotidine does not change semen parameters [25].

Lesions of the Prostate

These lesions can be produced by androgenic anabolic steroids or estrogens.

Androgenic steroids can increase the severity of prostate hyperplasia and can be a risk factor for prostate carcinoma. Estrogens can induce prostate infarction and squamous metaplasia [13].

IATROGENIC LESIONS DURING DIAGNOSTIC AND THERAPEUTIC PROCEDURES

Urethral Injuries can occur following urethral catheterization, cystourethroscopy and transurethral resection (TUR). Urethroplasty can be followed by bleeding, fistulae, wound dehiscence, hematoma, scrotal abscess, epididymitis, penile injuries (edema, numbness, skin ischemia), urosepsis, rectal injury, *etc.* [26].

Endoscopic Examination can be followed by hemorrhages, ascending infections, perforation of the urinary tract, fistulae and peritonitis. Special attention should be paid to diabetics and patients with low immunity. In diabetics, Klebsiella infection increases the risk of emphysematous prostatic abscess [27].

Transurethral Resection of the Prostate (TUR-P) is a relatively safe procedure with a complication rate of approximately 11%, increasing in patients with hyperplastic glands greater than 80 grams in size. The most common complications are hemorrhages, ascending infections, urethral stricture and TUR-P syndrome (acute salt and water retention). Urinary incontinence, bladder neck contracture, thrombosis and embolism are infrequently reported. Such complications are most frequent following monopolar as compared to bipolar TUR-P. Reoperation is necessary in 5% of cases and transfusions are required in 3%. The seeding of prostate cancer along a needle biopsy track is a rare but possible complication. Retrograde ejaculation occurs in half of patients. Patients' libidos and erections are not impacted [28 - 30].

Laparoscopic Radical or Robotic Prostatectomy can be followed by erectile dysfunctions, which can, in turn, be resolved *via* a minimally invasive infrapubic inflatable penile prosthesis implant [31]. However, laparoscopic resection of the prostate is the preferred method for large glands, with a lower complication rate and shorter catheterization time as compared to open prostatectomy [28, 29].

Testicular Biopsy has a low complication rate regarding hemorrhages, orchitis and periorchitis [13].

Orchiectomy can be accompanied by inflammation, pain, sexual dysfunctions (decreased libido, impotence), hot flashes, gynecomastia, osteoporosis (hyperestrogenism), fatigue, weight gain, muscular atrophy (decreasing number of ribosomes), depression, *etc.* Retroperitoneal lymph node dissection for testicular cancer can be associated with chylous ascites [32 - 34].

Circumcision is associated with a very low complication rate (0.2-0.6%). Bleeding, urethral lesions (fistulae, stricture of the meatus, iatrogenic hypospadias), wound infection, septicemia, hydrocele, and scrotal and lower limb lymphedema (especially in elderly patients with preexisting circulatory disorders) are the most common complications. Penile lesions refer, in adults, to pseudo-elephantiasis or giant elephantiasis. In children, radical circumcision can be followed by excessive penile skin denudation and the formation of circumferential scar tissue that pulls the penis proximally. This can lead to secondary phimosis, recurrent balanitis, voiding problems, sexual dysfunctions and social embarrassment. The most serious complication of neonatal circumcision is partial or complete glans amputation. The glans can be reattached in the first eight hours following amputation, but the risk of fistulae formation is a serious concern. In adults with neglected postoperative wound infections, chronic inflammation can lead to transformation into squamous cell carcinoma of the penis. Penile cancer surgery can be complicated by glans amputation [35 - 38].

Hypospadias Surgery is an intervention for which the complication rate depends on the age of the patient at surgery (the age recommended by the American Academy of Pediatrics is between six and 12 months), type of hypospadias, width of the urethral plate, type of stitch used for urethroplasty, surgical technique and type of urethral stent. Between 20% and 30% of patients undergoing this surgery present postoperative complications, such as urethrocutaneous fistulae, dehiscence of the neourethra and meatal disorders (stenosis, retraction and formation of urethral diverticulum) [39, 40].

Postoperative Genital Lymphedema is reported following biopsy or dissection of inguinal nodes and as a complication of aortobifemoral bypass grafting. Its manifestations are genitalia heaviness, hydrocele, preputial swelling, micturition disturbances and leakage of lymphatic fluid. Lower limb lymphedema with/without erysipelas can also be associated [41].

Iatrogenic Priapism can be induced by intracavernosal injection of vasoactive agents, such as alprostadil, that are used for diagnostic purposes or to treat erectile dysfunctions [42].

Hernia Repair Surgery can be complicated by damage to the femoral/epigastric/spermatic vessels. "Corona mortis" is an anatomical variant characterized by the presence of an anastomosis between the obturator and the external iliac or inferior epigastric arteries or veins, located behind the superior pubic ramus at a variable distance from the symphysis pubis. This can be accidentally cut and a severe hemorrhage with difficult hemostasis can occur. Other organs and structures, such as the bladder, testes, intestine and liver, can also be damaged. Postoperatively, wound infections, testicular edema, atrophy or necrosis, intestinal fistulae/ileus and formation of foreign body granulomas (involving surgical thread, mesh) are the most common complications [43].

CONFLICT OF INTEREST

The authors confirm that this chapter content has no conflict of interest.

ACKNOWLEDGEMENTS

Declared none.

REFERENCES

[1] Kastalli S, El Aïdli S, Lakhoua G, Daghfous R. Genital fixed drug eruption induced by miconazole with positive provocation test. Tunis Med 2014; 92(11): 703.
[PMID: 25867162]

[2] Eubel J, Diepgen TL, Weisshaar E. [Allergic diseases in the genital area]. Hautarzt 2015; 66(1): 45-52.
[http://dx.doi.org/10.1007/s00105-014-3561-1] [PMID: 25532902]

[3] Lonsdale-Eccles E, Wallett A, Ward AM. A case of fixed drug eruption secondary to quinine in tonic water presenting to a sexual health clinic. Sex Transm Infect 2014; 90(5): 356-7.
[http://dx.doi.org/10.1136/sextrans-2013-051458] [PMID: 24583965]

[4] Saka B, Kombaté K, Médougou BH, *et al.* [Fixed drug eruption in dermatology setting in Lomé (Togo): a retrospective study of 321 cases]. Bull Soc Pathol Exot 2012; 105(5): 384-7.
[http://dx.doi.org/10.1007/s13149-012-0237-x] [PMID: 22669581]

[5] Roett MA, Mayor MT, Uduhiri KA. Diagnosis and management of genital ulcers. Am Fam Physician 2012; 85(3): 254-62.
[PMID: 22335265]

[6] Ozel Coskun BD, Karaman A, Gorkem H, Buğday I, Poyrazoğlu OK, Senel F. Terlipressin-induced ischemic skin necrosis: a rare association. Am J Case Rep 2014; 15: 476-9.
[http://dx.doi.org/10.12659/AJCR.891084] [PMID: 25360696]

[7] Guerra JR, Suelves AM, Bella A, Lolo D. Hand, foot and scrotal blisters in a patient with cancer receiving oral chemotherapy. BMJ Case Rep 2014; 2014: bcr2013202822.
[http://dx.doi.org/10.1136/bcr-2013-202822] [PMID: 24842353]

[8] Narang T, Kumaran MS, Dogra S, Saikia UN, Kumar B. Red scrotum syndrome: idiopathic neurovascular phenomenon or steroid addiction? Sex Health 2013; 10(5): 452-5.
[http://dx.doi.org/10.1071/SH13052] [PMID: 24028828]

[9] Li W, Xin H, Ge L, Song H, Cao W. Induction of vitiligo after imiquimod treatment of condylomata acuminata. BMC Infect Dis 2014; 14: 329.
[http://dx.doi.org/10.1186/1471-2334-14-329] [PMID: 24928346]

[10] Tonini G, Intagliata S, Cagli B, *et al.* Recurrent scrotal hemangiomas during treatment with sunitinib. J Clin Oncol 2010; 28(35): e737-8.
[http://dx.doi.org/10.1200/JCO.2010.30.4865] [PMID: 20823408]

[11] Miller DG, Sweis RT, Toerne TS. Penile angioedema developing after 3 years of ACEI therapy. J Emerg Med 2012; 43(2): 273-5.
[http://dx.doi.org/10.1016/j.jemermed.2011.05.102] [PMID: 22560272]

[12] Lwo FS, Lee YJ. Insulin edema in a diabetic child. J Formos Med Assoc 1995; 94(8): 509-11. [PMID: 7549583]

[13] Jung J, Ed. Patologie iatrogenă. Tîrgu-Mureş, Romania: University Press 2006.

[14] Smith PJ, Talbert RL. Sexual dysfunction with antihypertensive and antipsychotic agents. Clin Pharm 1986; 5(5): 373-84. [PMID: 2872991]

[15] Labbate LA. Psychotropics and sexual dysfunction: the evidence and treatments. Adv Psychosom Med 2008; 29: 107-30. [http://dx.doi.org/10.1159/000126627] [PMID: 18391560]

[16] Zhu B, Zheng YF, Zhang YY, *et al.* Protective effect of L-carnitine in cyclophosphamide-induced germ cell apoptosis. J Zhejiang Univ Sci B 2015; 16(9): 780-7. [http://dx.doi.org/10.1631/jzus.B1500015] [PMID: 26365120]

[17] Amory JK. Drug effects on spermatogenesis. Drugs Today (Barc) 2007; 43(10): 717-24. [http://dx.doi.org/10.1358/dot.2007.43.10.1131829] [PMID: 17987224]

[18] Nuttall FQ, Warrier RS, Gannon MC. Gynecomastia and drugs: a critical evaluation of the literature. Eur J Clin Pharmacol 2015; 71(5): 569-78. [http://dx.doi.org/10.1007/s00228-015-1835-x] [PMID: 25827472]

[19] Lo Andal ZC, Lantion-Ang FL. Fluoxymesterone-induced gynaecomastia in a patient with childhood aplastic anaemia. BMJ Case Rep 2015 2015.

[20] Jung HS, Park CH, Park YT, *et al.* Gynecomastia induced by H1-antihistamine (ebastine) in a patient with idiopathic anaphylaxis. Asia Pac Allergy 2015; 5(3): 187-90. [http://dx.doi.org/10.5415/apallergy.2015.5.3.187] [PMID: 26240797]

[21] Köklü E, Arslan Ş, Yüksel IO, Bayar N, Demirci D. Nebivolol-induced gynecomastia. J Pharmacol Pharmacother 2015; 6(3): 166-8. [http://dx.doi.org/10.4103/0976-500X.162009] [PMID: 26312003]

[22] Reyes-Habito CM, Roh EK. Cutaneous reactions to chemotherapeutic drugs and targeted therapy for cancer: Part II. Targeted therapy. J Am Acad Dermatol 2014; 71(2): 217.e1-217.e11. [http://dx.doi.org/10.1016/j.jaad.2014.04.013] [PMID: 25037801]

[23] Asadi-Pooya A, Farazdaghi M, Ashjazadeh N. Effects of carbamazepine on semen parameters in men with newly diagnosed epilepsy. Iran J Neurol 2015; 14(3): 168-70. [PMID: 26622983]

[24] Kose-Ozlece H, Ilık F, Cecen K, Huseyınoglu N, Serım A. Alterations in semen parameters in men wıth epilepsy treated with valproate. Iran J Neurol 2015; 14(3): 164-7. [PMID: 26622982]

[25] Banihani SA. Histamine-2 Receptor Antagonists and Semen Quality. Basic Clin Pharmacol Toxicol 2016; 118(1): 9-13. [http://dx.doi.org/10.1111/bcpt.12446] [PMID: 26176290]

[26] Martins FE, Kulkarni SB, Joshi P, Warner J, Martins N. Management of long-segment and panurethral stricture disease. Adv Urol 2015; 2015: 853914. [http://dx.doi.org/10.1155/2015/853914]

[27] Lee CY, Tsai HC, Lee SS, Chen YS. Concomitant emphysematous prostatic and periurethral abscesses due to Klebsiella pneumoniae: a case report and review of the literature. Southeast Asian J Trop Med Public Health 2014; 45(5): 1099-106. [PMID: 25417511]

[28] Sivarajan G, Borofsky MS, Shah O, Lingeman JE, Lepor H. The role of minimally invasive surgical techniques in the management of large-gland benign prostatic hypertrophy. Rev Urol 2015; 17(3): 140-9.

[PMID: 26543428]

[29] Parker DC, Simhan J. Management of complications after surgical outlet reduction for benign prostatic obstruction. Can J Urol 2015; 22 (Suppl. 1): 88-92.
[PMID: 26497349]

[30] Johnson MH, Khani F, Schaeffer EM. Iatrogenic extraprostatic extension of prostate cancer from a needle biopsy. Urol Case Rep 2015; 3(3): 56-8.
[http://dx.doi.org/10.1016/j.eucr.2015.01.011] [PMID: 26793501]

[31] Antonini G, Busetto GM, De Berardinis E, *et al.* Minimally invasive infrapubic inflatable penile prosthesis implant for erectile dysfunction: evaluation of efficacy, satisfaction profile and complications. Int J Impot Res 2016; 28: 4-8.
[http://dx.doi.org/10.1038/ijir.2015.33]

[32] Baniel J, Foster RS, Rowland RG, Bihrle R, Donohue JP. Management of chylous ascites after retroperitoneal lymph node dissection for testicular cancer. J Urol 1993; 150(5 Pt 1): 1422-4.
[PMID: 8411415]

[33] Shah SS, Ahmed K, Smith R, Mallina R, Akhbari P, Khan MS. Chylous ascites following radical nephrectomy: a case report. J Med Case Reports 2008; 2: 3.
[http://dx.doi.org/10.1186/1752-1947-2-3] [PMID: 18190695]

[34] Incrocci L, Hop WC, Wijnmaalen A, Slob AK. Treatment outcome, body image, and sexual functioning after orchiectomy and radiotherapy for Stage I-II testicular seminoma. Int J Radiat Oncol Biol Phys 2002; 53(5): 1165-73.
[http://dx.doi.org/10.1016/S0360-3016(02)02849-3] [PMID: 12128117]

[35] Sylla C, Diao B, Diallo AB, Fall PA, Sankale AA, Ba M. [Complications of circumcision. Report of 63 cases]. Prog Urol 2003; 13(2): 266-72.
[PMID: 12765062]

[36] Prakash J, Kumar M, Singh V, Sankhwar S. Giant penile elephantiasis after circumcision: a devastating complication. BMJ Case Rep 2013; 2013: bcr2013200780.
[http://dx.doi.org/10.1136/bcr-2013-200780] [PMID: 24042209]

[37] Ziylan O, Acar Ö, Özden BC, Tefik T, Dönmez MI, Oktar T. A practical approach for the correction of iatrogenic penile skin loss in children: Scrotal embedding technique. Turk J Urol 2015; 41(4): 235-8.
[http://dx.doi.org/10.5152/tud.2015.17048] [PMID: 26623155]

[38] Nasr R, Traboulsi SL, Abou Ghaida RR, Bakhach J. Iatrogenic penile glans amputation: major novel reconstructive procedure. Case Rep Urol 2013; 2013: 741980.
[http://dx.doi.org/10.1155/2013/741980]

[39] Appeadu-Mensah W, Hesse AA, Glover-Addy H, Osei-Nketiah S, Etwire V, Sarpong PA. Complications of hypospadias surgery: Experience in a tertiary hospital of a developing country. Afr J Paediatr Surg 2015; 12(4): 211-6.
[http://dx.doi.org/10.4103/0189-6725.172538] [PMID: 26712282]

[40] Gozar H, Ardelean M, Gurzu S. One-stage repair of proximal hypospadias using lateral penile flap-preliminary results in a single-center experience. Indian J Surg 2014; 76(2): 171-3.
[http://dx.doi.org/10.1007/s12262-013-0951-z] [PMID: 24891792]

[41] Vignes S, Trévidic P. [Lymphedema of male external genitalia: a retrospective study of 33 cases]. Ann Dermatol Venereol 2005; 132(1): 21-5.
[http://dx.doi.org/10.1016/S0151-9638(05)79190-0] [PMID: 15746602]

[42] Jiang P, Christakos A, Fam M, Sadeghi-Nejad H. Prophylactic phenylephrine for iatrogenic priapism: a pilot study with Peyronies patients. Korean J Urol 2014; 55(10): 665-9.
[http://dx.doi.org/10.4111/kju.2014.55.10.665] [PMID: 25324950]

[43] Darmanis S, Lewis A, Mansoor A, Bircher M. Corona mortis: an anatomical study with clinical implications in approaches to the pelvis and acetabulum. Clin Anat 2007; 20(4): 433-9. [http://dx.doi.org/10.1002/ca.20390] [PMID: 16944498]

CHAPTER 12

Iatrogenic Pathology of Bone Marrow and Lymphoid Tissue

Simona Gurzu* and **Ioan Jung**

Department of Pathology, University of Medicine and Pharmacy, Tirgu-Mures, Romania

Abstract: Bone marrow and lymphoid tissue can be damaged by medications or radiation and are particularly susceptible to injury in bone marrow transplant recipients. Iatrogenic bone marrow suppression is a common in-hospital complication, the therapeutic management of which is difficult. In patients with cancer, aggressive treatment usually induces bone marrow damage, but this can be prevented using specific colony-stimulating factors. Heparin-induced thrombocytopenia is a distinct lesion with unusual clinical features. Its two types of manifestation are presented in this chapter, together with other lymphoid tissue-specific iatrogenic disorders.

Keywords: Adverse drug reaction, Bone marrow, Chemotherapeutics, Iatrogenic, Infection, Lymphoid tissue, Radiation, Sepsis, Thrombocytopenia, Thrombocytosis, Thromboembolism, Thrombosis, Transplant.

INTRODUCTION

Iatrogenic lesions of the bone marrow are primarily induced by medications, radiation and drugs that are administered before bone marrow transplantation. These can also be complications of diagnostic and therapeutic procedures (lymphography, silicone implant, *etc.*).

DRUG-INDUCED LESIONS

Similar to other organs and systems, drug-induced lesions of the bone marrow occur as a result of direct toxicity, immune mechanisms or idiosyncrasy. The most common ADR is bone marrow suppression and subsequent granulocytopenia, aplastic anemia, thrombocytopenia or pancytopenia. Thrombocytopenia and hemolytic anemia can emerge through immune-mediated formation of antiplatelets antibodies.

* **Corresponding author Simona Gurzu:** Department of Pathology, University of Medicine and Pharmacy, Tirgu-Mures, Romania; Tel: 0040-745-673550; Fax: 0040-372-653250; E-mail: simonagurzu@yahoo.com

Suppression of Hematopoiesis

Drug-induced bone marrow suppression is histologically characterized by hypoplasia, aplasia, panmyelophthisis or myelofibrosis (atrophy of bone marrow hematopoietic tissue and its replacement with connective tissue). The specific drug-related side effects are presented in Table **12-1**.

Chloramphenicol is the main drug known to induce myelotoxicity, which is more pronounced in the erythroid series. In most patients, this involves a dose-related anemia with reticulocytopenia, decreased erythrocytes and erythrocytes precursors production, infrequent leukopenia and thrombocytopenia. This effect is reversible and occurs during treatment. The erythroid cell precursors decrease until the first day of treatment and begin to regenerate from the seventh day of treatment. Dose-independent erythropoiesis inhibition leads to aplastic anemia. This reaction is reported in 1:24,000-1:40,000 of users, occurs within weeks or months of treatment and is often irreversible. Chloramphenicol also inhibits ribosomal protein synthesis [1, 2].

Phenylbutazone is the second drug known to demonstrate dose- and time-dependent myelotoxicity. This drug, which is primarily used to treat pain and fever in horses and was historically prescribed in sports medicine, is no longer available in the United States. Phenylbutazone-related myelotoxicity primarily refers to the inhibition of granulocytopoiesis, but myelophthisis and aplastic anemia can also be induced. Regarding its role in carcinogen-inducing blood dyscrasia, it has been proven that the cytogenetic effect is possible only in extremely high doses and phenylbutazone is thus not considered a carcinogenic substance in humans [3 - 5].

Chemotherapeutics induce dose-related leukopenia, emerging after the first or second cycle of administration. Thrombocytopenia and aplastic anemia can also be induced. The combination of chemotherapeutic drugs increases the risk of leukopenia and bone marrow aplasia with subsequent risk of infections, sepsis, hemorrhages, *etc*. (Fig. **12-1**). For example, the combination of paclitaxel and carboplatin induces anemia and neutropenia in about half of patients. Despite this, grade 3-4 toxicity occurs in fewer than 15% of such patients and can be prevented through administration of granulocyte colony-stimulating factor. Due to the fact that cisplatin is highly myelotoxic, there is a tendency to use carboplatin instead [1, 6].

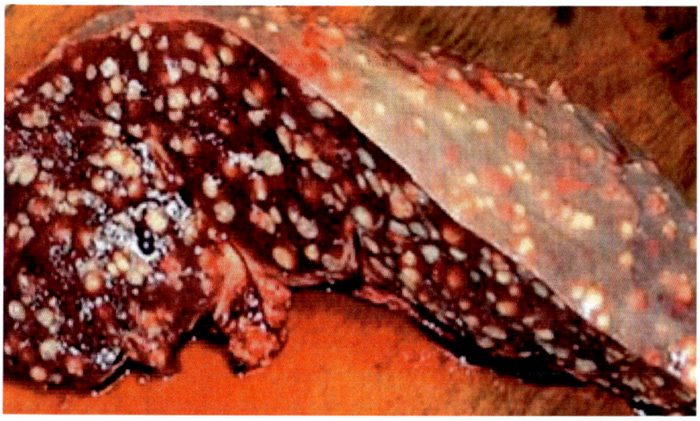

Fig. (12-1). Spleen mycotic granulomas in an immunosuppressed patient.

Antithyroid (thyreostatic) Drugs can produce leukopenia and, more rarely, anemia, thrombocytopenia, agranulocytosis (0.25-1.75% of patients) and myelophthisis. The side effects can be dose-dependent or induced through idiosyncrasy [7, 8].

Anticonvulsant/antiepileptic Drugs can induce myelotoxicity, but this dose- and time-dependent side effect is rare. Neutropenia, agranulocytosis and panmyelopathy have also been reported. The most common consequences are opportunistic infections (*e.g.,* Clostridium difficile) and sepsis [1, 9 - 13].

Besides the above-mentioned drugs, myelotoxicity can also be induced by heparin, PPIs, antidepressant drugs, *etc.* Some vitamin K antagonists, such as ***fluindione***, can lead to agranulocytosis within one month of the initiation of treatment [14]. ***Azathioprine***, used for inflammatory bowel diseases, may induce fatal myelotoxicity, even after standard dosing [15]. ***PPIs*** can induce thrombocytopenia and anemia in a dose-dependent manner [16, 17]. ***Antidepressant selective serotonin reuptake inhibitors,*** such as sertraline, can cause coagulation abnormalities [18].

Drug-Induced Hemolytic Anemia is uncommon in daily practice, but its incidence has increased in recent years as a result of the widening therapeutic arsenal. It can be produced by several drugs (Table **12-1**), including NSAIDs (*e.g.,* nimesulide), antibiotics (meropenem, dapsone, *etc.*), long-term adalimumab treatment (in patients with psoriasis), chloramphenicol, nitrofurantoin, furazolidone, phenacetin, phenothiazine, salicylates, sulfonamides, *etc.* [1, 19 - 21]. Dose-dependent hemolytic anemia is induced by intravenous immunoglobulin in fewer than 0.5% of patients [22].

Chemotherapeutics can induce immune-mediated hemolysis. A few cases are reported in the literature indicating the risk of hemolytic anemia following carboplatin- or paclitaxel-based regimens [23].

Thrombocytopenia is a consequence of drug-related myelotoxicity, and can also emerge as the result of immune-mediated interaction between drugs and platelets. It can be reversible following drug cessation, such as in the case of NSAIDs, or persistent after completion of treatment, such as in patients treated with gold salts. The most common consequences are hemorrhages and thrombocytopenic purpura [1, 19, 24].

Several drugs, including antibiotics, NSAIDs and hypolipidemic agents such as fenofibrate, can be responsible for *immune-mediated thrombocytopenia* (Table **12-1**). Some drugs, such as cephalothin and sulfamethoxazole, are bound by the platelet membrane, inducing synthesis of antiplatelets antibodies. Other substances, such as quinidine or alpha-methyldopamine, induce the formation of immune complexes that stimulate intrasplenic destruction of the platelets [1, 19, 24].

Aspirin induces thrombocytopenia through an irreversible inhibition of thromboxane synthesis and ADP-mediated platelet aggregation. Sulfinpyrazone, penicillin and cephalosporins inhibit platelet adhesion to the subendothelial structures. Dipyridamole is a phosphodiesterase inhibitor that inhibits platelet aggregation. Dextran inhibits the activity of platelets through their immune-mediated interaction with coagulation factor VIII and fibrin polymerization [1, 25].

Heparin-induced thrombocytopenia is a distinct lesion occurring as a rare complication of heparin therapy, with unusual clinical features. There are two types of this disorder. In some patients, a slight, reversible and asymptomatic decrease in the number of platelets can be seen in the first two days of treatment, as a result of the direct effect of heparin on platelets. The second type, which is also called *heparin-induced thrombocytopenia and thrombosis,* is rare but underrecognized, occurs between four and 10 days after exposure to heparin, and is primarily asymptomatic. The mechanism involves the transactivation of antibody-mediated platelets by monocytes linked with surface-bound platelet factor 4. The result is an aberrant risk of venous or arterial thromboembolism. In about 1% of heparin users, immune-mediated arterial and venous thrombosis (deep venous thrombosis, pulmonary embolism, myocardial infarction) are noted. Type 2 heparin-induced thrombocytopenia and thrombosis should be suspected in patients with platelet levels decreased to 50% of their normal value, even if the absolute platelet count remains above $150x10^9/L$. Clinically, such patients can present skin injuries at heparin injection sites or acute systemic reactions [26 - 31]. In one of our cases, a 63-year-old diabetic female who had undergone surgery for an umbilical hernia experienced delayed wound healing, and anticoagulant therapy with fraxiparine was thus initiated. After five weeks of treatment, sudden death occurred as a result of a massive thromboembolism of the right pulmonary artery trunk (Fig. **12-2**). All of the coagulation parameters and the serum platelets level were within normal limits.

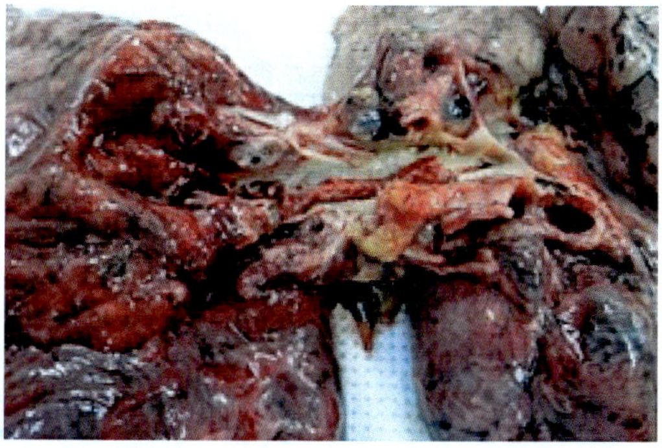

Fig. (12-2). Thromboembolism of the right pulmonary artery trunk in a patient receiving heparin-based therapy.

Reactive Thrombocytosis

Thrombocytosis involves a platelet count of over 450×10^9 platelets/L. Drug-induced thrombocytosis is a rare event that can occur in long-term corticosteroids users [32, 33] or induced by antibiotics, such as ceftazidime and amoxicillin with clavulanate [34]. It can also be a side effect of the antiviral ribavirin or can occur in patients receiving targeted therapy with erlotinib (an anti-EGFR agent used for lung and prostate cancer) or ruxolitinib (used in treatment of primary myelofibrosis and other hematological disorders) [35 - 37]. Transient thrombo- cytosis has also been reported in patients taking drugs for psychiatric disorders (*e.g.*, clozapine) [38]. In patients with psoriasis, efalizumab therapy can induce thrombocytosis [39]. *Heparin-related aberrant thrombocytosis* is a very rare event that has been reported in patients treated with enoxaparin [40].

Table 12-1. Drug-induced hematologic abnormalities.

ADR	Drugs
Aplastic anemia	Cytotoxic drugs (*e.g.*, cyclophosphamide, azathioprine, methotrexate), phenylbutazone, gold salts, anticonvulsants (hydantoin)

(Table 12-1) contd.....

ADR	Drugs
Hemolytic anemia	Methyldopa, penicillin, procainamide, hydralazine, augmentin (amoxicillin with clavulanate), meropenem, dapsone, NSAIDs (nimesulide), nitrofurantoin, chloramphenicol, adalimumab, serum sickness, furazolidone, phenacetin, phenothiazine, carboplatin, paclitaxel
Thrombocytopenia	Heparin, dipyridamole, aspirin, thyreostatic drugs, augmentin (amoxicillin with clavulanate), penicillin, sulfamethoxazole, sulfasalazine, cephalosporins, beta blockers, quinidine, alpha-methyldopamine, sulfinpyrazone, local anesthetics, antihistamines, antidepressants, corticosteroids, PPIs, NSAIDs (nimesulide, phenylbutazone, indomethacin), fenofibrate, gold salts, dextrans, serum sickness (thrombotic thrombocytopenic purpura)
Neutropenia/agranulocytosis	Cytotoxic drugs (cyclophosphamide, cisplatin), phenylbutazone, thyreostatic drugs (carbimazole, methimazole, propylthiouracil), antiepileptics (carbamazepine, pregabalin, levetiracetam, lamotrigine), vitamin K antagonists (fluindione)
Leukocytosis/leukopenia	Neuroleptic/antidepressant drugs (imipramine, haloperidol, benperidol, lithium), augmentin (amoxicillin with clavulanate), thyreostatic drugs, cytotoxic drugs (cisplatin, carboplatin, paclitaxel, cabazitaxel)
Bone marrow suppression – other drugs	Cytotoxic drugs, immunosuppressive drugs (azathioprine), sulfonamides, antidiabetics, analgesics, *etc*.
Polycythemia	Hematopoietic growth factors (dose-dependent effect)
Coagulopathy	Colloid expanders, antidepressants (sertraline)
Reactive thrombocytosis	Corticosteroids, augmentin (amoxicillin with clavulanate), ceftazidime, ciprofloxacin, antifungal agents, ribavirin, erlotinib, ruxolitinib, clozapine, heparin, efalizumab
Lymphadenopathy	Serum sickness, antiepileptic drugs (phenytoin, phenobarbital, carbamazepine), cytotoxic drugs, corticosteroids, sulfonamides, metronidazole, minocycline, allopurinol, antivirals (nevirapine, abacavir), polyvinylpyrrolidone
Lymphoproliferative disorders	Corticosteroids, azathioprine, methotrexate, cyclosporine, anticonvulsants, antidepressants, tamoxifen, amlodipine, dapsone, ACE inhibitors
Splenomegaly	Serum sickness
Sarcoid-like granulomatosis	TNF-α blockers (adalimumab, ipilimumab, etanercept), interferon, vildagliptin, cancer vaccines

Disorders of the Lymphatic System

Lymphadenopathy can be a side effect of several drugs (Table **12-1**) but is primarily associated with the consumption of anticonvulsants (phenytoin, phenobarbital, carbamazepine). It can be accompanied by cutaneous rash, gingival hyperplasia and bone marrow suppression, and primarily involves the cervical nodes, though generalized lymphadenopathy has also been noted. Under the microscope, normal lymph node architecture is replaced by the proliferation of reticulocytes and histiocytes, mixed with inflammatory infiltrate (neutrophils, plasmocytes and eosinophils), and necrotic and fibrotic areas. Noncaseating granulomatous lymphadenitis can also be observed. Differential diagnosis should take into account the infectious mononucleosis and angioimmunoblastic, as well as Hodgkin's lymphomas. Other substances, such as plasma expanders (*e.g.*, polyvinylpyrrolidone) or contrast agents (Fig. **12-3**), can be stored in the lymph nodes and induce formation of foreign body granulomas [1, 41, 42].

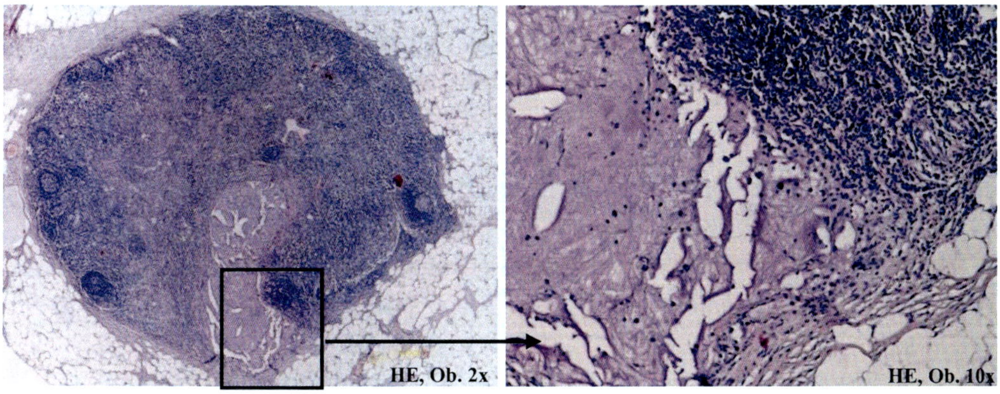

Fig. (12-3). Contrast agent stored in the perirectal lymph nodes after a contrast agent-based MRI scan.

Vaccine-Related Lesions of the Lymph Nodes are frequently reported after BCG vaccination. In most cases, asymptomatic lymphadenopathy is noted. The axillar, supraclavicular and inguinal lymph nodes can be involved. In infants receiving the vaccine a short time after birth, lymphadenopathy can be more pronounced. Accumulation of a large amount of caseous necrosis can initiate fistulae formation. Tuberculous granulomas can occur within between two and four months of BCG vaccination. In immunosuppressed patients, disseminated tuberculosis can emerge [1, 43].

Intranodal Necrosis accompanied by fibrotic areas and infrequent reticulocytes hyperplasia is a common lesion induced by chemotherapeutics [1].

Atrophy of Lymphatic Tissue can be induced by corticosteroids. Compensatory hyperplasia of macrophages is usually associated [1]. Thymus atrophy can be induced by cyclophosphamide [44].

Hyperplasia of the Splenic Germinal Centers and an increasing number of IgG-positive plasma cells in the splenic red pulp has been reported in experimental studies in animals treated with antithyroid drugs for 14 days [8].

Sarcoid-Like Granulomatosis can emerge in the cervical/axilar lymph nodes and in the bone marrow, with or without pulmonary involvement, months after administration of TNF-α blockers [45, 46], but also after vildagliptin, a lymphocyte inhibitor used in patients receiving hemodialysis [47].

Pseudolymphomas can be induced by anticonvulsants, antidepressants, cyclosporine, tamoxifen, amlodipine, dapsone and ACE inhibitors. Phenytoin-induced pseudolymphomas are usually T-cell predominant, involve the skin, and can mimic mycosis fungoides. B-cell lymphoproliferative disorders are primarily associated with antidepressants [48, 49].

IATROGENIC LESIONS DURING DIAGNOSTIC AND THERAPEUTIC PROCEDURES

Lymphography is a safety technique used extensively with a relatively low rate of complications. In oil-based lymphography, oleogranuloma formation in the lymph nodes can lead to intranodal hyalinization or reactive histiocytosis, usually without clinical impact. Differential diagnosis should consider Whipple's disease, sarcoid-like granulomatosis and idiopathic lipogranulomatosis [1, 45, 46]. Cerebral and renal lipid embolization are also reported [50].

Silicone Implants can be followed by migration of the silicone particles into the lymph nodes inducing foreign body granuloma formation. This lesion is known as silicone granulomatous lymphadenopathy, or siliconoma [51].

Heart Valve Implantation induces hemolysis, in fewer than 4% of cases, as a result of direct mechanic effect, structural deterioration or paravalvular leak. The process is usually asymptomatic but postoperative anemia can be associated [1, 52, 53].

General Anesthesia-Related Bone Marrow Suppression is an infrequent but severe lesion. Exposure to nitric oxide for more than six hours can induce temporary suppression of megaloblastic hematopoiesis [54].

Reactive (Secondary) Thrombocytosis occurs in more than 70% of patients undergoing *splenectomy,* but generally presents a spontaneous resolution without thrombotic complications. Severe thrombotic events involving the peripheral extremities, lungs, brain and myocardial arteries are infrequently reported. Retinal vein occlusion with subsequent loss of vision can also emerge [55]. During splenectomy, damage to blood vessels can induce hemorrhages and/or thrombosis. Intraoperative injuries of the surrounding organs (stomach, pancreas, intestine, kidney) can lead to pancreatitis, peritonitis, *etc*.

Self-limited reactive thrombocytosis is reported following *surgical procedures and delivery,* and can be followed by postoperative thromboembolic complications. The supposed mechanism involves the activation of platelets *via* increased levels of thrombopoietin, interleukin-6, interferon gamma and catecholamines [32, 56].

Because reactive thrombocytosis can be a consequence of severe tissue injuries, this lesion is also reported following *electrical injuries* [57]. In ICUs the long-term *insertion of indwelling catheters* (central venous catheter, pacemaker, defibrillator leads) causes tissue lysis, inflammation and sepsis, with subsequent thrombocytosis and thrombosis of the upper extremities [32].

CONFLICT OF INTEREST

The authors confirm that this chapter content has no conflict of interest.

ACKNOWLEDGEMENTS

Declared none.

REFERENCES

[1] Jung J, Ed. Patologie iatrogenă. Tîrgu-Mureş, Romania: University Press 2006.

[2] Turton JA, Fagg R, Sones WR, Williams TC, Andrews CM. Characterization of the myelotoxicity of chloramphenicol succinate in the B6C3F1 mouse. Int J Exp Pathol 2006; 87(2): 101-12. [http://dx.doi.org/10.1111/j.0959-9673.2006.00460.x] [PMID: 16623754]

[3] Black HM, Cox JS, Straughn WR. Use of phenylbutazone in sports medicine: understanding the risks. Am J Sports Med 1980; 8(4): 270-3. [http://dx.doi.org/10.1177/036354658000800411] [PMID: 7053221]

[4] Combes RD. Is phenylbutazone a genotoxic carcinogen? A weight-of-evidence assessment. Altern Lab Anim 2013; 41(3): 235-48. [PMID: 23971704]

[5] Lees P, Toutain PL. Pharmacokinetics, pharmacodynamics, metabolism, toxicology and residues of phenylbutazone in humans and horses. Vet J 2013; 196(3): 294-303. [http://dx.doi.org/10.1016/j.tvjl.2013.04.019] [PMID: 23721873]

[6] Yang L, Guo J, Shen Y, *et al.* Clinical efficacy and safety of paclitaxel plus carboplatin as neoadjuvant chemotherapy prior to radical hysterectomy and pelvic lymphadenectomy for Stage IB2-IIB cervical cancer. Int J Clin Exp Med 2015; 8(8): 13690-8. [PMID: 26550314]

[7] Zwaveling-Soonawala N, Veenhoven RH, Wolfs TF, Bokma JA. [Agranulocytosis induced by an antithyroid drug in a 14-year-old girl]. Ned Tijdschr Geneeskd 2005; 149(2): 89-92. [PMID: 15688841]

[8] Fukui M, Fukui N, Sakai K, *et al.* Spleen-specific development of germinal centers in rats treated with antithyroid drugs. J Toxicol Pathol 2013; 26(4): 375-84.
[http://dx.doi.org/10.1293/tox.2013-0012] [PMID: 24526810]

[9] Invernizzi R, Ambaglio C, Quaglia F. A case of feverish neutropenia. Clin Case Rep 2014; 2(6): 336-7.
[http://dx.doi.org/10.1002/ccr3.122] [PMID: 25548642]

[10] Taberner Bonastre MT, Peralta Muñoz S, Boza FM, Gumà I Padró J, Padro J. Neutropenia secondary to exposure to levetiracetam. Tumori 2015; 101(5): e145-6.
[PMID: 26045109]

[11] Kino H, Suzuki H, Nakamura K, *et al.* Clostridium difficile infection induced by pregabalin-associated agranulocytosis. Intern Med 2014; 53(18): 2149-52.
[http://dx.doi.org/10.2169/internalmedicine.53.2085] [PMID: 25224205]

[12] Thistleton S, Grandidge L, Sharlala H, Adebajo A. A hunt for the source of sepsis. BMJ Case Rep 2014; 2014: bcr2014204169.
[http://dx.doi.org/10.1136/bcr-2014-204169] [PMID: 24962485]

[13] Yasui-Furukori N, Hashimoto K, Tsuruga K, Nakamura K. Comorbidity of Stevens-Johnson syndrome and neutropenia associated with lamotrigine: a case report. Gen Hosp Psychiatry 2014; 36(6): 761.e9-761.e11.
[http://dx.doi.org/10.1016/j.genhosppsych.2014.07.010] [PMID: 25169759]

[14] Ngo S, Benhamou Y, Armengol G, *et al.* [Agranulocytosis related to fluindione: A case report]. Rev Med Interne 2016; 37(1): 58-61.
[http://dx.doi.org/10.1016/j.revmed.2015.05.013] [PMID: 26096756]

[15] Slanar O, Chalupná P, Novotný A, Bortlík M, Krska Z, Lukás M. Fatal myelotoxicity after azathioprine treatment. Nucleosides Nucleotides Nucleic Acids 2008; 27(6): 661-5.
[http://dx.doi.org/10.1080/15257770802143905] [PMID: 18600523]

[16] Ruiz de Angulo D, Ortiz MA, Martínez de Haro LF. Side effects of proton-pump inhibitors: another reason to indicate anti-reflux surgery for Barretts esophagus? Cir Esp 2014; 92(5): 303-4.
[http://dx.doi.org/10.1016/j.ciresp.2014.01.009] [PMID: 24625629]

[17] Wilhelm SM, Rjater RG, Kale-Pradhan PB. Perils and pitfalls of long-term effects of proton pump inhibitors. Expert Rev Clin Pharmacol 2013; 6(4): 443-51.
[http://dx.doi.org/10.1586/17512433.2013.811206] [PMID: 23927671]

[18] Bassotti G, Nzepa FS, de Roberto G, Fischer MJ, Morelli A. Symptomatic reversible duodenal compression due to iatrogenic retroperitoneal hematoma. Dig Liver Dis 2004; 36(1): 78-81.
[http://dx.doi.org/10.1016/j.dld.2003.06.003] [PMID: 14971820]

[19] Sathiasekar AC, Deepthi DA, Sathia Sekar GS. Drug-induced thrombocytopenic purpura. J Pharm Bioallied Sci 2015; 7 (Suppl. 2): S827-9.
[http://dx.doi.org/10.4103/0975-7406.163595] [PMID: 26538982]

[20] Oka S, Shiragami H, Nohgawa M. Intravascular hemolytic anemia in a patient with antibodies related to meropenem. Intern Med 2015; 54(10): 1291-5.
[http://dx.doi.org/10.2169/internalmedicine.54.3385] [PMID: 25986273]

[21] Harada Y, Yamamoto H, Sato M, Kodaira M, Kono T. Autoimmune hemolytic anemia during adalimumab treatment for plaque psoriasis. Intern Med 2015; 54(9): 1103-4.
[http://dx.doi.org/10.2169/internalmedicine.54.3433] [PMID: 25948357]

[22] Luban NL, Wong EC, Henrich Lobo R, Pary P, Duke S. Intravenous immunoglobulin-related hemolysis in patients treated for Kawasaki disease. Transfusion 2015; 55 (Suppl. 2): S90-4.
[http://dx.doi.org/10.1111/trf.13089] [PMID: 26174904]

[23] Leger RM, Jain S, Nester TA, Kaplan H. Drug-induced immune hemolytic anemia associated with

anti-carboplatin and the first example of anti-paclitaxel. Transfusion 2015; 55(12): 2949-54. [http://dx.doi.org/10.1111/trf.13255] [PMID: 26264449]

[24] Agapakis DI, Massa EV. A case of fenofibrate-induced immune thrombocytopenia: first report. P R Health Sci J 2015; 34(3): 170-3. [PMID: 26356743]

[25] Gresele P, Momi S, Falcinelli E. Anti-platelet therapy: phosphodiesterase inhibitors. Br J Clin Pharmacol 2011; 72(4): 634-46. [http://dx.doi.org/10.1111/j.1365-2125.2011.04034.x] [PMID: 21649691]

[26] Srinivasan AF, Rice L, Bartholomew JR, *et al.* Warfarin-induced skin necrosis and venous limb gangrene in the setting of heparin-induced thrombocytopenia. Arch Intern Med 2004; 164(1): 66-70. [http://dx.doi.org/10.1001/archinte.164.1.66] [PMID: 14718324]

[27] Noel E, Abbas N, Skaradinskiy Y, Schreiber Z. Heparin-induced thrombocytopenia in a patient with essential thrombocythemia: a case based update. Case Rep Hematol 2015; 2015: 985253. [http://dx.doi.org/10.1155/2015/985253]

[28] Tutwiler V, Madeeva D, Ahn HS, *et al.* Platelet transactivation by monocytes promotes the prothrombotic state in heparin-induced thrombocytopenia. Blood 2015; 127(4): 464-72. [http://dx.doi.org/10.1182/blood-2013-11-539262] [PMID: 26518435]

[29] Warkentin TE, Greinacher A. Heparin-induced thrombocytopenia: recognition, treatment, and prevention: the Seventh ACCP Conference on Antithrombotic and Thrombolytic Therapy. Chest 2004; 126(3) (Suppl.): 311S-37S. [http://dx.doi.org/10.1378/chest.126.3_suppl.311S] [PMID: 15383477]

[30] Warkentin TE, Roberts RS, Hirsh J, Kelton JG. An improved definition of immune heparin-induced thrombocytopenia in postoperative orthopedic patients. Arch Intern Med 2003; 163(20): 2518-24. [http://dx.doi.org/10.1001/archinte.163.20.2518] [PMID: 14609790]

[31] Eke S, May SK. Heparin-induced thrombocytopenia. 2016 [08th January 2016]; Available at: http://emedicine.medscape.com/article/1357846-overview

[32] Mishra SB, Bhoyer J, Gurjar M, Muzaffar N, Verma A. Deep vein thrombosis of upper extremities due to reactive thrombocytosis in septic patients. Indian J Crit Care Med 2014; 18(8): 540-2. [http://dx.doi.org/10.4103/0972-5229.138162] [PMID: 25136196]

[33] Thapa SD, Hadid H, Imam W, *et al.* Persistent reactive thrombocytosis may increase the risk of coronary artery disease among inflammatory bowel disease patients. Dig Dis Sci 2015; 60(10): 3062-8. [http://dx.doi.org/10.1007/s10620-015-3701-1] [PMID: 25972153]

[34] Chen HC, Wang CY, Wang CS. Marked thrombocytosis during treatment with ceftazidime for pulmonary infection. Pharm World Sci 2008; 30(1): 70-2. [http://dx.doi.org/10.1007/s11096-007-9145-8] [PMID: 17619167]

[35] Kobayashi T, Hige S, Terashita K, *et al.* Anemia and thrombocytosis induced by ribavirin monotherapy in patients with chronic hepatitis C. J Gastroenterol 2012; 47(11): 1228-37. [http://dx.doi.org/10.1007/s00535-012-0579-y] [PMID: 22460221]

[36] Uwagawa T, Misawa T, Fujiwara Y, *et al.* Erlotinib-induced thrombocytosis in patients with recurrence of pancreatic cancer after distal pancreatectomy. Pancreas 2013; 42(7): 1196-7. [http://dx.doi.org/10.1097/MPA.0b013e31828cf976] [PMID: 24048463]

[37] Polverelli N, Catani L, Vianelli N, Baccarani M, Cavo M, Palandri F. Ruxolitinib- but not fedratinib-induced extreme thrombocytosis: the combination therapy with hydroxyurea and ruxolitinib is effective in reducing platelet count and splenomegaly/constitutional symptoms. Ann Hematol 2015; 94(9): 1585-7. [http://dx.doi.org/10.1007/s00277-015-2397-9] [PMID: 25975976]

[38] Atmaca M, Kilic F, Temizkan A, Ustundag B. What about platelet counts in clozapine users? Rev

Recent Clin Trials 2013; 8(2): 74-7.
[http://dx.doi.org/10.2174/1574887111308999004l] [PMID: 23863033]

[39] Firmin D, Roguedas AM, Lemasson G, Abgrall JF, Misery L. Eczematous dermatosis and thrombocytosis induced by efalizumab: two new side effects. Dermatology (Basel) 2008; 217(3): 203-6.
[http://dx.doi.org/10.1159/000141958] [PMID: 18594143]

[40] Tonbul A, Uras N, Tayman C, Halici T, Polat A, Mansur Tatli M. Thrombocytosis associated with enoxaparin: A very rare cause in newborns. Platelets 2010; 21(4): 300-2.
[http://dx.doi.org/10.3109/09537101003649807] [PMID: 20367573]

[41] Santhamoorthy P, Alexander KJ, Alshubaili A. Intravenous immunoglobulin in the treatment of drug rash eosinophilia and systemic symptoms caused by phenytoin. Ann Indian Acad Neurol 2012; 15(4): 320-2.
[http://dx.doi.org/10.4103/0972-2327.104348] [PMID: 23349605]

[42] Ovallath S, Remya RK, Kumar C, Nayanar S. Granulomatous lymphadenopathy secondary to phenytoin therapy. Seizure 2013; 22(3): 240-1.
[http://dx.doi.org/10.1016/j.seizure.2012.12.005] [PMID: 23280271]

[43] Mahmoudi S, Khaheshi S, Pourakbari B, *et al.* Adverse reactions to Mycobacterium bovis bacille Calmette-Guérin vaccination against tuberculosis in Iranian children. Clin Exp Vaccine Res 2015; 4(2): 195-9.
[http://dx.doi.org/10.7774/cevr.2015.4.2.195] [PMID: 26273579]

[44] Zhang H, Yu R, Liu X, Guo X, Zeng Z. The expression of PAC1 increases in the degenerative thymus and low dose PACAP protects female mice from cyclophosphamide induced thymus atrophy. Peptides 2012; 38(2): 337-43.
[http://dx.doi.org/10.1016/j.peptides.2012.09.009] [PMID: 23000307]

[45] Kanellopoulou T, Filiotou A, Kranidioti H, Dourakis SP. Sarcoid-like granulomatosis in patients treated with anti-TNFα factors. A case report and review of the literature. Clin Rheumatol 2011; 30(4): 581-3.
[http://dx.doi.org/10.1007/s10067-010-1603-3] [PMID: 20972592]

[46] Tong D, Manolios N, Howe G, Spencer D. New onset sarcoid-like granulomatosis developing during anti-TNF therapy: an under-recognised complication. Intern Med J 2012; 42(1): 89-94.
[http://dx.doi.org/10.1111/j.1445-5994.2011.02612.x] [PMID: 22389903]

[47] Sada KE, Wada J, Morinaga H, Tuchimochi S, Uka M, Makino H. Sarcoid-like lung granulomas in a hemodialysis patient treated with a dipeptidyl peptidase-4 inhibitor. Clin Kidney J 2014; 7(2): 182-5.
[http://dx.doi.org/10.1093/ckj/sft172] [PMID: 25852868]

[48] Riyaz N, Sasidharanpillai S, Aravindan KP, Nobin BK, Raghavan NT, Nikhila PK. Phenytoin induced cutaneous B Cell pseudolymphoma. Indian J Dermatol 2015; 60(5): 522.
[http://dx.doi.org/10.4103/0019-5154.164437] [PMID: 26538730]

[49] Rim MY, Hong J, Yo I, *et al.* Cervical lymphadenopathy mimicking angioimmunoblastic T-cell lymphoma after dapsone-induced hypersensitivity syndrome. Korean J Pathol 2012; 46(6): 606-10.
[http://dx.doi.org/10.4132/KoreanJPathol.2012.46.6.606] [PMID: 23323115]

[50] Winterer JT, Blum U, Boos S, Konstantinides S, Langer M. Cerebral and renal embolization after lymphography in a patient with non-Hodgkin lymphoma: case report. Radiology 1999; 210(2): 381-3.
[http://dx.doi.org/10.1148/radiology.210.2.r99fe09381] [PMID: 10207418]

[51] Vaamonde R, Cabrera JM, Vaamonde-Martín RJ, Jimena I, Marcos Martín J. Silicone granulomatous lymphadenopathy and siliconomas of the breast. Histol Histopathol 1997; 12(4): 1003-11.
[PMID: 9302562]

[52] Shapira Y, Vaturi M, Sagie A. Hemolysis associated with prosthetic heart valves: a review. Cardiol Rev 2009; 17(3): 121-4

[http://dx.doi.org/10.1097/CRD.0b013e31819f1a83] [PMID: 19384085]

[53] Hing JX, Macys A, Elshiekh MA, Momin A, Koertzen M, Punjabi PP. Haemolysis: the harbinger of recurrent mitral regurgitation after mitral valve repair. Perfusion 2014; 29(2): 184-6. [http://dx.doi.org/10.1177/0267659113505638] [PMID: 24043273]

[54] OSullivan H, Jennings F, Ward K, McCann S, Scott JM, Weir DG. Human bone marrow biochemical function and megaloblastic hematopoiesis after nitrous oxide anesthesia. Anesthesiology 1981; 55(6): 645-9.
[http://dx.doi.org/10.1097/00000542-198155060-00008] [PMID: 6975588]

[55] Oncel Acir N, Borazan M, Dadaci Z. Acute central retinal vein occlusion secondary to reactive thrombocytosis after splenectomy. Case Rep Ophtalmol Med 2014; 2014: 930843. [http://dx.doi.org/10.1155/2014/930843]

[56] Madaan GB, Jairajpuri ZS, Hajini FF, Jetley S. Postoperative thrombocytosis: An unusual case report. Int J Appl Basic Med Res 2015; 5(3): 225-7. [http://dx.doi.org/10.4103/2229-516X.165372] [PMID: 26539380]

[57] Katiyar R, Patne SC, Pankaj P. Post electric shock reactive thrombocytosis. J Clin Diagn Res 2015; 9(4): ED10-1.
[PMID: 26023559]

CHAPTER 13

Iatrogenic Pathology of the Skin and Subcutaneous Tissue

Simona Gurzu* and **Ioan Jung**

Department of Pathology, University of Medicine and Pharmacy, Tirgu-Mures, Romania

Abstract: The skin and liver are the most common organs affected by the side effects of drugs. Drug-related damage to the skin and subcutaneous tissue is presented in detail in this chapter. Benign lesions include contact dermatitis and eczematous eruptions. Severe drug-induced injuries include Stevens-Johnson syndrome (SJS), toxic epidermal necrolysis, drug reaction with eosinophilia and systemic symptoms (DRESS syndrome), acute generalized exanthematous pustulosis, bullous dermatoses and other hypersensitivity syndromes. The specific characteristics and responsible agents of these conditions are offered in tables in this chapter, and particular types of drug-induced lesions are also presented. A significant part of the chapter focuses on the effects of targeted cancer therapies on the skin and subcutaneous tissue. Granulomas and vaccine-induced lesions are also examined.

Keywords: Adverse drug reaction, Allergy, Antibody, Contact dermatitis, Dermatosis, DRESS syndrome, Eczema, eruption, Hyperpigmentation, Hypersensitivity, Iatrogenic, Pustulosis, Stevens-Johnson syndrome, Toxic epidermal necrolysis, Vitiligo.

DRUG-INDUCED LESIONS

Of all the organs and tissue of the human body, the skin and cutaneous annexes are the systems most commonly affected by ADRs. The incidence of CU-ADRs is 2-3% of all hospitalized patients and even higher in females and elderly patients [1 - 3]. In pediatric emergency departments, the incidence is about 1% [4].

Most CU-ADRs are induced through hypersensitivity reactions, but direct toxicity, idiosyncrasy, metabolic enzymatic deficiencies and other mechanisms can also be involved.

About 98% of CU-ADRs are benign lesions (Tables **13-1** and **13-2**), with only 2% showing severe evolution (Tables **13-3** and **13-4**). In pediatric emergency

* **Corresponding author Simona Gurzu:** Department of Pathology, University of Medicine and Pharmacy, Tirgu-Mures, Romania; Tel: 0040-745-673550; Fax: 0040-372-653250; E-mail: simonagurzu@yahoo.com

departments, 53% of CU-ADRs are benign. These benign lesions occur primarily in children between two and 11 years of age, whereas severe CU-ADRs are more common in children between the ages of 12 and 15. The severe CU-ADRs of childhood are commonly induced by drug overdose [4].

Benign lesions include maculopapular and eczematous eruptions, exanthema, urticaria, erythema multiforme, erythroderma, lichenoid and lupus-like reactions, vesicular lesions, necroses, hemorrhages, hyperpigmentation, atrophy, alopecia, *etc.* [5].

Severe CU-ADRs are known to have potential lethality or to produce lifelong sequelae [5, 6]. They are immune-mediated by the drug-antigen/HLA-T-cell receptor complex and genetic susceptibility is a major component of their occurrence [6, 7]. Elderly patients and carriers of HLA-B*15:02, HLA-B*58:01, HLA-B*59:01 and HLA-B*13:01 present an increased expression of cytotoxic cytokines in serum and tissues, thereby being more predisposed to develop severe CU-ADRs [3, 8]. Severe CU-ADRs include Stevens-Johnson syndrome (SJS), toxic epidermal necrolysis (TEN), drug reaction with eosinophilia and systemic symptoms (DRESS syndrome), linear immunoglobulin A (IgA) bullous dermatosis, acute generalized exanthematous pustulosis (AGEP), and the risk of pseudolymphoma, lymphoma and other tumors [7, 9 - 11].

Benign Lesions

Allergic Contact Dermatitis can be induced by cosmetics, drugs, laboratory chemicals, ultrasound gel, colophony, balsam of Peru, propolis, nickel sulfate, lanolin, pyocyanin, butylhydroquinone, surgical preparations of chlorhexidine and povidone-iodine, medical adhesives, topical neomycin/bacitracin, *etc.* [11 - 15].

Antiseptic bath emollients are frequently used in patients with eczema, which can induce local irritant reactions without significant clinical impact. In a few cases, large benzalkonium chloride-related ulcerations of the external genitalia were reported in young males, mimicking Fournier's gangrene [16].

In patients with carcinoma of the urinary bladder, granulomatous ulcerations at the base of the penis were reported one month following injection of intravesical BCG. In other patients, gangrene of the penis and perineum were seen within 24 hours of intravesical administration of mitomycin C, and penectomy was necessary three months after injection. The pathomechanism was the allergic contact reaction [17].

Eczematous Eruptions are primarily self-limited or present benign behavior. They can be induced by several drugs, including antimicrobial agents, NSAIDs, antihypertensives and anticonvulsants (Tables **13-1** and **13-2**). Exanthema (42%), erythema multiforme (10.5%) and vasculitis (9.5%) are the most common manifestations and are more severe in patients showing peripheral eosinophilia [18, 19].

Of all CU-ADRs produced by anti-infective drugs, radiographic contrast substances and NSAIDs, morbilliform exanthema (40%) and urticaria (23%) are predominant [2].

Eczematous dermatosis has been reported in patients with psoriasis treated with efalizumab [20], whereas acneiform eruptions can be induced by corticosteroids, iodides, bromides, anticonvulsants, isoniazid and immunosuppressants [21].

Table 13-1. Benign drug-related cutaneous lesions. Part I. Data from references [1-36].

Lesion	Drug class	Drug name
Eczematous eruptions	Antibiotics	Penicillins, Cephalosporins, Sulfonamides
	Diuretics	Thiazides
	Antihypertensives	Methyldopa, Beta blockers
	Anticonvulsants	Phenytoin, Phenobarbital, Carbamazepine
	Antidiabetics	Sulfonylurea
	Antipsychotics	Chlorpromazine Hydrochloride
	Other drugs	Quinidine, Bleomycin, Statins
Maculopapular eruptions	Antibacterial	Sulfonamides, Penicillins, Isoniazid
	Anticonvulsants	Phenytoin, Carbamazepine, Barbiturates
	Anti-inflammatory	NSAIDs, Sulfasalazine, Gold salts
	Antidiabetics	Sulfonylurea
	Antihypertensives	Captopril, Beta blockers
	Other drugs	Allopurinol, Bismuth, Carbimazole,
Urticaria	Anti-infective	Sulfonamides, Penicillins, Aminoglycosides, Cephalosporins, Vancomycin, Antifungals
	Anti-inflammatory	NSAIDs, Salicylates
	Antihypertensives	ACE inhibitors
	Contrast substances	Iodine-based radiographic contrast substances
	Vaccines	Animal serum, Desensitizing agents
	Other drugs	Anesthetic agents, Myorelaxants, Opiates, Dextrans

(Table 13-1) contd.....

Lesion	Drug class	Drug name
Erythema multiforme/ erythroderma	Anti-infective	Penicillins, Tetracyclines, Sulfonamides, Isoniazid, Nitrofurantoin
	Anticonvulsants	Phenytoin, Carbamazepine, Barbiturates
	Antipsychotics	Chlorpromazine, Phenothiazines, Lithium
	Other drugs	NSAIDs, Aspirin, Codeine phosphate, Thiazides, Omeprazole, Captopril, Cimetidine, Quinine, Sulfonylurea

Table 13-2. Benign drug-related cutaneous lesions. Part II. Data from references [1-36].

Lesion	Drug class	Drug name
Lichenoid reaction	Antihypertensive /Antiarrhythmics	Beta blockers, methyldopa, captopril, quinidine
	Anti-infective	P-aminosalicylic acid, tetracyclines, isoniazid, ethambutol, dapsone
	Anticonvulsants	Phenytoin, carbamazepine
	Immunosuppressives	Hydroxyurea, penicillamine, gold salts, bleomycin
	Antipsychotics	Phenothiazines, chloral hydrate
	Antimalarials	Mepacrine, chloroquine
	Other drugs	Sulfonylurea, iodides, quinine
Iatrogenic discoid/systemic lupus erythematosus	Diuretics	Thiazides (hydralazine)
	Antiarrhythmics	Procainamide, quinidine
	Tuberculostatics	Isoniazid
	Contraceptive pills	NS
Lipodystrophy	Subcutaneous injections	Insulin
Permanent alopecia	Oncologic regimens	Anthracycline with cyclophosphamide, docetaxel with carboplatin and trastuzumab, paclitaxel or docetaxel alone

Severe Lesions

Stevens-Johnson Syndrome (SJS) and Toxic Epidermal Necrolysis (TEN) are induced through HLA-related delayed type immune reactions and are characterized by widespread keratinocyte apoptosis [6 - 8]. SJS is defined as the presence of skin lesions over the whole body cutaneous area, covering less than 10% of the surface area, with lesion severity spanning from erythematous patches to large ulcerations and skin detachment. In cases of skin detachment involving more than 30% of the whole body surface area, the lesion is known as TEN. The SJS/TEN overlap is common and indicates skin detachment greater than 10% but less than 30% of the body surface area. These lesions occur between two and three weeks following drug use [22 - 25]. SJS/TEN can be induced by several drugs, including anticonvulsants, acetaminophen (Fig. **13-1**), allopurinol and anti-inflammatory agents (Tables **13-3** and **13-4**). The mortality rate is 5-10% for SJS, about 30% for SJS/TEN overlap, and 50% for TEN [8, 23 - 28].

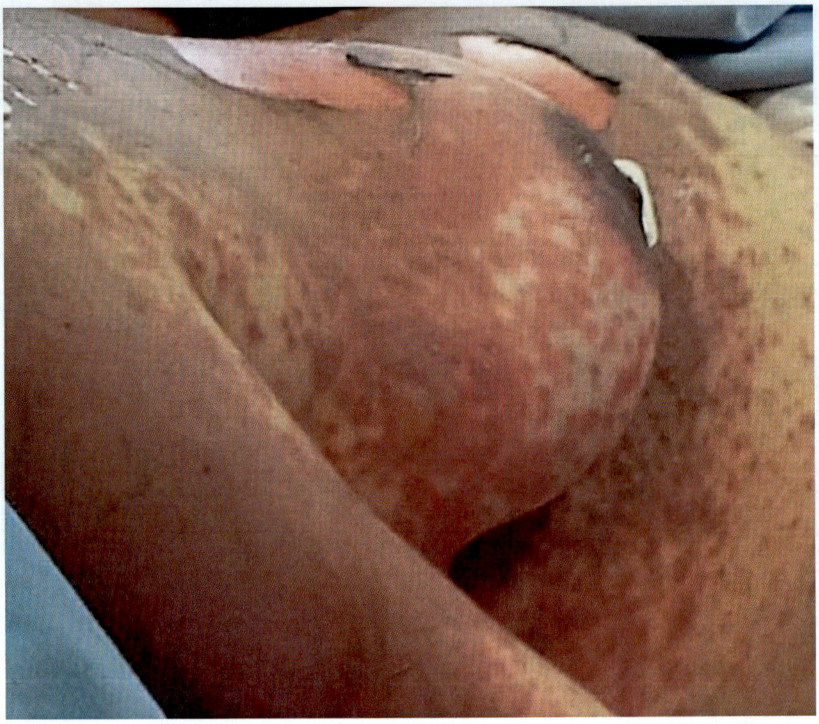

Fig. (13-1). Erythematous patches and large skin detachment areas induced by acetaminophen (courtesy of Prof. Tivadar Bara).

Drug Reaction with Eosinophilia and Systemic Symptoms (DRESS syndrome) refers to the association of cutaneous rash with systemic lesions, such as fever, hematologic abnormalities (eosinophilia, thrombocytopenia, atypical lymphocytes), lymphadenopathy, pseudolymphomas and visceral organ involvement. In patients with fixed drug eruptions, the immune-mediated DRESS syndrome mechanism involves viral reactivation and the presence of tissue resident memory T-cells in recurrent site-specific lesions [6, 7, 29]. DRESS syndrome can be induced by anticonvulsants, antibacterial agents, allopurinol, antivirals, *etc*. (Table **13-4**). It is a rare but life-threatening lesion with a mortality rate of about 10% [10, 19, 22, 29 - 31].

Table 13-3. Severe types of drug-related cutaneous lesions. Part I. Data from references [1-36].

Cutaneous lesion	Drug class	Drug name
Stevens-Johnson syndrome (SJS)	Anti-infective	Augmentin (amoxicillin with clavulanate), penicillins, D-penicillamine, ampicillin, sulfonamides, nitrofurantoin, tuberculostatics
	Anti-inflammatory	Aspirin, salazopyrin, phenylbutazone, methimazole, ibuprofen
	Analgesics/antipyretics	Acetaminophen
	Anticonvulsants	Phenytoin, phenobarbital, carbamazepine, lamotrigine, clozapine, barbiturates
	Antipsychotics	Phenothiazines
	Anti-hyperuricemia	Allopurinol

Table 13-4. Severe types of drug-related cutaneous lesions. Part II. Data from references [1 - 36].

Cutaneous lesion	Drug class	Drug name
Toxic epidermal necrolysis (TEN)	Anti-infective	Sulfonamides, penicillins, tetracyclines nitrofurantoin, chloramphenicol
	Analgesics/antipyretics	Opiates, codeine phosphate, acetaminophen
	Anti-inflammatory	NSAIDs, aspirin, gold salts
	Cytotoxics	Cyclophosphamide, methotrexate, adriamycin, mithramycin
	Anticonvulsants	Phenytoin, carbamazepine, barbiturates
	Antidiabetics	Sulfonylurea
	Anti-hyperuricemia	Allopurinol
Drug reaction with eosinophilia and systemic symptoms (DRESS syndrome)	Anticonvulsants	Phenytoin, phenobarbital, carbamazepine, levetiracetam
	Antibacterial	Sulfonamides, sulfasalazine, metronidazole, minocycline
	Antivirals	Nevirapine, abacavir
Acute generalized exanthematous pustulosis (AGEP)	Antibiotics	Amoxicillin, ampicillin, vancomycin, pristinamycin, ceftriaxone, macrolides, quinolones
	Analgesics/antipyretics	Acetaminophen
	NSAIDs	Celecoxib
	Antifungal	Fluconazole
	Calcium channel blockers	Diltiazem

(Table 13-4) contd.....

Cutaneous lesion	Drug class	Drug name
Linear immunoglobulin A (IgA) bullous dermatosis	Anti-inflammatory	Sulfasalazine, NSAIDs (diclofenac, piroxicam)
	Antibacterial	Vancomycin, penicillin, cefamandole trimethoprim-sulfamethoxazole
	Diuretics	Furosemide
	Anticonvulsants	Phenytoin, vigabatrin
	Antiarrhythmics	Amiodarone, captopril
	Antidiabetics	Glibenclamide
	Antipsychotic	Lithium
	Hormones	Somatostatin
Allopurinol hypersensitivity syndrome	Antihyperuricemic	Allopurinol
Pseudolymphoma	Anticonvulsants	Phenytoin

Acute Generalized Exanthematous Pustulosis (AGEP) is a rare (between one and five cases/1,000,000/year) but severe drug-induced disorder characterized by acute development of nonfollicular sterile pustular eruptions, erythematous edema, fever and leukocytosis. The cutaneous lesions occur between two and three days after drug exposure. The rash typically begins in the intertriginous area or on the face, with further diffuse spreading accompanied by an itching sensation. In severe cases, the involvement of mucous membranes (*e.g.,* oral mucosa) and visceral organs can mimic septic shock. AGEP is particularly, but not exclusively, induced by antibiotics (Table **13-4**). Ordinarily, this lesion self-limits upon drug cessation, but steroids are sometimes necessary [4, 25, 32 - 34].

Linear Immunoglobulin A (IgA) Bullous Dermatosis is a severe immune-mediated bullous disease characterized by linear deposits of IgA along the basal membrane. It can be induced by several drugs, including sulfasalazine, vancomycin, trimetoprim-sulfametoxazol, amiodarone, captopril, cefamandole, NSAIDs (diclofenac, piroxicam), furosemide, glibenclamide, lithium, penicillin, phenytoin, somatostatin, vigabatrin, *etc*. (Table **13-4**). In some cases, DRESS syndrome or TEN can be associated [19].

Allopurinol Hypersensitivity Syndrome is reported in patients with hyper-uricemia-related disorders, such as recurrent acute gouty arthritis, tophi, urate nephropathy, urate lithiasis and tumor lysis syndrome. It is characterized by association with cutaneous lesions (maculopapular rash, bullae, TEN and/or erythema multiforme), fever, decreased renal function, hepatocellular injury, leukocytosis and eosinophilia. The mortality rate is about 32% [28, 35].

Other Particular Types of Drug-Induced Lesions

Fixed Drug Eruptions represent recurrent well-defined lesions appearing in the same mucocutaneous site each time the causative agent is taken. Under the microscope, basal cell vacuolization, dermal melanophages and superficial perivascular lymphocytic infiltrate are characteristic. These lesions preferentially occur on the external genital organs, oral mucosa, extremities and trunk. The most common drugs that can present this side effect, upon oral or systemic administration, are antifungals (*e.g.,* ketoconazole), antiparasitic agents (*e.g.,* metronidazole, miconazole), quinine, antibacterial sulfonamides, NSAIDs, antimalarial drugs, antibiotics, antihistamines and steroids. The lesion disappears following drug cessation and reoccurs upon readministration [37 - 40].

Vitiligo-Like Hypopigmentation can emerge after local application of creams, such as imiquimod 5%. This cream is used for HPV-related condylomata accuminata, Bowen's disease, common and plantar warts, molluscum contagiosum, herpes simplex, Paget's disease, basal cell carcinoma and superficial squamous cell carcinoma. White patches occur on the penis, scrotum, pubic area, perianal area, perineum, *etc.* [41].

CU-ADRs of Steroids occur as a result of steroids-induced decrease of epidermal mitotic rate and collagen synthesis. The result is cutaneous atrophy that can be complicated by the formation of striae distensae [42]. These reactions are also responsible for hypersecretion of the sweat glands and hyperplasia of the sebaceous glands, accompanied by formation of acneiform eruptions [21].

CU-ADRs of Cytotoxic Drugs range from mild to life-threatening lesions. The most common reported lesions are the following: urticaria (asparaginase, cisplatin, melphalan), acral erythema (doxorubicin, 5-FU, cytosine arabinoside), photosensitivity (dacarbazine, vinblastine, 5-FU, mitomycin), alopecia (cyclophosphamide), hand-foot skin reaction (cisplatin), excessive hair growth (cyclosporine), hyperpigmentation (bleomycin, cyclophosphamide, busulfan, doxorubicin), eccrine hidradenitis (bleomycin, cyclophosphamide, busulfan, doxorubicin), dermatomyositis-like lesions (hydroxyurea), dermatitis (mitomycin), Raynaud phenomenon (cisplatin), *etc.* [9, 43, 44].

CU-ADRs of Targeted Cancer Therapies are reported in patients taking the following drug types: monoclonal antibodies, cancer vaccines, growth factors inhibitors, immunotherapies (interferon, interleukins), antiangiogenic drugs (bevacizumab, temozolomide), kinase inhibitors (erlotinib, gefitinib, imatinib, nilotinib, dasatinib, sunitinib, sorafenib, pazopanib, lapatinib, everolimus, cabozantinib, regorafenib), hedgehog pathway inhibitors (vismodegib) and gene therapy agents. The following growth factors can be therapeutically inhibited: epidermal growth factor (EGF) and its receptor (EGFR), VEGF, platelet-derived endothelial growth factor (PDGF) and fibroblast growth factor (FGF). Multikinase inhibitors act against protein kinases and the receptors of the following genes: VEGF, tyrosine kinase with Ig, EGF homology domains-2, and the proto-oncogenes of mesenchymal-epithelial transition (MET) and rearranged during transfection (RET). Although biological therapy is considered to have a lower rate of side effects than conventional chemotherapeutics, some specific CU-ADRs have been reported [45 - 50].

- *EGFR inhibitors* (cetuximab, panitumumab, erlotinib, lapatinib, *etc.*) can cause maculopapular/papulopustular rash, lichenoid or acneiform eruptions, hair and nail changes, itching, xerosis and oral mucositis [47, 49]. The CU-ADRs of EGFR inhibitors are known as PRIDE syndrome (paronychia, papulopustular rash, itching and dryness) [49]. In one of our cases, skin bioptic specimens from red patches occurring on the limbs of a female with lung cancer treated with erlotinib indicated a cutaneous leukocytoclastic vasculitis (Fig. **13-2**). This type of vasculitis had previously been reported in a patient with hepatocellular carcinoma and bone metastasis treated with bevacizumab-erlotinib therapy [45].
- *Kinase inhibitors* can induce edema, maculopapular rash (imatinib, bortezomib, sorafenib, regorafenib, *etc.*), urticaria (sorafenib), facial erythema (sorafenib), splinter subungual hemorrhages (sorafenib), hemangiomas development (sorafenib), acneiform eruptions (dasatinib, radotinib, nilotinib), alopecia and hand-foot skin reactions (erlotinib, sorafenib, sunitinib, regorafenib). Severe lesions, including ulcerations, vasculitis and purpura (sorafenib or sunitinib) and DRESS syndrome (imatinib) have been reported in 17% of patients. These severe lesions are more common in females and primarily occur within the first two months of treatment [46, 49, 51 - 55]. The multikinase inhibitor, cabozantinib, which is used in the treatment of metastatic medullary thyroid cancer and other solid malignancies, presents a dose-limiting hand-foot skin reaction in about 35% of patients [48]. A sorafenib-related risk of development of a squamous cell carcinoma was also reported [52].
- *Antiangiogenic drugs* can produce rash, skin discoloration, hand-foot skin reactions, exfoliative dermatitis and xerosis, and induce risk of wound dehiscence, delayed wound healing and skin ulcerations [42, 50]. The association of bevacizumab with carboplatin therapy increases the severity of hand-foot skin reactions [44]. In patients with steroids-induced striae, ulcerations within striae are seen in patients also receiving bevacizumab. This is why long-term association of bevacizumab with dexamethasone should be avoided [42].
- *Monoclonal antibodies* that are used for melanoma treatment, such as ipilimumab, can cause dermatitis and pruritus [49].

- *BRAF inhibitors,* such as vemurafenib and dabrafenib, which are used for melanoma treatment, can produce exanthema and lead to an increased risk of squamous cell carcinoma [49].
- *mTOR inhibitors* that are used in transplant recipients for their immune suppressive effect, but also as targeted cancer therapeutics, can be responsible for delayed wound healing and leg edema [56].

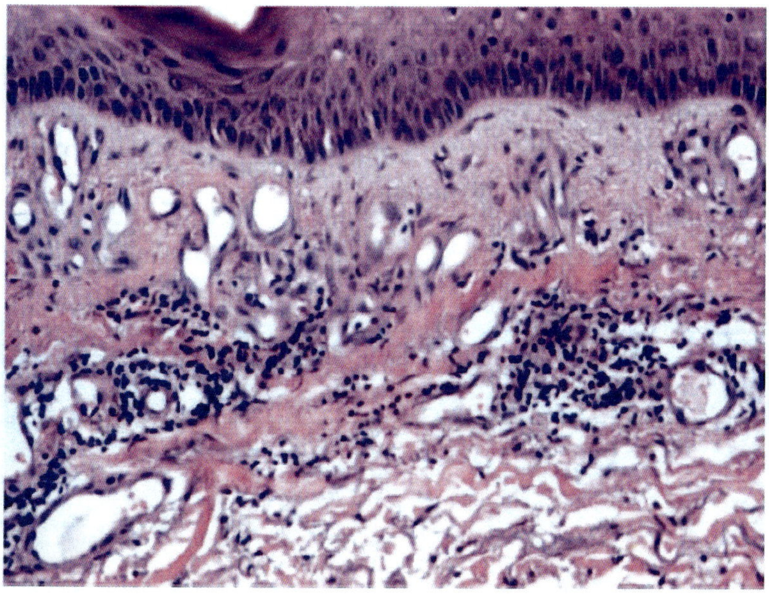

Fig. (13-2). Leukocytoclastic vasculitis of the superficial dermis in a patient with lung cancer treated with erlotinib. HE, Ob. 10x.

Cutaneous Lipomatosis onset coinciding with drug treatment has been reported in patients receiving chemotherapy (*e.g.,* cisplatin, bortezomib), especially in combined regimens and associated steroids (*e.g.,* mechlorethamine with vincristine, procarbazine and prednisolone; bortezomib with dexamethasone). Subcutaneous fat development has also been seen to be associated with steroids-only and anti-HIV treatment. In diabetics, lipomatosis is associated with peroxisome proliferator-activated receptor (PPAR) gamma agonists, such as rosiglitazone and pioglitazone [43, 57].

Thrombocytopenic Purpura (Moschcowitz syndrome) is reported to be induced by drugs that stimulate the formation of antiplatelets antibodies, such as *NSAIDs* (*e.g.,* nimesulide) [58]. Nimesulide use has also been associated with urticaria, maculopapular rash and toxic pustuloderma, being withdrawn from the market in many countries [58]. Purpura can also be induced by *hypolipidemic drugs,* such as fenofibrate, *serum sickness* (*e.g., rituximab*) and *allergic reactions,* or can be a side effect of *anti-BCG vaccination*, together with skin ulcerations and lymphadenitis [59, 60].

Necrotic Lesions

- *Anticoagulants* can be responsible for inducing the diffuse hemorrhagic necrosis of the dermis and hypodermis, which is more characteristic than localized ulcerations. The most common involved areas are the thigh, calf, buttock, abdominal wall and breast skin [9]. *Heparin-induced thrombocytopenia* can be associated with skin necrosis and venous limb gangrene [61], especially in diabetic patients using warfarin (Fig. **13-3**). *Coumarin-type anticoagulants* produce severe necroses in 0.1-0.5% of patients, more frequently in females, on the skin of the breast [9].
- *Other drugs* that can produce vasculitis, leg ulcers or leg gangrene are dopamine, cytotoxic agents and vitamin K antagonists [62, 63].

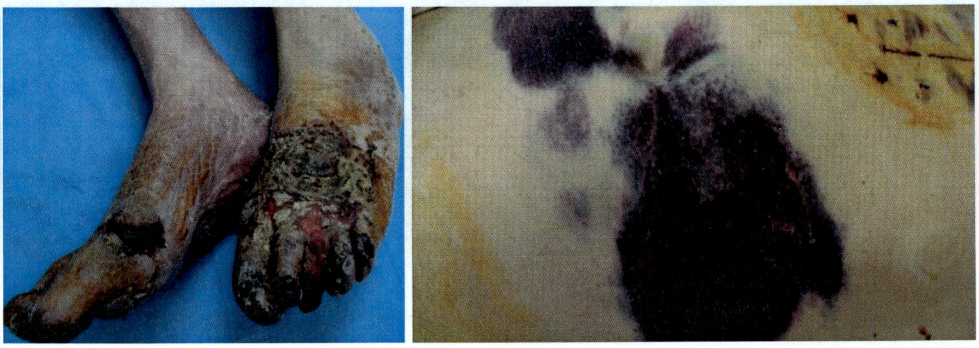

Fig. (13-3). Heparin-induced gangrene (left) and post-injection subcutaneous hematoma (right) in a diabetic patient.

Calcinosis Cutis is a benign lesion characterized by storage of calcium in the dermis and hypodermis. The forearm is primarily affected in patients receiving long-term intravenous administration of calcium gluconate [64]. The main complications are skin necrosis (*calciphylaxis*), cellulitis, osteomyelitis and compartment syndrome, which is more common in neonates [65]. Heparin-induced calciphylaxis is reported in patients receiving subcutaneous warfarin [66].

Iatrogenic Anetoderma is a benign dermatosis characterized by focal loss of dermal elastic fibers and multiple macular depressions. It can be an idiopathic or secondary lesion related to autoimmune, inflammatory and infectious diseases. Anetoderma can also be induced by penicillamine and anti-hepatitis B vaccination. In premature infants, this dermatosis has been related to the placement of monitoring devices on the skin [11, 67].

Aquagenic Palmoplantar Keratoderma is characterized by whitish edematous papules and an itchy or painful sensation upon immersion of the palms and/or soles in water (*e.g.*, after bathing), followed by fine desquamation of the skin of the palms and soles. It was recently reported in a patient with Langerhans cell histiocytosis, which was treated for six months with vinblastine in conjunction with mercaptopurine and oral corticosteroids. In other cases, anti-inflammatory drugs have been involved in its occurrence. Hyperhidrosis and *CFTR* gene mutations seem to be predisposing factors [68].

Bromoderma is a rare skin disorder caused by long-term intake of bromide-containing sedatives. It is characterized by the presence of single or multiple papillomatous nodules and pustules on the face or limbs. Hyperchloremia and neurological or psychiatric symptoms can be associated. Clinically, it should be differentiated from pyoderma gangrenosum. Although this type of sedative has been banned by the US FDA, they are still used in some countries [69].

Iatrogenic Skin Lesions in Preterm Infants occur due to the immature skin barrier of neonates younger than 32 weeks of gestational age. They can be induced by ventilation techniques, central/umbilical venous catheters, electrodes, disinfectants, dressing, *etc.* [70, 71]. The incidence of CU-ADRs is about 57% at gestational ages between 24 and 27 weeks, and 3% in infants at term [72]. Aside from age and indwelling catheters, other causal factors are low birth weight, increased length of hospital stay, staphylococcal scalded skin syndrome, atopic dermatitis, drug eruptions and inherited or acquired blistering disorders [71].

Embolia Cutis Medicamentosa or Nicolau Syndrome was first reported in 1924 following intragluteal injection of bismuth salts for the treatment of syphilis. It refers to hyperemia, skin discoloration, livedoid dermatitis and a hemorrhagic patch occurring at the injection site following intramuscular drug administration. A deep necrosis is then developed and death is a possible outcome. The supposed mechanism is the injection of the substance into an arterial lumen or wall, leading to immune-mediated vessel thrombosis and necrosis of subcutaneous tissue and muscles. Nowadays, this syndrome is reported in children below three years of age and in adults receiving NSAIDs injections, such as diclofenac sodium (Voltaren®) [73].

Necrotizing Fasciitis is reported to infrequently occur following use of sunitinib [74] or NSAIDs [75]. It can also be a consequence of injection (*e.g.*, morphine), infiltration or placement of indwelling devices, such as central venous catheters [76].

Arsenicosis and Arsenical Keratosis can be induced by herbal medications in patients with refractory chronic eczema long-term treated with realgar. This is an arsenic-based drug used in traditional Chinese medicine for detoxification, elimination of dampness, relief of itching and removal of putrefaction. Peripheral neuritis can be associated [77].

Functional skin disorders include dysphoria and can be induced by first and second generation antipsychotic agents [78].

Skin Granulomas

- *Lipogranuloma is a lesion that* can occur postoperatively as a result of fatty tissue necrosis or as a complication of intramuscular injections. It is microscopically composed of foamy macrophages and infrequent giant cells. It is primarily a benign lesion with further subcutaneous fibrosis and formation of scarring tissue [9, 79].
- *Oleogranuloma* is formed surrounding unabsorbed oily drops in soft tissue following oil-based intramuscular injections. These granulomas are composed of oily cysts, foamy macrophages and multinucleated giant cells [9, 79].
- *Granuloma formed surrounding nonabsorbable suture material,* such as polyglactin, braided polyethylene-polyester and Ethibond, is usually a benign lesion [80]. In some cases, multiple small granulomatous nodules might be seen at the suture line (Fig. **13-4**).

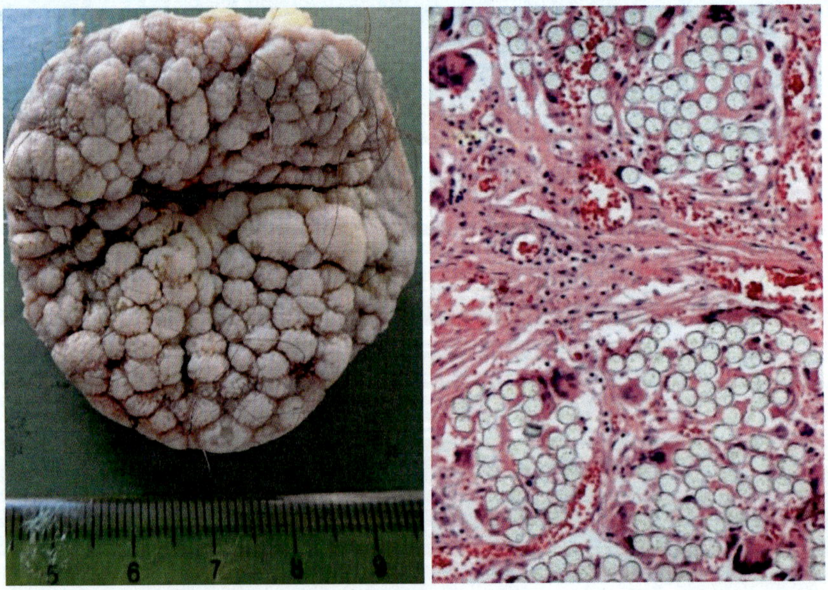

Fig. (13-4). Post-laparotomy foreign body granuloma on the skin (left) and soft tissue (right). The multinucleated giant cells surround the suture material (right).

Angiolymphoid Hyperplasia with Eosinophilia Induced by Vaccination is a rare granulomatous lesion of the subcutaneous tissue that can occur at months following vaccination (*e.g.,* antituberculosis, antipolio, tetanus toxoid) [81]. In one of our cases, it was surgically excised from the right upper arm (deltoid region) of a six-year-old girl. A progressively growing encapsulated bluish painless nodule of 30 mm in diameter, it was clinically thought to be a hemangioma. Under the microscope, it involved proliferation, in the dermis and subcutaneous tissue, of small and large vessels lined by elongated cells with well-defined cytoplasm and vesicular nuclei, without cytological atypia. Among these vessels, solid areas of CD68 positive cells with epithelioid architecture were seen. Scattered lymphoid follicles with germinal centers and mixed inflammatory infiltrate (eosinophils, lymphocytes and plasma cells) were also noted (Fig. **13-5**). Differential diagnosis (regarding Kimura's disease, tuberculosis, hemangio-endothelioma, Kaposi's sarcoma and histiocytes-derived tumors) is very difficult and is primarily based on clinical history and absence of atypical cells.

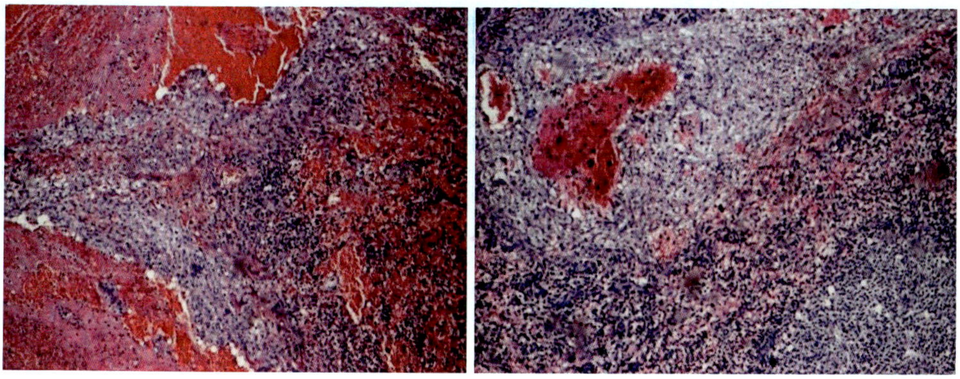

Fig. (13-5). Microscopic features of post-vaccination reactive angiolymphoid hyperplasia. HE, Ob. 4x.

CONFLICT OF INTEREST

The authors confirm that this chapter content has no conflict of interest.

ACKNOWLEDGEMENTS

Declared none.

REFERENCES

[1] Hussein MR. Drug-induced skin reactions: a pathologist viewpoint. Cutan Ocul Toxicol 2015; 26: 1-13.
[PMID: 26113029]

[2] Tian XY, Liu B, Shi H, *et al.* Incidence of adverse cutaneous drug reactions in 22,866 Chinese inpatients: a prospective study. Arch Dermatol Res 2015; 307(9): 829-34.

[http://dx.doi.org/10.1007/s00403-015-1589-4] [PMID: 26246330]

[3] Heng YK, Lim YL. Cutaneous adverse drug reactions in the elderly. Curr Opin Allergy Clin Immunol 2015; 15(4): 300-7.
[http://dx.doi.org/10.1097/ACI.0000000000000181] [PMID: 26110679]

[4] Darnis D, Mahé J, Vrignaud B, Guen CG, Veyrac G, Jolliet P. Adverse drug reactions in pediatric emergency medicine. Ann Pharmacother 2015; 49(12): 1298-304.
[http://dx.doi.org/10.1177/1060028015602904] [PMID: 26324354]

[5] Basilio FM, Brenner FM, Werner B, Rastelli GJ. Clinical and histological study of permanent alopecia after bone marrow transplantation. An Bras Dermatol 2015; 90(6): 814-21.
[http://dx.doi.org/10.1590/abd1806-4841.20154013] [PMID: 26734861]

[6] Dao RL, Su SC, Chung WH. Recent advances of pharmacogenomics in severe cutaneous adverse reactions: immune and nonimmune mechanisms. Asia Pac Allergy 2015; 5(2): 59-67.
[http://dx.doi.org/10.5415/apallergy.2015.5.2.59] [PMID: 25938070]

[7] Hoetzenecker W, Nägeli M, Mehra ET, *et al.* Adverse cutaneous drug eruptions: current understanding. Semin Immunopathol 2016; 38(1): 75-86.
[http://dx.doi.org/10.1007/s00281-015-0540-2] [PMID: 26553194]

[8] Yang F, Yang Y, Zhu Q, *et al.* Research on susceptible genes and immunological pathogenesis of cutaneous adverse drug reactions in chinese hans. J Investig Dermatol Symp Proc 2015; 17(1): 29-31.
[http://dx.doi.org/10.1038/jidsymp.2015.6] [PMID: 26067314]

[9] Jung J, Ed. Patologie iatrogenă. Tîrgu-Mureş, Romania: University Press 2006.

[10] Riyaz N, Sasidharanpillai S, Aravindan KP, Nobin BK, Raghavan NT, Nikhila PK. Phenytoin induced cutaneous B cell pseudolymphoma. Indian J Dermatol 2015; 60(5): 522.
[http://dx.doi.org/10.4103/0019-5154.164437] [PMID: 26538730]

[11] Cheng CE, Kroshinsky D. Iatrogenic skin injury in hospitalized patients. Clin Dermatol 2011; 29(6): 622-32.
[http://dx.doi.org/10.1016/j.clindermatol.2011.08.006] [PMID: 22014984]

[12] de Groot AC. New contact allergens: 20082015. Dermatitis 2015; 26(5): 199-215.
[http://dx.doi.org/10.1097/DER.0000000000000144] [PMID: 26367204]

[13] Chasset F, Soria A, Moguelet P, *et al.* Contact dermatitis due to ultrasound gel: A case report and published work review. J Dermatol 2015; 43(3): 318-20.
[http://dx.doi.org/10.1111/1246-8138.13066] [PMID: 26346708]

[14] Lee B, Warshaw E. Lanolin allergy: history, epidemiology, responsible allergens, and management. Dermatitis 2008; 19(2): 63-72.
[PMID: 18413106]

[15] Mahler V. [Contact allergies in the elderly]. Hautarzt 2015; 66(9): 665-73.
[http://dx.doi.org/10.1007/s00105-015-3668-z] [PMID: 26285897]

[16] Saw NK, Hindmarsh JR. Acute irritant reaction to an antiseptic bath emollient. Postgrad Med J 2005; 81(952): 131-2.
[http://dx.doi.org/10.1136/pgmj.2003.018564] [PMID: 15701748]

[17] Kureshi F, Kalaaji AN, Halvorson L, Pittelkow MR, Davis MD. Cutaneous complications of intravesical treatments for bladder cancer: granulomatous inflammation of the penis following BCG therapy and penile gangrene following mitomycin therapy. J Am Acad Dermatol 2006; 55(2): 328-31.
[http://dx.doi.org/10.1016/j.jaad.2005.07.041] [PMID: 16844523]

[18] Drago F, Cogorno L, Agnoletti AF, Ciccarese G, Parodi A. A retrospective study of cutaneous drug reactions in an outpatient population. Int J Clin Pharm 2015; 37(5): 739-43.
[http://dx.doi.org/10.1007/s11096-015-0134-z] [PMID: 26050251]

[19] Hernández N, Borrego L, Soler E, Hernández J. Sulfasalazine-induced linear immunoglobulin A

bullous dermatosis with DRESS. Actas Dermosifiliogr 2013; 104(4): 343-6.
[http://dx.doi.org/10.1016/j.adengl.2011.11.022] [PMID: 23562401]

[20] Firmin D, Roguedas AM, Lemasson G, Abgrall JF, Misery L. Eczematous dermatosis and thrombocytosis induced by efalizumab: two new side effects. Dermatology (Basel) 2008; 217(3): 203-6.
[http://dx.doi.org/10.1159/000141958] [PMID: 18594143]

[21] Mackesy MM, Selhorst C, Raza S. Immunosuppressant-induced acneiform eruption of the breast. Breast J 2014; 20(6): 650-2.
[http://dx.doi.org/10.1111/tbj.12339] [PMID: 25229395]

[22] Bocquet H, Bagot M, Roujeau JC. Drug-induced pseudolymphoma and drug hypersensitivity syndrome (Drug Rash with Eosinophilia and Systemic Symptoms: DRESS). Semin Cutan Med Surg 1996; 15(4): 250-7.
[http://dx.doi.org/10.1016/S1085-5629(96)80038-1] [PMID: 9069593]

[23] Wu MK, Chung W, Wu CK, Tseng PT. The severe complication of Stevens-Johnson syndrome induced by long-term clozapine treatment in a male schizophrenia patient: a case report. Neuropsychiatr Dis Treat 2015; 11: 1039-41.
[PMID: 25914536]

[24] Yasui-Furukori N, Hashimoto K, Tsuruga K, Nakamura K. Comorbidity of Stevens-Johnson syndrome and neutropenia associated with lamotrigine: a case report. Gen Hosp Psychiatry 2014; 36(6): 761.e9-761.e11.
[http://dx.doi.org/10.1016/j.genhosppsych.2014.07.010] [PMID: 25169759]

[25] Mawri S, Jain T, Shah J, Hurst G, Swiderek J. Vancomycin-induced acute generalized exanthematous pustulosis (AGEP) masquerading septic shock-an unusual presentation of a rare disease. J Intensive Care 2015; 3: 47.
[http://dx.doi.org/10.1186/s40560-015-0114-3] [PMID: 26561525]

[26] Pereira FA, Mudgil AV, Rosmarin DM. Toxic epidermal necrolysis. J Am Acad Dermatol 2007; 56(2): 181-200.
[http://dx.doi.org/10.1016/j.jaad.2006.04.048] [PMID: 17224365]

[27] Borchers AT, Lee JL, Naguwa SM, Cheema GS, Gershwin ME. Stevens-Johnson syndrome and toxic epidermal necrolysis. Autoimmun Rev 2008; 7(8): 598-605.
[http://dx.doi.org/10.1016/j.autrev.2008.06.004] [PMID: 18603022]

[28] Min HK, Lee B, Kwok SK, *et al.* Allopurinol hypersensitivity syndrome in patients with hematological malignancies: characteristics and clinical outcomes. Korean J Intern Med 2015; 30(4): 521-30.
[http://dx.doi.org/10.3904/kjim.2015.30.4.521] [PMID: 26161019]

[29] Bayram AK, Canpolat M, Cinar SL, *et al.* Drug reaction with eosinophilia and systemic symptoms syndrome induced by levetiracetam in a pediatric patient. J Emerg Med 2016; 50(2): e61-6.
[http://dx.doi.org/10.1016/j.jemermed.2015.10.004] [PMID: 26597350]

[30] Santhamoorthy P, Alexander KJ, Alshubaili A. Intravenous immunoglobulin in the treatment of drug rash eosinophilia and systemic symptoms caused by phenytoin. Ann Indian Acad Neurol 2012; 15(4): 320-2.
[http://dx.doi.org/10.4103/0972-2327.104348] [PMID: 23349605]

[31] Cacoub P, Musette P, Descamps V, *et al.* The DRESS syndrome: a literature review. Am J Med 2011; 124(7): 588-97.
[http://dx.doi.org/10.1016/j.amjmed.2011.01.017] [PMID: 21592453]

[32] Szatkowski J, Schwartz RA. Acute generalized exanthematous pustulosis (AGEP): A review and update. J Am Acad Dermatol 2015; 73(5): 843-8.
[http://dx.doi.org/10.1016/j.jaad.2015.07.017] [PMID: 26354880]

[33] Lee SK, Lee DY, Kim DJ, Kim MS, Lee UH, Hahm JH. Acute generalized exanthematous pustulosis induced by celecoxib. J Cutan Pathol 2016; 43(1): 80-1.
[http://dx.doi.org/10.1111/cup.12604] [PMID: 26488335]

[34] Barcik K, Protas-Drozd F, Weiss-Rostkowska W, Flis E, Placek W. [Acute generalised exanthematosus pustulosis (AGEP) due to diltiazem a case report]. Kardiol Pol 2009; 67(8): 887-91.
[PMID: 19784887]

[35] Singer JZ, Wallace SL. The allopurinol hypersensitivity syndrome. Unnecessary morbidity and mortality. Arthritis Rheum 1986; 29(1): 82-7.
[http://dx.doi.org/10.1002/art.1780290111] [PMID: 3947418]

[36] Lupton GP. Adverse drug reactions in the skin. Adverse dug reactions and other topics Handout XXII International Congress of the International Academy of Pathology . 1998; 58-6

[37] Eubel J, Diepgen TL, Weisshaar E. [Allergic diseases in the genital area]. Hautarzt 2015; 66(1): 45-52.
[http://dx.doi.org/10.1007/s00105-014-3561-1] [PMID: 25532902]

[38] Kastalli S, El Aïdli S, Lakhoua G, Daghfous R. Genital fixed drug eruption induced by miconazole with positive provocation test. Tunis Med 2014; 92(11): 703.
[PMID: 25867162]

[39] Lonsdale-Eccles E, Wallett A, Ward AM. A case of fixed drug eruption secondary to quinine in tonic water presenting to a sexual health clinic. Sex Transm Infect 2014; 90(5): 356-7.
[http://dx.doi.org/10.1136/sextrans-2013-051458] [PMID: 24583965]

[40] Saka B, Kombaté K, Médougou BH, *et al.* [Fixed drug eruption in dermatology setting in Lomé (Togo): a retrospective study of 321 cases]. Bull Soc Pathol Exot 2012; 105(5): 384-7.
[http://dx.doi.org/10.1007/s13149-012-0237-x] [PMID: 22669581]

[41] Li W, Xin H, Ge L, Song H, Cao W. Induction of vitiligo after imiquimod treatment of condylomata acuminata. BMC Infect Dis 2014; 14: 329.
[http://dx.doi.org/10.1186/1471-2334-14-329] [PMID: 24928346]

[42] Farber SA, Samimi S, Rosenbach M. Ulcerations within striae distensae associated with bevacizumab therapy. J Am Acad Dermatol 2015; 72(1): e33-5.
[http://dx.doi.org/10.1016/j.jaad.2014.09.023] [PMID: 25497948]

[43] Bracaglia R, DEttorre M, Gentileschi S, Mingrone G, Tambasco D. Multiple lipomatosis after stem cell transplant and chemotherapy: a case report. Eur Rev Med Pharmacol Sci 2014; 18(3): 413-5.
[PMID: 24563443]

[44] Yokokawa T, Kawakami K, Mae Y, *et al.* Risk factors exacerbating hand-foot skin reaction induced by capecitabine plus oxaliplatin with or without bevacizumab therapy. Ann Pharmacother 2015; 49(10): 1120-4.
[http://dx.doi.org/10.1177/1060028015594451] [PMID: 26160973]

[45] Brandi G, Venturi M, Dika E, Maibach H, Patrizi A, Biasco G. Cutaneous leukocytoclastic vasculitis due to erlotinib: just an adverse event or also a putative marker of drug efficacy? Cutan Ocul Toxicol 2013; 32(4): 336-8.
[http://dx.doi.org/10.3109/15569527.2013.780179] [PMID: 23534992]

[46] Faye E, Bondon-Guitton E, Olivier-Abbal P, Montastruc JL. Spontaneous reporting of serious cutaneous reactions with protein kinase inhibitors. Eur J Clin Pharmacol 2013; 69(10): 1819-26. [http://dx.doi.org/10.1007/s00228-013-1532-6] [PMID: 23748749]

[47] Lupu I, Voiculescu VM, Bacalbasa N, Prie BE, Cojocaru I, Giurcaneanu C. Cutaneous adverse reactions specific to epidermal growth factor receptor inhibitors. J Med Life 2015; 8(Spec Issue): 57-61.
[PMID: 26361513]

[48] Belum VR, Serna-Tamayo C, Wu S, Lacouture ME. Incidence and risk of hand-foot skin reaction with

cabozantinib, a novel multikinase inhibitor: a meta-analysis. Clin Exp Dermatol 2016; 41(1): 8-15. [http://dx.doi.org/10.1111/ced.12694] [PMID: 26009777]

[49] Reyes-Habito CM, Roh EK. Cutaneous reactions to chemotherapeutic drugs and targeted therapy for cancer: Part II. Targeted therapy. J Am Acad Dermatol 2014; 71(2): 217.e1-217.e11. [http://dx.doi.org/10.1016/j.jaad.2014.04.013] [PMID: 25037801]

[50] Hummel TR, Salloum R, Drissi R, *et al.* A pilot study of bevacizumab-based therapy in patients with newly diagnosed high-grade gliomas and diffuse intrinsic pontine gliomas. J Neurooncol 2016; 127(1): 53-61. [http://dx.doi.org/10.1007/s11060-015-2008-6] [PMID: 26626490]

[51] Musri FY, Mutlu H, Kivrak Salim D, *et al.* Sorafenib-induced severe urticaria in a patient with hepatocellular cancer. J Oncol Pharm Pract 2016; 22(2): 350-3. [http://dx.doi.org/10.1177/1078155214565126] [PMID: 25567520]

[52] Lynch MC, Straub R, Adams DR. Eruptive squamous cell carcinomas with keratoacanthoma-like features in a patient treated with sorafenib. J Drugs Dermatol 2011; 10(3): 308-10. [PMID: 21369650]

[53] Jung YS, Kim M, Lee JH, Cho BK, Kim DW, Park HJ. Acneiform eruptions caused by various second-generation tyrosine kinase inhibitors in patients with chronic myeloid leukaemia. Br J Dermatol 2016; 174(2): 456-8. [http://dx.doi.org/10.1111/bjd.14185] [PMID: 26399382]

[54] Guerra JR, Suelves AM, Bella A, Lolo D. Hand, foot and scrotal blisters in a patient with cancer receiving oral chemotherapy. BMJ Case Rep 2014; 2014: bcr2013202822. [http://dx.doi.org/10.1136/bcr-2013-202822] [PMID: 24842353]

[55] Tonini G, Intagliata S, Cagli B, *et al.* Recurrent scrotal hemangiomas during treatment with sunitinib. J Clin Oncol 2010; 28(35): e737-8. [http://dx.doi.org/10.1200/JCO.2010.30.4865] [PMID: 20823408]

[56] Carenco C, Faure S, Ursic-Bedoya J, Herrero A, Pageaux GP. Solid, non-skin, post-liver transplant tumors: Key role of lifestyle and immunosuppression management. World J Gastroenterol 2016; 22(1): 427-34. [http://dx.doi.org/10.3748/wjg.v22.i1.427] [PMID: 26755888]

[57] Miraglia E, Calvieri S, Giustini S. A case of iatrogenic cutaneous lipomatosis. Acta Dermatovenerol Croat 2015; 23(3): 220-1. [PMID: 26476909]

[58] Sathiasekar AC, Deepthi DA, Sathia Sekar GS. Drug-induced thrombocytopenic purpura. J Pharm Bioallied Sci 2015; 7 (Suppl. 2): S827-9. [http://dx.doi.org/10.4103/0975-7406.163595] [PMID: 26538982]

[59] Agapakis DI, Massa EV. A case of fenofibrate-induced immune thrombocytopenia: first report. P R Health Sci J 2015; 34(3): 170-3. [PMID: 26356743]

[60] Fajt ML, Petrov AA. Desensitization protocol for rituximab-induced serum sickness. Curr Drug Saf 2014; 9(3): 240-2. [http://dx.doi.org/10.2174/1574886309666140509154056] [PMID: 24861993]

[61] Srinivasan AF, Rice L, Bartholomew JR, *et al.* Warfarin-induced skin necrosis and venous limb gangrene in the setting of heparin-induced thrombocytopenia. Arch Intern Med 2004; 164(1): 66-70. [http://dx.doi.org/10.1001/archinte.164.1.66] [PMID: 14718324]

[62] Park JY, Kanzler M, Swetter SM. Dopamine-associated symmetric peripheral gangrene. Arch Dermatol 1997; 133(2): 247-9. [http://dx.doi.org/10.1001/archderm.133.2.247] [PMID: 9041849]

[63] Chabli H, Hocar O, Akhdari N, Amal S, Hakkou M, Hamdaoui A. [Necrotic leg ulcer revealing

vasculitis induced by vitamin K antagonists]. J Mal Vasc 2015; 40(6): 402-5.
[http://dx.doi.org/10.1016/j.jmv.2015.10.002] [PMID: 26548536]

[64] Moss J, Syrengelas A, Antaya R, Lazova R. Calcinosis cutis: a complication of intravenous administration of calcium gluconate. J Cutan Pathol 2006; 33 (Suppl. 2): 60-2.
[http://dx.doi.org/10.1111/j.1600-0560.2006.00519.x] [PMID: 16972958]

[65] Chen TK, Yang CY, Chen SJ. Calcinosis cutis complicated by compartment syndrome following extravasation of calcium gluconate in a neonate: a case report. Pediatr Neonatol 2010; 51(4): 238-41.
[http://dx.doi.org/10.1016/S1875-9572(10)60045-9] [PMID: 20713289]

[66] Hafiji J, Deegan P, Brais R, Norris P. Warfarin-induced calciphylaxis successfully treated with sodium thiosulphate. Australas J Dermatol 2013; 54(2): 133-5.
[http://dx.doi.org/10.1111/j.1440-0960.2011.00861.x] [PMID: 23581997]

[67] Maffeis L, Pugni L, Pietrasanta C, *et al.* Iatrogenic anetoderma of prematurity: a case report and review of the literature. Case Rep Dermatol Med 2014; 2014: 781493.
[http://dx.doi.org/10.1155/2014/781493] [PMID: 25374702]

[68] Bonhomme A, Barbaud A, Schmutz JL, Bursztejn AC. [Aquagenic palmoplantar keratoderma during treatment of Langerhans cell histiocytosis]. Ann Dermatol Venereol 2015; 142(3): 197-200.
[http://dx.doi.org/10.1016/j.annder.2015.01.009] [PMID: 25683007]

[69] Oda F, Tohyama M, Murakami A, Kanno K, Sonobe N, Sayama K. Bromoderma mimicking pyoderma gangrenosum caused by commercial sedatives. J Dermatol 2016; 43(5): 564-6.
[http://dx.doi.org/10.1111/1346-8138.13162] [PMID: 26507105]

[70] Roche-Kubler B, Puzenat E, Mariet AS, Thiriez G, Aubin F, Humbert P. [Iatrogenic skin lesions: a prospective study in premature infants born at less than 33 weeks of amenorrhea at Besançon university hospital]. Ann Dermatol Venereol 2015; 142(1): 3-9.
[http://dx.doi.org/10.1016/j.annder.2014.09.001] [PMID: 25600788]

[71] Reddy K, Kogan S, Glick SA. Procedures and drugs in pediatric dermatology: iatrogenic risks and situations of concern. Clin Dermatol 2011; 29(6): 633-43.
[http://dx.doi.org/10.1016/j.clindermatol.2011.08.028] [PMID: 22014985]

[72] Sardesai SR, Kornacka MK, Walas W, Ramanathan R. Iatrogenic skin injury in the neonatal intensive care unit. J Matern Fetal Neonatal Med 2011; 24(2): 197-203.
[http://dx.doi.org/10.3109/14767051003728245] [PMID: 20540679]

[73] Kılıç İ, Kaya F, Özdemir AT, Demirel T, Çelik İ. Nicolau syndrome due to diclofenac sodium (Voltaren®) injection: a case report. J Med Case Reports 2014; 8: 404.
[http://dx.doi.org/10.1186/1752-1947-8-404] [PMID: 25471251]

[74] Piszczek J, Dalton B, Peters T, Ruether D, Urbanski S. Extensive necrotizing fasciitis associated with sunitinib therapy. Clin Genitourin Cancer 2014; 12(2): e47-9.
[http://dx.doi.org/10.1016/j.clgc.2013.11.017] [PMID: 24445249]

[75] Kahn LH, Styrt BA. Necrotizing soft tissue infections reported with nonsteroidal antiinflammatory drugs. Ann Pharmacother 1997; 31(9): 1034-9.
[PMID: 9296245]

[76] Leibig N, Hirche C, Schmidt VJ, Bigdeli AK, Kneser U, Kremer T. Necrotizing fasciitis after central venous catheter placement. Surg Infect (Larchmt) 2014; 15(6): 850-2.
[http://dx.doi.org/10.1089/sur.2014.074] [PMID: 25493536]

[77] Zhou S, Zhou J, Liu S, Wang R, Wang Z. Arsenical keratosis caused by medication: a case report and literature. Int J Clin Exp Med 2015; 8(1): 1487-90.
[PMID: 25785160]

[78] Wu HE, Okusaga OO. Antipsychotic medication-induced dysphoria: its meaning, association with typical *vs.* atypical medications and impact on adherence. Psychiatr Q 2015; 86(2): 199-205.
[http://dx.doi.org/10.1007/s11126-014-9319-1] [PMID: 25164199]

[79] Gurzu S, Jung I, Eds. Basic concepts of Pathology. University Press, Tîrgu-Mureş 2011.

[80] Kara A, Celik H, Seker A, Uysal MA, Uzun M, Malkoc M. Granuloma formation secondary to Achilles tendon repair with nonabsorbable suture. Int J Surg Case Rep 2014; 5(10): 720-2. [http://dx.doi.org/10.1016/j.ijscr.2014.07.026] [PMID: 25212905]

[81] Jeon EK, Cho AY, Kim MY, *et al.* Angiolymphoid hyperplasia with eosinophilia that was possibly induced by vaccination in a child. Ann Dermatol 2009; 21(1): 71-4. [http://dx.doi.org/10.5021/ad.2009.21.1.71] [PMID: 20548862]

CHAPTER 14

Iatrogenic Lesions in Neurology

Rodica Balasa*

Department of Neurology, University of Medicine and Pharmacy, Tirgu-Mures, Romania

Abstract: Iatrogenic neurological disorders can be induced by several factors, such as pharmacological agents prescribed for treatment or prevention (drug-induced neurological disorders [DIND]), complications of diagnostic and treatment procedures, like cerebral angiography or lumbar puncture, organ transplantation (related to the surgical procedure of transplantation, post-transplant immunosuppression, opportunistic infection or the inherent disorders that lead to transplantation), radiation therapy, *etc*. Iatrogenic neurological effects may be devastating due to the higher potential irreversibility of central nervous system, peripheral nervous system, neuromuscular junction (NMJ) and/or muscular system involvement. DIND represent the majority of iatrogenic neurological disorders. Drugs may directly induce neurological damage (through primary neurotoxicity, such as damage to the blood-brain barrier [BBB], disturbances of brain energy metabolism, ion channels/neurotransmitters disturbances, mitochondrial dysfunction, metabolite-mediated toxins, drug-induced selective cell death) or do so indirectly (cardiovascular, hematological or renal effects). Identification of DIND is important because early recognition and drug withdrawal can prevent irreversible damage. The numerous intrinsic risk factors for DIND should be well known by medical practitioners.

Keywords: Anticholinergic syndrome, Choreoathetosis, Dyskinesia, Dystonia, Encephalopathies, Intracranial hypertension, Meningitis, Myoclonus, Myopathies, Neuroleptic malignant syndrome, Neuromuscular junction, Neurotoxicity, Organ transplantation, Parkinsonism, Polyneuropathy, Radiation therapy, Serotonin syndrome, Sympathomimetic syndrome, Tremor.

INTRODUCTION

Iatrogenic neurological disorders (iatrogenic neurological adverse effects, iatrogenic neurology) are induced by: a) the administration of pharmacological agents prescribed for treatment or prevention (drug-induced neurological disorders); b) utilization of diagnostic and treatment procedures; c) organ transplantation. Iatrogenic neurological adverse effects may be devastating due to

* **Corresponding author Rodica Balasa:** Department of Neurology, University of Medicine and Pharmacy, Tirgu-Mures, Romania; Tel: 0040-265-212111; Fax: 0040-372-653250; E-mail: rodica.balasa@umftgm.ro

Simona Gurzu & Ioan Jung (Eds.)

the higher potential irreversibility of central nervous system (CNS), peripheral nervous system (PNS), neuromuscular junction (NMJ) and/or muscular system (MS) involvements.

DRUG-INDUCED NEUROLOGICAL DISORDERS

The term "drug-induced neurological disorders" (DIND) refers to unintended/undesirable effects on the CNS, PNS, NMJ and/or MS caused by drugs or associated with drug use (inappropriate use, overdose of a drug or interaction with other drugs). DIND are important because early recognition and drug withdrawal can prevent irreversible damage. The drug may act directly (primary neurotoxicity) or indirectly *via* other systemic disturbances caused by the drug (secondary neurotoxicity).

The primary mechanisms of neurotoxicity are: a) damage to blood-brain barrier (BBB), facilitating the passage of drugs that normally do not cross the BBB; b) disturbances of brain energy metabolism (ATP synthetase inhibition, uncoupling/dissociation of oxidative phosphorylation, disturbances of oxygen consumption, enzymatic dysfunction, selective vulnerability of the nervous system); c) products of brain energy metabolism disturbances (calcium ions entry into the cells, oxygen free radical formation, excitatory amino acids); d) ion channels/neurotransmitters disturbances; e) mitochondrial dysfunction; f) metabolite-mediated toxins; g) drug-induced selective cell death.

Secondary neurotoxicity is the condition in which the CNS, PNS, NMJ and/or MS are affected by ADR-induced disorders in other organs/systems, such as the cardiovascular, respiratory, hepatic, renal, hematological and endocrine systems. Drug-related metabolic disorders and vitamin deficiencies are also common.

The main DIND-related mechanisms of neurotoxicity include oxidative stress, excitotoxicity, neuroinflammation, ubiquitin proteasome system, dysfunction of mitochondrial and/or neurotrophic factors.

The risk factors for DIND are patient-related (genetic predisposition, old age, history of neurological disorders, degenerative brain disease, intracranial space-occupying lesions, brain damage, systemic diseases, pregnancy) or drug-related (high doses, drug-drug interaction, drug-disease interaction, rate of drug delivery, route of drug administration, drug withdrawal).

The treatment of DIND involves the immediate discontinuation of the suspected drug [1 - 4].

Drug-Induced Disorders of Consciousness

Consciousness (CN) is a state of awareness, or of being aware of an external object or something within oneself. Its disturbance includes the following main clinical consequences [3]:

Syncope (SN) is a sudden transient loss of CN and postural tone, usually lasting no more than 15 seconds. Drug-induced SN represents 2-9% of all patients with SN. It is a common event, reported as an ADR, and its relation to the drug is difficult to determine in most cases. SN and falls are often two concomitant side effects of drugs reported in elderly patients. The most common drugs inducing SN include analgesics, antineoplastics, cytokines (interferon-alpha), digitalis, drugs that produce postural hypotension, vasodilators, drugs and combinations that prolong the QT interval, hypnotic sedatives (depressants of the CNS), antidepressants, antipsychotics, antiparkinsonian drugs, antidiabetics, selective serotonin reuptake inhibitors and vaccines.

Somnolence (SM) is a state of a strong desire for sleep, or sleeping for unusually long periods.

Lethargy (LG) is a state of sleepiness, deep unresponsiveness, listless, tiredness, lack of energy, apathy and inactivity.

Stupor (ST) is the lack of critical mental functions and a level of consciousness wherein a sufferer is almost entirely unresponsive, only responding to base stimuli such as pain.

SM, LG or ST may be due to overdose of a drug that does not produce any impairment of consciousness at therapeutic doses. The most common drugs that can induce SM, LG or ST include antidepressants, antiepileptics, antihistaminics, neuroleptics, analgesics and hypnotic sedatives.

Coma is a state of unconsciousness associated with neurological disorders in which the patient cannot be awakened, fails to respond normally to stimuli (pain, light, sound), lacks a normal sleep-wake cycle and does not initiate voluntary actions. Coma is a serious condition and a medical emergency. The most common drugs that can induce coma include hypnotic sedatives, anesthetics (propofol), antidiabetics (insulin, oral hypoglycemic agents) and drug-inducing encephalopathies (presented later in this chapter). Coma can also be a direct effect of prolonged use or overdose of barbiturates, benzodiazepines, opioids, tricyclic antidepressants, antiepileptics, *etc.*

Drug-Induced Encephalopathies

Encephalopathy (EP) refers to a wide variety of permanent/reversible, acute/chronic brain disorders with different etiologies and prognoses. Leukoencephalopathy is a particular type of encephalopathy characterized by lesions of the white matter. The most common neurological symptoms of EP are loss of cognitive function, subtle personality changes, inability to concentrate, lethargy, cortical blindness, depressed consciousness, myoclonus, tremor, nystagmus, seizures and autonomic disorders. The mechanisms of drug-induced EP include cytotoxic and neurotoxic disorders, electrolytic disturbances (hyponatremia, hypopotassemia), hepatic enzyme interactions and hyperammonemia, drug effects upon cerebral receptors (GABA receptors), and drug-induced vasogenic and cytotoxic brain edema [3, 5].

Primary Drug-Induced EP occurs as a result of direct drug effects upon the brain. The most common drugs that can produce primary encephalopathy are analgesics, anesthetics, antibiotics, antivirals, antiepileptics, antineoplastics, immunosuppressants, immunomodulators, neuroleptics and mood stabilizers [3, 5].

EP Secondary to Drug-Induced Metabolic Disorders can be a secondary effect of drug-induced hepatic, renal, metabolic or cardiovascular toxicity [3, 5 - 7]:

- *Hepatic EP* occurs in patients using hepatotoxic drugs, such as acetaminophen, acetylsalicylic acid, anesthetics, antineoplastics, benzodiazepines, narcotics, antiepileptics and diuretics.
- *Vitamin B12 deficiency-related dementia* is a dose-dependent lesion of patients taking proton pump inhibitors (PPIs).
- *Uremic EP* occurs secondary to the nephrotoxic effect of NSAIDs, antibiotics/antivirals, benzodiazepines, antidepressants/mood stabilizers, antihistamines, antineoplastics, cardiovascular agents, diuretics, proton pump inhibitors (PPIs) and illicit drugs (cocaine, heroin, methadone).
- *Hypoglycemic EP* can emerge in diabetic patients taking insulin, oral hypoglycemic agents, insulin-like growth factor, ACE inhibitors or beta blockers.
- *Hypertensive EP* can emerge in patients with malignant hypertension taking mineralocorticoids or catecholamines.

Iatrogenic Spongiform EP is also known as Creutzfeldt-Jakob disease. It can be a sporadic, familial or transmissible spongiform EP caused by pathogenic prions. The clinical signs and symptoms are rapidly progressive dementia, memory loss, profound personality changes, hallucinations, speech impairment, myoclonus, ataxia, rigid posture and seizures. The two main sources of prion infection are transplantation of contaminated cadaveric tissues (cornea, dura mater, pituitary gland) and utilization of contaminated devices (stereotactic electroencephalography [EEG] electrodes, neurosurgical instruments) [8].

Progressive Multifocal Leukoencephalopathy (PML) is a rare demyelinating and usually fatal virus-related disease of the white matter of the CNS. It is caused by the reactivation of ubiquitous John Cunningham polyomavirus (JCV), which is present in 50-60% of healthy adults between 20 and 50 years of age, the percentage increasing with age. JCV is normally kept under control and is harmless except in cases of weakened immune system.

Iatrogenic PML can be linked to treatment with several drugs, especially immunosuppressive agents and monoclonal antibodies. It is considered a multi-symptomatic condition, often with cognitive disturbances accompanying deficits in motor and sensory function. PML has a mortality rate of 30-50% in the first few months if the patients remain immunocompromised, and those who survive can present varying degrees of neurological disabilities [9, 10].

Posterior Reversible EP Syndrome is typically developed in organ transplantation (~0.5% of organ recipients). Patients with this syndrome develop headaches, visual disturbances, altered mentation and often seizures. Severe hypertension is commonly present, but a quarter of such patients are normotensive [11].

Drug-Induced Movement Disorders

Several groups of drugs may induce abnormalities of movement, posture and muscle tone that resemble primary extrapyramidal disorders [3, 12].

Parkinsonism is a clinical syndrome characterized by tremor, bradykinesia, rigidity and postural instability. The prevalence of drug-induced parkinsonism is about 20% of total Parkinson's disease patients and can be classified according to the following groups [13, 14]:

- *High-risk drugs*: dopamine receptor-blocking agents (DRBA, neuroleptics), dopamine depleters and drugs reducing dopamine levels.
- *Drugs with intermediate risk*: calcium channel blockers, anticonvulsants and mood stabilizers (lithium).
- *Low-risk drugs*: antihypertensives, antiarrhythmics, immunosuppressants, selective serotonin reuptake inhibitors, tricyclic antidepressants, monoamine oxidase inhibitors, antifungals, antibiotics, antivirals, antineoplastics, statins and hormones.

Dystonia is a neurological movement disorder in which sustained muscle contractions cause twisting and repetitive movement or abnormal posture. It can be an early or late drug-related effect [15]:

- *Acute dystonia* occurs shortly after use of DRBA in 2.3-94% of patients. The main risk factors are male gender, young age (under 30 years of age), high potency and dose of DRBA, underlying psychiatric illness, mental retardation and familial predisposition.
- *Tardive dystonia* develops after weeks or years of DRBA exposure and involves (but is not necessarily limited to) orofacial muscles.

Akathisia is a neurological movement disorder characterized by a feeling of inner restlessness and compelling need to be in constant motion. It can be an early or late drug-related effect [15]:

- *Acute akathisia* starts within hours or days (first two weeks) of initiation or increase in DRBA dosage. The incidence ranges from 21% to 31%. Use of atypical neuroleptics decreases the risk of this lesion.
- *Tardive akathisia* is defined as being present for at least one month when the patient is on a constant dose of a DRBA. It occurs with an incidence of 20-40%.

Dyskinesia refers to a category of acute or tardive movement disorders characterized by involuntary muscle movement (especially stereotypic orobuccolingual dyskinesia) and diminished voluntary movements. *Tardive dyskinesia* is defined as an abnormal involuntary movement following a minimum of three months of neuroleptic treatment in a patient with no other known etiology for movement disorders. It occurs in 24% of patients taking neuroleptics, butyrophenones, phenothiazines, thioxanthenes, anticholinergics, antidepressants, antiemetics, anxiolytics, antiepileptics, antiparkinsonian agents or mood stabilizers. The main risk factors for tardive dyskinesia are affective disorders, old age, female gender, total cumulative drug exposure, diabetes mellitus, alcohol abuse and cocaine intake [15].

Tremor is an involuntary, somewhat rhythmic muscle contraction and relaxation involving twitching movements of one or more body parts. It can be induced by the following drugs: beta-adrenergic agonists, sympathomimetics, anticonvulsants, neuroleptics, dopamine depleters, antidepressants, selective serotonin reuptake inhibitors, mood stabilizers, antiarrhythmics, antineoplastics, immunosuppressants, amphetamines, xanthines, precursors of catecholamines, hormones (tyrosine) and illicit drugs (cocaine, alcohol, nicotine) [12, 16].

Choreoathetosis is an abnormal involuntary movement disorder characterized by a combination of chorea (rapid, brief, irregular, nonrepetitive, randomly distributed movements involving both proximal and distal muscles, unstable with a "dance-like" gait) and athetosis (slow, convoluted, writhing movements of the fingers, hands, toes, feet and, in some cases, arms, legs, neck and tongue). It can be induced by the following drugs: anticonvulsants, anticholinergics, tricyclic antidepressants, amphetamines, antihistamines, selective serotonin reuptake inhibitors, xanthenes, antiemetics (metoclopramide) and precursors of catecholamines (levodopa) [12].

Myoclonus is a sudden, abrupt, brief, "shock-like" involuntary movement caused by muscular contractions or a sudden brief lapse of muscle tonus in active postural muscles. It can be induced by the following drugs: antiparkinsonian agents, cyclic antidepressants, atypical antipsychotics, hypnotics, opioids, antiepileptics, antibiotics and calcium channel blockers [12, 17].

Neuroleptic Malignant Syndrome is a life-threatening neurological disorder (with a mortality rate of 4-22%) that occurs in 0.1-1.8% of patients taking neuroleptic drugs. The main risk factors are use of high-potency drugs, rapid increase in dosage, long-acting forms of neuroleptics and combination of neuroleptics with lithium and antidepressants. It is more common in young adults (under 40 years of age) and in men as compared to women (1.5-2.1 ratio).

The clinical signs and symptoms are severe muscular rigidity, fever (above 39°C), tremor, diaphoresis, symptoms of autonomic system instability (incontinence, tachycardia, tachypnea, labile blood pressure, incontinence), mutism and alterations in mental status (agitation, delirium or coma). Leukocytosis and elevated serum levels of creatinine phosphokinase are associated. This syndrome has a primarily hyperacute presentation (occurring in the first 24-72 hours after drug administration). In patients taking oral neuroleptics, the syndrome can emerge after 10-13 days, and even later following administration of depot agents [3, 12, 15].

Serotonin Syndrome is a potentially life-threatening condition induced by increased serotoninergic activity in the CNS. It can be induced by the following drugs: selective serotonin reuptake inhibitors, serotonin-norepinephrine reuptake inhibitors, dopamine-norepinephrine reuptake inhibitors, serotonin modulators and tricyclic antidepressants. Moreover, drug-drug interaction increases the severity of serotonin toxicity.

Serotonin syndrome emerges between six and 24 hours after initiation of treatment. The clinical symptoms include hyperthermia (above 38°C), agitated delirium, ocular clonus (slow, continuous, horizontal movement), dilated pupils, tremor, myoclonus, akathisia, deep tendon hyperreflexia, inducible/spontaneous muscle clonus, incoordination, muscle rigidity, bilateral Babinski signs, dry membranes, flushed skin and diaphoresis. Elevated serum levels of leukocytes and creatinine phosphokinase, along with low levels of serum bicarbonate concentration, are associated [3, 18].

Drug-Induced Seizures

A seizure is defined as "a paroxysmal clinical event characterized by an altered state of consciousness, with or without presence of motor activity or abnormal motor activity accompanied by epileptic EEG activity". About 0.08-1.7% of all seizures are drug-induced. Moreover, 9% of patients with status epilepticus presenting to an emergency department do so as a result of drug toxicity.

Seizures can be induced by the following drugs: anesthetics, antidepressants, antipsychotics, antiepileptics, antihistamines, antibiotics, antineoplastics, CNS stimulants, immunosuppressives, antidiabetics, narcotics/analgesics, NSAIDs, contrast agents and vaccines.

Drug-induced seizures occur as a result of direct (disturbances of cerebral energy metabolism, stimulation of the CNS, neurotransmitter disturbances, cerebral cortical irritation, toxic effects on neurons, *etc.*) or indirect effects on the CNS (cerebral blood flow disturbances, cerebral hypoxia, cardiac rhythm disturbances, electrolyte or metabolic disorders, *etc.*). They can also be the result of drug overdose, drug interactions or sedative drug withdrawal. The main patient-related risk factors are family history of epilepsy, previous seizures, preexisting CNS disorders, extreme ages (infants and elderly patients), associated systemic diseases affecting drug metabolism, alcohol abuse and high fever [3, 12].

Drug-Induced Cerebrovascular Disorders

These disorders occur as a result of the direct or indirect effects of drugs on cerebral vessels, extracerebral vascular systems or coagulation cascade, and include the following lesions [3, 4, 12, 19, 20]:

Hypertension can be induced by sympathomimetics, mineralocorticoids, erythropoietin, amphetamines, NSAIDs and cocaine. It is a major risk factor for stroke, particularly cerebral hemorrhage.

Cerebral Thromboembolic Disorders are caused by procoagulant drugs, heparin (heparin-induced thrombocytopenia), contraceptives, antineoplastics, *etc.*

Cerebral Hemorrhage can occur in patients taking anticoagulants (9-23% of users), thrombolysis agents (1.5% of patients) or platelets antiaggregation drugs (7.3% of users). Prolonged use of platelets antiaggregation drugs, particularly aspirin, is associated with a high risk of brain hemorrhage, notably microbleeds.

Cerebral Vasculitis can be induced by sympathomimetics, amphetamines, antineoplastics, ergot alkaloids, vaccines, *etc.*

Cerebral Vasoconstriction/Vasospasm can occur in patients taking ergot alkaloids, nitrogen monoxide (NO) synthase inhibitors, serotoninergic drugs or antineoplastics. Hyperbaric oxygen therapy is a causal factor.

Iatrogenic Benign Intracranial Hypertension is characterized by increased intracranial pressure in the absence of a tumor or other diseases. It can be induced by the following drugs: antiarrhythmics, antibiotics/antimicrobial agents, withdrawal of corticosteroids, antineoplastics, synthetic steroid ethisterone, growth hormone, NSAIDs, mood stabilizers, oral contraceptives, antiepileptics, retinoids and excess or deficiency of vitamin A. Signs and symptoms are headaches (worse in the morning), nausea, vomiting, pulsatile tinnitus, paresis of the abducens nerve (the sixth cranial nerve) and papilledema or optic atrophy with visual disorders.

Drug-Induced Cerebellar Disorders

These disorders include ataxia, dysmetria, dyssynergia, dysarthria, dysdiadochokinesia, cerebellar nystagmus, intention tremor and muscular hypotonia. They can be induced by the following drugs: antidepressants, antineoplastics, antiepileptics, mood stabilizers, histamine-H2 receptor antagonists, sedatives and vaccines [3, 12, 21].

Drug-Induced Disorders of Cranial Nerves

These primarily relate to optic and vestibular nerve injuries, dysgeusia and dysosmia [3, 12, 19, 22, 23]:

Optic Neuropathy can be induced by antiarrhythmics, antibiotics, antineoplastics, antiepileptics, ergot alkaloids, NSAIDs, immunosuppressants, oral contraceptives, phosphodiesterase type 5 inhibitors, vaccines and chelators. The main symptoms are visual changes, which can also be induced by hyperbaric oxygen therapy.

Ophthalmoplegia is the paralysis of one or more of the six muscles that hold the eye in place and control its movements. External ophthalmoplegia can occur in patients taking antiepileptics, barbiturates, tricyclic antidepressants or antineoplastics. Internal ophthalmoplegia can be induced by benzodiazepines, mood stabilizers or antineoplastics.

Ototoxicity is known to be induced by over 100 drugs that can cause acoustic and vestibular damage to the inner ear and/or to the cochleovestibular nerve. They include aminoglycoside antibiotics, anesthetics, antiepileptics, antihistaminics, antimalarial drugs, antineoplastics, antacids, anxiolytics, CNS stimulants, diuretics, NSAIDs, opioids, neuroleptics, sedatives and tricyclic antidepressants. The acoustic symptomatology refers to tinnitus and hypo-/anacusis, whereas vestibular injuries induce vertigo, nystagmus and balance impairment. Otic barotrauma can also be induced by hyperbaric oxygen therapy.

Smell and Taste Disorders are also known as dysosmia and dysgeusia. Drugs can produce injuries of receptors (90%), disorders of sensory neural transmission (5%) or disturbances of CNS perception (5%). They include the following agents: analgesics, anesthetics, anorectics, antiasthmatics, antihistamines, antibiotics, antifungals, antivirals, antineoplastics, chelators, ACE inhibitors, calcium channel inhibitors, angiotensin II receptor antagonists, antiarrhythmics, hypolipemiant drugs, alpha-adrenergic agonists, antithyroid drugs, antidiabetics, antiparkinsonian drugs, antiepileptics, psychotropic drugs, antimigraine drugs, NSAIDs and nasal decongestants.

Drug-Induced Aseptic Meningitis

Iatrogenic aseptic meningitis can occur following lumbar puncture or as an immune-mediated ADR-related complication. It can also be the result of irritation of the meninges by intrathecal instillation of a certain agent. The most common drugs involved in its etiology are antivirals (valacyclovir), antibiotics/sulfonamides (amoxicillin, ciprofloxacin, isoniazid, sulfamethoxazole, trimethoprim, metronidazole), allopurinol, anticonvulsants (lamotrigine), antineoplastics, monoclonal antibodies, NSAIDs (ibuprofen), immunomodulators (immunoglobulin IV, muromonab-CD3), vaccines and contrast agents. Its clinical signs and symptoms are headaches, photophobia, myalgia, nausea, vomiting, fever and neck stiffness. Cerebrospinal fluid examination reveals neutrophilic pleocytosis, high levels of proteins, normal levels of glucose and lactic acid and negative Gram stain and cultures [3, 24, 25].

Drug-Induced Spinal Cord Disorders

Intrathecal Toxicity can be induced by those drugs introduced into the intrathecal space for diagnostic or therapeutic purposes. The clinical consequences are spinal cord disorders. The main myelotoxic drugs are antineoplastics, corticosteroids, lidocaine, morphine and radiological contrast agents [3, 12].

Myelopathy describes any neurological deficit related to the spinal cord. It can be induced by antineoplastics, corticosteroids, penicillin, vaccines and illicit drugs (heroin, use of NO for recreational purposes). Signs and symptoms depend on the affected spinal level (cervical, thoracic or lumbar) and include upper motor neuron signs (weakness, spasticity, hyperreflexia, and pathological reflexes), lower motor neuron signs (weakness, muscle hypotonicity, muscle atrophy, fasciculations in the innervated muscle), sensory deficits (global/partial hypo-/anesthesia) and autonomic disturbances (bowel/bladder disorders, sexual dysfunctions) [3, 12].

Drug-Induced Peripheral Neuropathies

Polyneuropathy encompasses a wide range of disorders in which the peripheral nerves are damaged. About 2-4% of all polyneuropathies are drug-induced. The most common drugs involved in its etiology are antineoplastics, antibiotics/antifungals/antivirals, antiarrhythmics, neuroleptics, tricyclic antidepressants, mood stabilizers, serotonin reuptake inhibitors and miscellaneous drugs (allopurinol, anticoagulants, botulinum toxin, cimetidine, colchicine, disulfiram, interferon-alpha, hypolipemiants, oral contraceptives, D-penicillamine, pyridoxine abuse, sulfasalazine, vaccines, *etc*.).

The mechanisms involved in the genesis of drug-related polyneuropathy include drug-induced vitamin deficiencies, interference with metabolic processes within nerves, immune mechanisms and direct injuries to nerves or vessels.

The clinical signs and symptoms are related to the peripheral somatosensory system (pain, hyperalgesia, hyperpathia, hyperesthesia, paresthesia, dysesthesia, allodynia, hypo-/anesthesia) or somatomotor system (paresis/paralysis, muscle hypotonia, muscular atrophy, hypo-/areflexia) [3, 26 - 28].

Polyradiculoneuropathy (Guillain-Barré syndrome) is an acute inflammatory demyelinating polyradiculoneuropathy characterized by concomitant occurrence of polyneuropathy and polyradiculopathy. It can be induced by corticosteroids, antimalarial drugs, parenteral gangliosides, gold salts, quinolone antibiotics, oxytocin, D-penicillamine, streptokinase and vaccines. Its clinical signs and symptoms are similar to those described in polyneuropathy, but respiratory failure and hypotension are also associated. Elevated protein levels with low numbers of white blood cells (albuminocytological dissociation) are specific changes in the cerebrospinal fluid [3, 26 - 28].

Disorders of the Autonomic Nervous System can be associated with the following neurological disorders [3, 12].

- *Cholinergic syndrome* can be induced by cholinomimetics and anti-cholinesterases, and is characterized by confusion, weakness, hypersalivation, urinary and fecal incontinence, vomiting, sweating, muscle fasciculations, miosis, pulmonary edema and bradycardia.
- *Anticholinergic syndrome* can be a consequence of anesthesia or administration

of drugs such as antiemetics, antihistamines with anticholinergic activity, medications used for urinary incontinence, antiparkinsonian medications, antipsychotics, tricyclic antidepressants, antispasmodics for the GI tract, and herbal medications. Clinical signs and symptoms of anticholinergic syndrome are delirium, cognitive impairment, agitation, hallucinations (visual, auditory and tactile), poor coordination, dry mouth, low sweating, pupil dilatation, tachycardia, respiratory depression, urinary retention, diminished bowel movements, orthostatic hypotension, seizures and coma.

- *Sympathomimetic syndrome* can be induced by amphetamine, beta-adrenoceptor stimulants, ephedrine, theophylline, caffeine overdose and cocaine. Its clinical signs and symptoms are bronchospasm, hyperthermia, extreme hypertension, cardiac arrhythmias, myocardial ischemia, seizures, mydriasis, diaphoresis, acute psychosis and bruxism.
- *Autonomic neuropathy* is a term used for various conditions characterized by disorders of the autonomic nervous system. Autonomic dysfunctions are well recognized as complications of peripheral neuropathy, but can also be produced by drugs such as antineoplastics and ergot compounds. The clinical signs/symptoms/consequences of such conditions are excessive fatigue, polydipsia, dizziness (often associated with orthostatic hypotension and even syncope), blood pressure or heart rate fluctuations, mydriasis, neurogenic bladder dysfunctions, gastroparesis, constipation, excessive or lack of sweating, and sexual dysfunctions.

Drug-Induced Muscle Disorders

Disorders of Neuromuscular Junctions (NMJs) relate to disturbances of the synapses at the point of contact between nerve terminals and muscular fibers, which specialize in conversion of presynaptic nervous influx into postsynaptic action potential. The neurotransmitter acetylcholine is responsible for its integrity. Drugs that impair neuromuscular transmission include anesthetics (general and local), antibiotics, antiepileptics, botulinum toxin, benzodiazepines, anti-arrhythmics, calcium channel blockers, beta-adrenergic blockers, neuromuscular blocking agents and miscellaneous drugs (chloroquine, D-penicillamine, corticosteroids, interferon-alpha, psychotropic drugs, diuretics, magnesium sulfate, sodium lactate, statins, tetanus antitoxin and iodinated contrast substances). Disorders of NMJs are first characterized by muscle weakness. The above-mentioned drugs exacerbate myasthenia gravis or induce myasthenic syndromes that can spontaneously resolve following drug cessation [3, 12, 29, 30].

Iatrogenic Myopathies can be induced by anesthetic agents, ACE inhibitors, calcium channel blockers, diuretics, antibiotics, antifungals, antiparasitics, antiretroviral agents, anticholinesterase medications, antineoplastics, depolarizing muscle relaxants, beta-adrenergic agonists, hypolipemiants, corticosteroids, immunomodulators, alcohol intoxication and miscellaneous drugs (amiodarone, D-penicillamine, lithium, L-tryptophan, procainamide, retinoids, riluzole, interferon-alpha, iodinated contrast agents, cocaine, *etc.*). These drugs present direct myotoxicity, immune-mediated inflammatory myopathy or indirect muscle damage (*e.g.,* drug-induced hypokalemia).

The clinical signs/symptoms/consequences are myalgia (muscle pain, stiffness or cramps), myotonia (delayed relaxation of skeletal muscle after voluntary contraction), painless proximal myopathy (proximal muscle weakness), polymyositis (muscle pain, stiffness, muscle weakness), myokymia (rhythmic muscle rippling), hypokalemic myopathy (severe muscle weakness), depressed tendon reflexes, high serum levels of creatine kinase, mitochondrial myopathy with ragged-red fibers (myalgia, proximal generalized muscle weakness, high serum levels of creatine kinase), rhabdomyolysis (muscle pain, tenderness, severe muscle weakness, muscle swelling, serum electrolytes disturbances, myoglobinuria, high serum levels of creatine kinase), malignant hyperthermia (severe muscular rigidity, hyperpyrexia, metabolic acidosis, myoglobinuria) and focal myopathy (fibrous myopathy after drug injection) [3, 12, 31, 32].

NEUROLOGICAL COMPLICATIONS DURING DIAGNOSTIC AND THERAPEUTIC PROCEDURES

Cerebral Angiography

Cerebral angiography is performed for diagnosis or therapeutic purposes in patients with cerebral aneurysms, brain arteriovenous malformations, dural arteriovenous fistulae, cryptogenic intracerebral hemorrhage, carotid/vertebral arteries dissections, high-grade intracranial stenosis, cerebral arteries thrombolysis/thrombectomy, cerebral vasculitis, preoperative cerebral tumor embolization or cerebral venous thrombosis.

The most common angiography-related neurological complication is cerebral ischemia, which occurs in 2% of cases (transient in 0.7%, reversible in 0.2% and permanent in 0.5% of patients). Iodinated contrast encephalopathy with persistent neurological deficit is another rare but reported complication. A higher rate of complications occurs in patients over 55 years of age and in patients with associated morbidities (cardiovascular disorders, atherosclerotic cerebrovascular disease, subarachnoid hemorrhage, transient ischemic attack, *etc.*) [33 - 35].

Lumbar Puncture

In daily practice, diagnosis of lumbar puncture is indicated to be performed either urgently (suspected CNS bacterial/viral/fungal infections and suspected subarachnoid hemorrhage in a patient with a negative CT scan) or non-urgently (carcinomatous meningitis, tuberculous meningitis, sarcoidosis, normal pressure hydrocephalus, CNS vasculitis). In other cases, it is non-mandatory for diagnosis (multiple sclerosis, Guillain-Barré syndrome, chronic inflammatory demyelinating polyneuropathy, leukoencephalopathies and paraneoplastic syndromes). It is also performed for spinal anesthesia, intrathecal administration of antibiotics or contrast agents for myelography/cisternography, and intrathecal chemotherapy. It is contraindicated in patients with high intracranial pressure, coagulopathy or brain abscesses, or when there is infected skin over the needle entry site.

The most common neurological complication of lumbar puncture is headache. This occurs in 40% of patients, more frequently in women, worsens 15 minutes after sitting/standing, and can be accompanied by stiffness, tinnitus, hyperacusis, photophobia and nausea. A severe and uncommon complication is supra/infratentorial brain herniation. Other complications include bleeding (epidural/subdural hematoma or subarachnoid/intracranial hemorrhage), subarachnoid block and spinal coning (when the puncture is performed below the level of spinal compression), cranial neuropathies, disorders of nerve root irritation, lower back pain and intracranial low pressure.

Infections (meningitis) are rare and can be the result of contaminated needles, disseminating skin flora without adequate disinfection, performing a puncture in an area of infection, or introducing blood into the subarachnoid space in the presence of bacteremia. A few years ago (2012-2013), epidemic fungal meningitis (Aspergillus fumigatus, Exserohilum rostratum) was reported in the USA, caused by injection of contaminated methylprednisolone into the epidural compartment of more than 150 patients [36 - 38].

Organ Transplantations

Early and delayed neurological complications may develop in 30-60% of recipients of solid organs. These can be related to the surgical procedure, post-transplant immunosuppression or opportunistic infections. Details regarding the immunopathology of transplantation are presented in Chapter 3. Drug-related neurotoxicity is a dose-dependent lesion that is primarily induced by calcineurin inhibitors, such as cyclosporine and tacrolimus (10-30% of patients). Other drugs, such as mycophenolate mofetil, rapamycin (sirolimus, everolimus), azathioprine, corticosteroids and monoclonal/polyclonal antibodies, can also induce neurological disorders. Monoclonal/polyclonal antibodies can cause aseptic meningitis in 5-10% of patients.

Opportunistic infections of the CNS affect 5-7% of transplanted patients, with a reported mortality rate of 75-90%. Moreover, neurological complications are the primary cause of death in approximately 20% of transplant recipients. Bacterial infections primarily occur within the first two months, whereas viral and fungal infections occur at about six months post-transplant [39, 40].

Neurological Complications of Liver Transplantation

About 13-47% of patients receiving liver transplantation present neurological complications. The most common complications are tonic-clonic seizures, which emerge in 40% of patients. Central pontine myelinolysis is reported in 1-8% of recipients (usually in alcoholic and malnourished patients). Other complications include mononeuropathies (2-13%), acute myopathy (7%), brachial plexopathy (1-5.8%), polyneuropathies (1.5-10%), cerebrovascular disorders (3-6.5%), CNS opportunistic bacterial/viral meningitis/meningoencephalitis (5%), and post-transplant encephalopathy (caused by the presence of pre-transplant encephalopathy, complex metabolic disturbances, medication toxicity or CNS infections) [41].

Neurological Complications of Heart Transplantation

In heart transplanted patients, the rate of neurological complications varies from 23% in the perioperative period to 13% in the first month and 18% in the first 10 years following surgery. The main risk factors are previous morbidities, such as stroke, transient ischemic attack, diabetes mellitus, and renal failure.

Perioperative complications include cerebrovascular disorders that occur in 4-42% of patients (ischemic stroke is the most common complication, but hemorrhagic stroke, post-anoxic encephalopathy, seizures and transient ischemic attacks can also appear) and peripheral nervous system complications (brachial plexopathy, peroneal nerve neuropathy, vocal cord paralysis).

Postoperative complications are cerebrovascular disorders that occur in 9% of patients (ischemic stroke – 60%, transient ischemic attacks – 28%, hemorrhagic stroke – 12%), depression (28%), polyneuropathy (18%) and seizure (4%). Neurological-related death emerges in 8% of patients who die in the first year following intervention [42 - 44].

Neurological Complications of Renal Transplantation

The incidence of neurological complications in kidney transplanted patients is about 10-20% more common in elderly patients (over 65 years of age) and patients with diabetes mellitus. Bacterial/fungal/viral infections of the CNS occur in 5-10% of patients, being associated with a high rate of mortality. Other complications include cerebrovascular disorders (8%), peripheral neuropathy (uremic polyneuropathy improves after transplantation, but may persist in patients who have been on dialysis for years prior to transplant), metabolic disorders (uremia, hyperglycemia, hypercalcemia, hypo-/hypernatremia, hypo-/hyper-potassemia, hypomagnesemia), posterior reversible encephalopathy syndrome (0.5%) and genesis of brain malignant tumors (lymphomas and brain metastases of immunosuppression-related cancers) [45 - 47].

Post-Transplant Lymphoproliferative Disorders of the CNS

These are uncommon (2-7% of recipients) but severe complications of the CNS that develops in immunosuppressed recipients of solid organs, bone marrow and stem cells. The spectrum of diseases ranges from EBV-driven polyclonal proliferations to EBV+ or EBV- malignant lymphomas, most of which having B-cell phenotypes [48, 49]. Details regarding these disorders are presented in Chapter 3.

Radiation Therapy

Radiation therapy, which was explored in Chapter 2, may induce dose/volume/time-dependent damage to the nervous system. This can involve direct neurological damage or the consequences of radiation-induced injuries of the blood vessels supplying the brain or the endocrine organs necessary for normal nervous system functioning. The most common radiation-induced neurological complications are the following [50 - 52]:

- *Acute encephalopathy* occurs within hours or days of large radiation fractions given to patients with high intracranial pressure. It usually emerges after the first radiation session, presenting as headache and nausea and gradually becoming less severe.
- *Early delayed encephalopathy*, which is thought to be the result of demyelination, usually begins in the second or third month after irradiation. If the patient has a glioblastoma, the symptoms can simulate tumor progression ("pseudoprogression"). A rare and serious form of this lesion is brainstem encephalopathy, occurring as a result of radiation of posterior fossa tumors. This presents as ataxia, diplopia, dysarthria and nystagmus.
- *Late delayed radiation necrosis* usually begins one to two years following completion of radiotherapy for a brain or head and neck tumor. The clinical picture can mimic a tumor recurrence.
- *Cerebral atrophy* often follows prophylactic whole-brain irradiation (in acute

leukemia) and may be accompanied by periventricular leukoencephalopathy, presenting with memory loss, gait abnormalities and urge urinary incontinence.

- *Early delayed radiation myelopathy* is common following irradiation of the neck and starts within weeks after the initiation of radiotherapy. Symptoms (an electrical sensation that runs down the back and into the limbs) are thought to be attributable to demyelination of the posterior columns of the spinal cord (Lhermitte's sign).
- *Late delayed radiation myelopathy* appears in two forms. The first and most common form is characterized by progressive myelopathy, which appears between months and years following radiotherapy. Myelopathy progresses subacutely over weeks or months as spastic paraparesis or quadriparesis (transverse myelopathy). The second form is a rare motor neuron syndrome that follows pelvic irradiation. It occurs between months and years following irradiation and is characterized by flaccid paraparesis.
- *Cranial nerves injuries* present as smell and taste disorders (following cranial radiotherapy), optic neuropathy (progressive monocular or bilateral blindness occurring between seven and 26 months after cranial radiotherapy), and hearing loss. The hypoglossal nerve can be injured following neck irradiation, with damage to the recurrent laryngeal nerve and sympathetic fibers being associated in some cases.
- *Peripheral nerves injuries* can be early or late effects of radiotherapy. For example, delayed radiation brachial or lumbosacral plexopathies can occur months to years after radiotherapy performed for breast or testicular malignancies.
- *Radiation-induced cerebral tumors* such as meningiomas, gliomas or lymphomas can appear years to decades after irradiation of nervous tissue.
- *Cerebrovascular abnormalities* include the narrowing of large intracranial or extracranial blood vessels (radiation arteriopathy, occurring months to years after radiotherapy), vascular anomalies development (cavernous hemangiomas), transient ischemic attacks and cerebral infarction.

CONFLICT OF INTEREST

The authors confirm that this chapter content has no conflict of interest.

ACKNOWLEDGEMENTS

Declared none.

REFERENCES

[1] Grosset KA, Grosset DG. Prescribed drugs and neurological complications. J Neurol Neurosurg Psychiatry 2004; 75 (Suppl. 3): iii2-8. [http://dx.doi.org/10.1136/jnnp.2004.045757] [PMID: 15316038]

[2] Mark RB, Don JM. Drug-induced disorders of the nervous system. Clin Med (Lond) 2007; 7(2): 170-6.
[http://dx.doi.org/10.7861/clinmedicine.7-2-170] [PMID: 17491507]

[3] Jain KK. Drug-induced neurological disorders. 3rd. Hogrefe Publishing, Göttingen 2012; pp. 1-388.

[4] Sposato LA, Fustinoni O. Iatrogenic neurology. In: Biller J, Ferro JM, Eds. Handbook of clinical neurology: Neurologic aspects of systemic disease, Part III. Elsevier, Amsterdam 2014; vol 121 (3rd series).
[http://dx.doi.org/10.1016/B978-0-7020-4088-7.00107-3]

[5] Hansen N. Drug-induced encephalopathy. In: Tanasescu R, Ed. Miscellanea on encephalopathies – a second look. InTech 2012; pp. 39-59.
[http://dx.doi.org/10.5772/31172]

[6] Ruiz de Angulo D, Ortiz MA, Martínez de Haro LF. Side effects of proton-pump inhibitors: another reason to indicate anti-reflux surgery for Barretts esophagus? Cir Esp 2014; 92(5): 303-4.
[http://dx.doi.org/10.1016/j.ciresp.2014.01.009] [PMID: 24625629]

[7] Wilhelm SM, Rjater RG, Kale-Pradhan PB. Perils and pitfalls of long-term effects of proton pump inhibitors. Expert Rev Clin Pharmacol 2013; 6(4): 443-51.
[http://dx.doi.org/10.1586/17512433.2013.811206] [PMID: 23927671]

[8] Brown P, Brandel J-P, Sato T, *et al.* Iatrogenic Creutzfeldt-Jakob disease, final assessment. Emerg Infect Dis 2012; 18(6): 901-7.
[http://dx.doi.org/10.3201/eid1806.120116] [PMID: 22607808]

[9] Keene DL, Legare C, Taylor E, Gallivan J, Cawthorn GM, Vu D. Monoclonal antibodies and progressive multifocal leukoencephalopathy. Can J Neurol Sci 2011; 38(4): 565-71.
[http://dx.doi.org/10.1017/S0317167100012105] [PMID: 21672696]

[10] Melis M, Biagi C, Småbrekke L, *et al.* Drug-induced progressive multifocal leukoencephalopathy: A comprehensive analysis of the WHO adverse drug reaction database. CNS Drugs 2015; 29(10): 879-91.
[http://dx.doi.org/10.1007/s40263-015-0286-3] [PMID: 26507833]

[11] Bartynski WS, Tan HP, Boardman JF, Shapiro R, Marsh JW. Posterior reversible encephalopathy syndrome after solid organ transplantation. AJNR Am J Neuroradiol 2008; 29(5): 924-30.
[http://dx.doi.org/10.3174/ajnr.A0960] [PMID: 18272559]

[12] O'Connor KD, Mastaglia FL. Drug-induced disorders of nervous system. In: Aminoff MJ, Josephson SA, Eds. Aminoff's neurology and general medicine. 5th ed. Amsterdam: Elsevier 2014; pp. 685-711.
[http://dx.doi.org/10.1016/B978-0-12-407710-2.00032-1]

[13] Shin HW, Chung SJ. Drug-induced parkinsonism. J Clin Neurol 2012; 8(1): 15-21.
[http://dx.doi.org/10.3988/jcn.2012.8.1.15] [PMID: 22523509]

[14] Bohlega SA, Al-Foghom NB. Drug-induced Parkinsons disease. A clinical review. Neurosciences (Riyadh) 2013; 18(3): 215-21.
[PMID: 23887211]

[15] Sethi KD, Morgan JC. Drug-induced movement disorders. In: Jankovic J, Tolosa E, Eds. Parkinson's disease & movement disorders. 5th ed. Philadelphia: Lippincott Williams & Wilkins 2007; pp. 394-408.

[16] Morgan JC, Sethi KD. Drug-induced tremors. Lancet Neurol 2005; 4(12): 866-76.
[http://dx.doi.org/10.1016/S1474-4422(05)70250-7] [PMID: 16297844]

[17] Jiménez-Jiménez FJ, Puertas I, de Toledo-Heras M. Drug-induced myoclonus: frequency, mechanisms and management. CNS Drugs 2004; 18(2): 93-104.
[http://dx.doi.org/10.2165/00023210-200418020-00003] [PMID: 14728056]

[18] Boyer EW, Shannon M. The serotonin syndrome. N Engl J Med 2005; 352(11): 1112-20.

[http://dx.doi.org/10.1056/NEJMra041867] [PMID: 15784664]

[19] Obiagwu C, Paul V, Chadha S, Hollander G, Shani J. Acute pulmonary edema secondary to hyperbaric oxygen therapy. Oxf Med Case Rep 2015; 2015: 183-4.
[http://dx.doi.org/10.1093/omcr/omv002]

[20] Stiebel-Kalish H, Eyal S, Steiner I. The role of aquaporin-1 in idiopathic and drug-induced intracranial hypertension. Med Hypotheses 2013; 81(6): 1059-62.
[http://dx.doi.org/10.1016/j.mehy.2013.10.002] [PMID: 24169407]

[21] van Gaalen J, Kerstens FG, Maas RP, Härmark L, van de Warrenburg BP. Drug-induced cerebellar ataxia: a systematic review. CNS Drugs 2014; 28(12): 1139-53.
[http://dx.doi.org/10.1007/s40263-014-0200-4] [PMID: 25391707]

[22] Cianfrone G, Pentangelo D, Cianfrone F, *et al.* Pharmacological drugs inducing ototoxicity, vestibular symptoms and tinnitus: a reasoned and updated guide. Eur Rev Med Pharmacol Sci 2011; 15(6): 601-36.
[PMID: 21796866]

[23] Naik BS, Shetty N, Maben EV. Drug-induced taste disorders. Eur J Intern Med 2010; 21(3): 240-3.
[http://dx.doi.org/10.1016/j.ejim.2010.01.017] [PMID: 20493431]

[24] Hopkins S, Jolles S. Drug-induced aseptic meningitis. Expert Opin Drug Saf 2005; 4(2): 285-97.
[http://dx.doi.org/10.1517/14740338.4.2.285] [PMID: 15794720]

[25] Cascella C, Naushheen S, Cunha BA. A differential diagnosis of drug-induced aseptic meningitis. Infect Med 2008; 25: 331-4.

[26] Weimer LH. Medication-induced peripheral neuropathy. Curr Neurol Neurosci Rep 2003; 3(1): 86-92.
[http://dx.doi.org/10.1007/s11910-003-0043-8] [PMID: 12507417]

[27] Diezi M, Buclin T, Kuntzer T. Toxic and drug-induced peripheral neuropathies: updates on causes, mechanisms and management. Curr Opin Neurol 2013; 26(5): 481-8.
[http://dx.doi.org/10.1097/WCO.0b013e328364eb07] [PMID: 23995278]

[28] Vilholm OJ, Christensen AA, Zedan AH, Itani M. Drug-induced peripheral neuropathy. Basic Clin Pharmacol Toxicol 2014; 115(2): 185-92.
[http://dx.doi.org/10.1111/bcpt.12261] [PMID: 24786912]

[29] Ahmed A, Simmons Z. Drugs which may exacerbate or induce myasthenia gravis: clinician's guide. Internet J Neurol 2008; 10: 1-8.

[30] Howard JF Jr. Toxic neuromuscular transmission disorders. In: Kaminski HJ, Ed. *Myasthenia gravis* and related disorders. 2nd ed. Totowa: Humana Press 2009; pp. 255-77.
[http://dx.doi.org/10.1007/978-1-59745-156-7_16]

[31] Klopstock T. Drug-induced myopathies. Curr Opin Neurol 2008; 21(5): 590-5.
[http://dx.doi.org/10.1097/WCO.0b013e32830e2774] [PMID: 18769254]

[32] Dalakas MC. Toxic and drug-induced myopathies. J Neurol Neurosurg Psychiatry 2009; 80(8): 832-8.
[http://dx.doi.org/10.1136/jnnp.2008.168294] [PMID: 19608783]

[33] Willinsky RA, Taylor SM, TerBrugge K, Farb RI, Tomlinson G, Montanera W. Neurologic complications of cerebral angiography: prospective analysis of 2,899 procedures and review of the literature. Radiology 2003; 227(2): 522-8.
[http://dx.doi.org/10.1148/radiol.2272012071] [PMID: 12637677]

[34] Kaufmann TJ, Huston J III, Mandrekar JN, Schleck CD, Thielen KR, Kallmes DF. Complications of diagnostic cerebral angiography: evaluation of 19,826 consecutive patients. Radiology 2007; 243(3): 812-9.
[http://dx.doi.org/10.1148/radiol.2433060536] [PMID: 17517935]

[35] Leong S, Fanning NF. Persistent neurological deficit from iodinated contrast encephalopathy following intracranial aneurism coiling. Interv Neuroradiol 2012; 18: 33-41.

[http://dx.doi.org/10.1177/159101991201800105] [PMID: 22440599]

[36] Moghtaderi A, Alvi-Naini R, Sanatinia S. Lumbar puncture: techniques, complications and CNS analyses. In: Blaivas M, Ed. Emergency medicine – an international perspective. InTech 2012; pp. 43-62.
[http://dx.doi.org/10.5772/29511]

[37] Doherty CM, Forbes RB. Diagnostic lumbar puncture. Ulster Med J 2014; 83(2): 93-102.
[PMID: 25075138]

[38] Mutarelli EG, Adoni T. Iatrogenic meningitis. Arq Neuropsiquiatr 2013; 71(9B): 659-60.
[http://dx.doi.org/10.1590/0004-282X20130145] [PMID: 24141499]

[39] Senzolo M, Ferronato C, Burra P. Neurologic complications after solid organ transplantation. Transpl Int 2009; 22(3): 269-78.
[http://dx.doi.org/10.1111/j.1432-2277.2008.00780.x] [PMID: 19076332]

[40] Pruitt AA, Graus F, Rosenfeld MR. Neurological complications of solid organ transplantation. Neurohospitalist 2013; 3(3): 152-66.
[http://dx.doi.org/10.1177/1941874412466090] [PMID: 24167649]

[41] Guarino M, Benito-Leon J, Decruyenaere J, *et al.* Neurological problems in liver transplantation. European Handbook of Neurological Management. 2nd Edition. Willey-Blackwell, Oxford 2011; Vol I: pp. 491-9.

[42] Malheiros SM, Almeida DR, Massaro AR, *et al.* Neurologic complications after heart transplantation. Arq Neuropsiquiatr 2002; 60(2-A): 192-7.
[http://dx.doi.org/10.1590/S0004-282X2002000200002] [PMID: 12068344]

[43] Pérez-Miralles F, Sánchez-Manso JC, Almenar-Bonet L, Sevilla-Mantecón T, Martínez-Dolz L, Vílchez-Padilla JJ. Incidence of and risk factors for neurologic complications after heart transplantation. Transplant Proc 2005; 37(9): 4067-70.
[http://dx.doi.org/10.1016/j.transproceed.2005.09.162] [PMID: 16386628]

[44] Heroux A, Pamboukian SV. Neurologic aspects of heart transplantation. In: Biller J, Ferro JM, Eds. Handbook of clinical neurology: Neurologic aspects of systemic disease, Part III. Elsevier, Amsterdam 2014; vol 121 (3rd series): pp. 1229-36.
[http://dx.doi.org/10.1016/B978-0-7020-4088-7.00082-1]

[45] Ce P, Koskderelioglu A, Coban G, Gedizlioglu M, Nart A, Uslu A. Neurologic complications of renal transplant. Exp Clin Transplant 2012; 10(3): 243-6.
[http://dx.doi.org/10.6002/ect.2011.0130] [PMID: 22631060]

[46] Basso G, Cristelli M, Bichuetti D, *et al.* Major neurological complications following renal transplantation. Am J Transplant 2013; 13: C1379.

[47] Potluri K, Holt D, Hou S. Neurological complications in renal transplantation. In: Biller J, Ferro JM, Eds. Handbook of clinical neurology: Neurologic aspects of systemic disease, Part III. Elsevier, Amsterdam 2014; vol 121 (3rd series): pp. 1246-55.

[48] Castellano-Sanchez AA, Li S, Qian J, Lagoo A, Weir E, Brat DJ. Primary central nervous system posttransplant lymphoproliferative disorders. Am J Clin Pathol 2004; 121(2): 246-53.
[http://dx.doi.org/10.1309/N82CTQ1J0XEVEFQB] [PMID: 14983939]

[49] Kempf C, Tinguely M, Rushing EJ. Posttransplant lymphoproliferative disorder of the central nervous system. Pathobiology 2013; 80(6): 310-8.
[http://dx.doi.org/10.1159/000347225] [PMID: 24013167]

[50] Cross NE, Glantz MJ. Neurologic complications of radiation therapy. Neurol Clin 2003; 21(1): 249-77.
[http://dx.doi.org/10.1016/S0733-8619(02)00031-2] [PMID: 12690652]

[51] Rogers LR. Neurologic complications of radiation. Continuum (Minneap Minn) 2012; 18(2): 343-54.

[http://dx.doi.org/10.1212/01.CON.0000413662.35174.a8] [PMID: 22810131]

[52] Deutsch MB, DeAngelis LM. Neurologic complications of chemotherapy and radiation therapy. In: Aminoff MJ, Josephson SA, Eds. Aminoff's neurology and general medicine. 5th. Amsterdam: Elsevier 2014; pp. 591-609.
[http://dx.doi.org/10.1016/B978-0-12-407710-2.00028-X]

CHAPTER 15

The Endocrinology and Iatrogenesis

Imre Kun*

Department of Endocrinology, University of Medicine and Pharmacy, Tirgu-Mures, Romania

Abstract: Iatrogenicity is inherent to endocrinology, being a consequence of treatment (*e.g.*, use of thyroid hormones in large doses to suppress thyroid stimulating hormone [TSH] in thyroid cancer) or occurring due to a lack of patient compliance (*e.g.*, lack of adequate controls in chronic diseases, such as Hashimoto's chronic thyroiditis). Quite often, it is induced as a side effect of medicines (*e.g.*, long-lasting use of antithyroid agents or glucocorticoids). In this chapter, we review the most important iatrogenic effects, according to the main features of endocrinology. We present certain drugs that can trigger particular syndromes, such as the syndrome of inappropriate antidiuretic hormone secretion (SIAHS), along with preparations with pitressin and complications of treatment performed for pituitary adenomas, potential complications of drugs used to treat pituitary insufficiency in children and other specific features constituting required knowledge for medical practitioners. All therapeutic modalities of hyperthyroidism (medical, surgical, radioiodine) can cause iatrogenic pathology. For example, the euthyroid state is a sine qua non condition of thyroid surgery (except the thyrotoxic storm in advanced stages). Radioiodine treatment, in turn, has its own contraindications. Iodine-containing preparations can activate thyroid autonomies and aggravate autoimmune thyroiditis and overt hyperthyroidism. In hypothyroid elderly and cardiac patients, the thyroid hormone substitution must be applied only after initial cardiovascular treatment, in small, gradually increasing doses. In Addison's disease, indication of dietary salt reduction alongside glucocorticoid substitution, or the lack of increase in glucocorticoid dose in acute injuries, are serious iatrogenic complications.

Keywords: Acromegaly, Adrenal glands, Amiodarone, Antithyroid agents, Gonads, Hypercalcemia, Hyperthyroidism, Hypothyroidism, Octreotide, Thyroiditis.

INTRODUCTION

In endocrinology, iatrogenic lesions are inherent to the treatment of disease (*e.g.*, administration of large doses of thyroid hormones to substitute and suppress thyroid stimulating hormone [TSH] in the treatment of thyroid cancer), while in other circumstances, lesions appear due to lack of patient compliance (*e.g.*, lack of

* **Corresponding author Imre Kun:** Department of Endocrinology, University of Medicine and Pharmacy, Tirgu-Mures, Romania; Tel: 0040-265-212111; Fax: 0040-372-653250; E-mail: kunimre@gmail.com

Simona Gurzu & Ioan Jung (Eds.)

regular controls during treatment of diseases requiring long surveillance, as in the case of Hashimoto's chronic thyroiditis). Quite often, such lesions are induced as side effects of medicines (*e.g.,* long-lasting use of antithyroid agents or glucocorticoids), or by other therapeutic measures used in endocrinology or in associated diseases. In this chapter, the most important iatrogenic effects from the perspective of endocrinology will be reviewed.

IATROGENIC PATHOLOGY OF THE HYPOTHALAMIC-PITUITARY AXIS

Schwartz-Bartter Syndrome

Also known as inappropriate ADH secretion or as the syndrome of inappropriate antidiuretic hormone secretion (SIADH), this condition can be triggered by drugs such as vincristine, digitalis, some diuretics, morphine, carbamazepine, chlorpropamide, clofibrate, clozapine, cyclophosphamide, phenothiazines, tricyclic antidepressants, anesthetics, serotonin reuptake inhibitors, oxytocin, prostaglandin synthesis inhibitors, nicotine, omeprazole, ACE-inhibitors and 3,4-methylenedioxymethamphetamine (MDMA or "ecstasy", a psychostimulant and hallucinogenic drug). An iatrogenic disorder can develop when during the treatment of this syndrome (in its acute or chronic form), hyponatremia is corrected too quickly, triggering osmotic demyelination syndrome (spastic tetraparesis due to pontine demyelination, pseudobulbar palsy, dyskinesia) and diffusing the brain injury [1].

ADRs in Patients with Diabetes Insipidus

In the treatment of diabetes insipidus, rarely used preparations including pitressin (Pitressin^R, Pitressin tannate^R) can trigger, *via* a direct vasoconstrictor effect, coronary artery spasm, hypertension or abdominal colics. The primarily preferred drug is desmopressin, a synthetic analog of vasopressin in the form of nasal drops (Adiuretin^R, Minirin^R), or sublingual tablets (Minirin Melt^R). Chlorpropamide, carbamazepine and clofibrate are active in partial forms of central diabetes insipidus, but they are today considered outdated for this purpose (weak action, danger of hypoglycemia after chlorpropamide).

Complications Occurring in Patients with Pituitary Adenomas

Therapy-Related Complications

The general management of pituitary adenomas raises therapeutic problems related to neurosurgical, radiological and conservative treatments. Each of these can be associated with specific complications.

Neurosurgical Treatment – in addition to more complete removal of adenomas, the main objective of this treatment is to minimize pituitary and brain injuries related to intervention, realizing selective removal of adenomas. Therefore, total nonselective hypophysectomy is currently only practiced exceptionally, even in advanced forms, in preference for subtotal hypophysectomy in nonselective or even selective forms. The ideal solution is a selective adenomectomy. Regarding the surgical approach, the transsphenoidal method and microsurgery are expected, and only in forms in which the upper (to the hypothalamus) or lateral extension transcranial (transfrontal) approach is the treatment of choice.

Radiation Therapy exerts its pituitary effects very slowly (for 0.5-10 years and over) and induces many adverse events, primarily pituitary insufficiency and secondary brain tumors (glioma, meningioma). More recently, an increased incidence of cerebrovascular disease has been reported after radiotherapy, increasing the mortality rate of irradiated patients (in cases of acromegaly). Therefore, irradiation is only practiced in selected cases, whether or not combined with other therapeutics, the treatment details of which are beyond the scope of this work.

Stereotactic Radiosurgery is used to avoid adjacent brain tissue injury *via* more precise targeting. The radiation source may be a linear accelerator (linac), or cobalt (gamma-knife). Irradiation with heavy particles (*e.g.*, proton radiosurgery) can be achieved only in a few specialized centers, requiring a cyclotron. Radiosurgery may be applied when the tumor is relatively small and radiosensitive structures (optical pathways, the brainstem) are not in the vicinity of the lesion. The ideal target of radiosurgery is a small residual tumor, located in the cavernous sinus. If the tumor cannot be precisely located, fractional radiotherapy must be applied to the entire likely tumoral area.

Conservative Treatment for any histological type of pituitary adenomas will be discussed below.

ADRs and Other Complications

Prolactinoma and Hyperprolactinemic States – the dopaminomimetic *bromocriptine* is the most commonly used drug for patients with prolactinoma. We must take care that its dose is increased gradually, starting with low doses – typically 1.25 mg/day (in oral administration, after going to bed in the evening) – which may be increased to 5-7.5 mg/day. If this requirement is not met, a number of side effects will occur (these will be discussed below, in the section regarding treatment of acromegaly, which involves use of this drug in much higher doses, reaching 10-30 mg/day). These doses are very difficult for patients to support, and are not even tolerated by many patients. *Cabergoline* (Dostinex^{R}) is another D_2-

receptor agonist used in prolactinoma, having much higher and longer-lasting efficacy, and much fewer gastrointestinal side effects than bromocriptine. After a period of time, a *resistance to bromocriptine* may be developed (in this case cabergoline may be chosen), but resistance to the other dopaminergic agonists, including cabergoline, can also appear. Although the criteria for resistance put forth by several authors are different, its incidence is estimated to be about 24-36% (for bromocriptine) and 4-11% (for cabergoline) regarding their prolactin (PRL) and tumor size reducing effect, respectively [2]. The *quinagolide* (Norprolac^R) has an efficacy comparable to that of bromocriptine; its side effects are similar but of lower intensity, and it may be used in cases of bromocriptine resistance. Potentially causing congenital malformations, it is contraindicated during pregnancy (when necessary – for instance, in evolutive macro-prolactinomas – bromocriptine is mainly used, and cabergoline can also be administered to pregnant women). Very rarely, *hypophysis apoplexia* is induced by dopamine agonists. After cessation of their use, a rebound phenomenon can occur. Besides prolactinomas, *hyperprolactinemic states* can be determined by many other factors, among these being antidopaminergic medicines, neuroleptics and antidepressants. These drugs can induce amenorrhea-galactorrhea syndrome. The cessation of antipsychotics results in the normalization of PRL levels – within three or four days for phenothiazines, but only after long periods in the case of some antidepressants. There are also exceptions, such as clozapine, ziprasidone and aripiprazole, that do not provoke hyperprolactinemia [3].

Acromegaly is commonly induced by pituitary acidophilic adenomas secreting GH and the first choice of treatment is *neurosurgery*. The efficacy of this treatment is 70-80% for microadenomas, 65-70% for well-defined macroadenomas, but only 30% for invasive forms. In young people who require conservation of procreative capacity (knowing that the surgery can lead to pituitary insufficiency), and in patients who do not accept intervention, it is recommended that conservative treatment be first pursued, preferring preparations with long-acting octreotide. *Radiotherapy* has the disadvantage of acting only after a long latency period, ranging from six months to 10 years. For this reason, radiation therapy is typically used only in combination with neurosurgical and/or conservative treatment. *Conservative* treatment with octreotide and its analogs (lanreotide, octreotide-LAR, pasireotide) is usually well tolerated, the most common side effect being the risk of gallstone formation. *Resistance* to these drugs is infrequently reported. It has already been mentioned that dopamine agonists are also used in acromegaly, *e.g., bromocriptine*, but in much higher doses (10-30 mg/day) than in prolactinoma treatment. These doses cause important side effects, including orthostatic hypotension and even collapse, gastric irritation phenomena (nausea, vomiting), Raynaud syndrome and sometimes psychotic manifestations. *Cabergoline* (used in acromegaly in higher doses of 1-4 mg/week) is thought to be the strongest dopaminomimetic in acromegaly, being effective in 20-25% of patients. While in lower doses it can cause adverse effects, such as hypotension, in higher doses after long-lasting use (as in Parkinsonism and acromegaly, *e.g.,* total doses of 280 and 400 mg), it can provoke tricuspid regurgitation and valvular lesions, respectively [2]. In some cases, cabergoline aggravates optochiasmatic syndrome, which disappears after its cessation or continuation of treatment with bromocriptine. The explanation for this is not clear, though it is possibly attributable to a rapid reduction of tumor size and consecutive traction of the chiasm, or a toxic effect of cabergoline. In such cases, not only should the PRL level and tumor size be evaluated, but also the visual field should be examined.

Cushing's Disease is induced, in the vast majority of cases (85-90%), by a pituitary microadenoma. In these cases, the first treatment of choice is usually neurosurgery, which has 65-90% postoperative efficacy. In the case of macroadenomas (about 10% cases), only partial tumor resection or debulking is usually possible, the remission rate of patients being under 15%. In specialized institutes, neurosurgical complications are rare: early mortality is about 0-3%, pituitary insufficiency may appear in 2-41% of cases, permanent diabetes insipidus in 3-9%, cerebrospinal fluid leak in 0-8%, meningitis in 0-3%, new neurological deficit symptoms in 0-2%, thromboembolic and ear-nose-throat complications in 0-4%, and SIADH in the later postoperative periods [2]. Regarding conservative treatment, *cabergoline* (1-3 mg weekly) reduces not only ACTH and cortisol secretion, but also tumor size, being effective in about 25-30% of patients. The type 5 somatostatin receptor is highly expressed in corticotroph tumors, and this fact explains the efficacy of the new octreotide analog, *pasireotide*, acting mainly on these receptors. About 25-40% of patients respond with clinical and biochemical impairment. Besides gastrointestinal side effects (diarrhea in 58%, nausea in 52%), *hyperglycemia* is often provoked (40%), which can require treatment [4, 5]. The use of *ketoconazole* (Nizoral^R), an imidazole-derived antimycotic acting predominantly on the adrenal cortex, is restricted because it is noted for *hepatotoxicity* [6]. Of the adrenolytics, *o, p'-DDD* (Mitotane^R, Lysodren^R) is very toxic (its side effects include gastrointestinal problems in 70-80% of cases, neurological effects in 45-60%, gynecomastia, dermatological lesions and adrenocortical failure), and is used mainly in adrenal carcinomas and ectopic ACTH secretion. *Metyrapone* (Metyrapone^R, Metopirone^R) blocks the enzyme 11β-hydroxylase, has a prompt but short duration effect, and is today relatively rarely used (in surgical non-cure contexts). Similarly, *etomidate* (Amidate^R) has a rapid action, being a general anesthetic with an intravenous route of administration. It is indicated for seriously ill patients who cannot take medicines orally. In these patients, *etomidate* can be a lifesaver. The steroid receptor antagonist *mifepristone* also has a rapid effect, being important in the treatment of acute psychosis induced by hypercortisolism. Reducing the initial cortisol level may result in hypersecretion of ACTH and lead to hypercortisolism. These high levels of cortisol, through stimulation of mineralocorticoid receptors, may induce hypokalemia [6].

In the treatment of Cushing's disease, bilateral adrenalectomy is rarely used today. This method is reserved for cases in which all other treatment methods have proven ineffective, especially in emergency situations. The adrenalectomized patient requires adequate substitution treatment and is permanently exposed to acute adrenal insufficiency, so it is very important to apply the corresponding prevention methods (rigorous control of the patient's medical documents, including the interventions required in the case of intercurrent diseases). Following total bilateral adrenalectomy, Nelson's syndrome can emerge. This syndrome is also called corticotroph tumor progression (CTP), presumably because the tumor existed before the adrenalectomy. The operation promotes only the progression of adenoma, through a lack of negative feedback (*e.g.,* the absence of the ACTH-suppressing effect of an adequate cortisol level). It is a very aggressive macroadenoma, associated with symptoms of adrenal failure. In 25-50% of cases, it may be prevented through postoperative pituitary irradiation and adequate corticosteroid substitution [7].

Thyrotroph Adenomas are very rare, and the majority secret only thyroid stimulating hormone (TSH). The first treatment of choice is neurosurgery, but this resolves only 40% of cases. *Octreotide* and its long-acting derivatives (lanreotide SR or Autogel, octreotide-LAR) are effective in about 80% of patients. The presence of dopaminergic receptors permits the therapeutic action of *cabergoline*, it being preferred in mixed, TSH- and PRL-secreting tumors. In some therapeutically resistant cases, thyroidectomy, radioiodotherapy or antithyroid agents are used. The treatment aims to reduce the thyroid hormone levels, excluding or reducing the negative feedback mechanism exerted on the TSH secretion, and promoting the growth and aggression of TSH-secreting adenoma [8].

Gonadotropin-Secreting and Clinically Nonfunctioning Pituitary Adenomas can cause hypogonadism and other manifestations of pituitary failure. In macroadenomas and in progressive cases, neurosurgical intervention and hormonal correction of pituitary insufficiency are necessary. Octreotide, its analogs and dopamine agonists are only rarely efficacious. In microadenomas and non-evolutive tumors, the "wait and see" principle may be respected.

Pituitary Insufficiency in Children (pituitary dwarfism) – the main treatment for this condition involves recombinant human-type growth hormone (rhGH) preparations. For a long time, GH pituitary extracts obtained from cadavers were used in clinical practice. These often caused infection with prions, such as Creutzfeldt-Jakob disease (spongiosus encephalitis), and are therefore strictly contraindicated under present conditions. The preparations used today contain rhGH, obtained *via* genetic engineering methods (*e.g.*, Genotropin^R, Norditropin^R, Humatrope^R, Saizen^R, *etc.*). These preparations do not represent such a risk, but their contraindications must also be respected, as they can cause diabetes mellitus, may promote malignant cell proliferation, and very rarely can lead to epiphysiolysis capitis femoris. In situations of this kind, the mentioned preparations are contraindicated. Preparations containing IGF-I (*e.g.*, Increlex^R containing mecasermin), used for the treatment of primary IGF-I deficiency due to GH-resistance and some cases of GH-deficient dwarfism, can induce hypertrophy of the thymus and tonsils, headache, hypoacusis, sleep apnea, hypoglycemia, local lipodystrophy and cardiovascular complications. If there is polytope pituitary insufficiency, peripheral hormones, which are hyposecreted or absent, must also be substituted in addition to administration of preparations containing GH. However, care should be taken to ensure these are administered in doses small enough to avoid premature closure of growth plates. When polytope pituitary insufficiency and hypothyroidism coexists, treatment must be initiated with thyroid hormones because these favor the secretion and action of GH. Similarly, when T_4 levels are found to be in the lower third of the normal range, this must be consistently monitored and, if the level falls below the normal limit, T_4 must be associated. Taking into account the fact that glucocorticoids reduce the secretion and action of GH in children, in the majority of cases, before the closure of growth plates, they must be avoided, excepting emergencies (in cases of stress and intercurrent infections). This recommendation is also valid for their therapeutic use (*e.g.*, in chronic obstructive pulmonary disease [COPD], nephrotic syndrome, rheumatoid polyarthritis). If central hypogonadism is also present, the administration of sexual hormones must be postponed until after the patient reaches the age of 12-13 years, to avoid the premature closure of growth plates. Due to the imperfections of methods used for the diagnosis of pituitary insufficiency in children, the diagnosis cannot yet be confirmed for a large portion of patients treated with rhGH for long periods, and these patients much be reexamined post-puberty.

Pituitary Insufficiency of Adults – in these patients, it is mandatory to respect the order in which various peripheral hormones are introduced. The order of their introduction is the reverse of the usual emergence sequence of adenohypophysial hormones' hyposecretion – that is to say, it starts with glucocorticoid substitution, continues with thyroid hormones, and only then (and not always) with the replacement of sex hormones. If this order is not followed, the premature administration of thyroid hormone (before glucocorticoids) may lead to the decompensation of adrenocortical insufficiency. It should also be noted that the use of estrogens is contraindicated in prolactinomas, as these hormones may promote the proliferation of prolactinoma cells.

Pituitary GH Deficiency in Adults is a very real problem. Two categories of patients are enrolled: the first represents those who, in their childhoods, were treated with rhGH for pituitary insufficiency, while the second represents those whose diagnosis was made in adulthood (having "somatopause"). For the first category, upon reaching 18 years of age, the doses of rhGH must be reduced (to 0.01 mg/kg/day) in the majority of cases (after a transition period of rhGH interruption for six months, and retesting the patient to confirm the diagnosis), to avoid the side effects of GH. In the second "somatopause" group, presenting asthenia, hypoglycemia, reducing the muscular mass and increasing that of adipose tissue, impairment of quality of life, initial doses of 0.15-0.3mg/day must be applied (the doses can later be increased to a maximum of 0.66-1.0 mg/day). In cases of overdose, fluid retention, edema, myalgia, polyarthritic pain and other complications can develop. The contraindications of rhGH are the following: malignant tumors (and their suspicion), proliferative diabetic retinopathy, intracranial hypertension (irrespective of its etiology), pregnancy, alcoholism, drug dependency and poor compliance. States that evidently reduce the use of rhGH are: severe chronic illness, lactation period, untreated or resistant hypertension, treatment with glucocorticoids for pharmacodynamic purposes, age greater than 70 years and treatment for acromegaly (unless controlled).

Peripheral Endocrine Glands Extirpation leads to loss of negative feedback mechanisms, intensification of secretion of pituitary tropic hormones and pituitary cell proliferation. This especially occurs when the substitution treatment is not properly applied. Thus, after thyroidectomy with long-term untreated hypothyroidism, hyperplasia and, rarely, reactive TSH-secreting pituitary adenoma can develop. Following castration and other peripheral hypogonadisms, pituitary gonadotropin-producing "castration cells" proliferate. After bilateral adrenalectomy, aggressive ACTH-secreting adenoma (Nelson's syndrome) can occur.

Empty Sella (Turkish saddle) Syndrome gives rise to two iatrogenic problems. The first is the need to differentiate this condition from pituitary adenoma, which presents similar imaging, and the incorrect diagnosis of which could lead to inadequate treatment (surgery or radiation). A second problem is that, in a third of patients with empty sella syndrome, pituitary failure emerges. In these patients, substitution treatment is required.

IATROGENIC PATHOLOGY IN THYROIDOLOGY

Hyperthyroidism

In this area, iatrogenic pathology is more common considering the high prevalence of thyroid diseases. Thus, in the treatment of hyperthyroidism (including Basedow-Graves' disease) each form of treatment (conservative, surgery and radioiodine) can lead to iatrogenic side effects.

Conservative treatment – ADRs – the antithyroid agents *thioamides* produce many side effects, including allergic reactions and hematopoietic disorders (primarily leukopenia, which can sometimes lead to agranulocytosis, anemia and thrombocytopenia). Thioamides can also cause gastric disorders (pain, reduced appetite), liver lesions, headache, muscular pain, *etc*. Other antithyroid agents, such as *perchlorates*, are mainly used for the short treatment special forms of hyperthyroidism (*e.g.,* in iodine-induced forms), and can sometimes cause nephrotic syndrome and irreversible aplastic anemia.

Lithium has important potential therapeutic value in some severe forms of Basedow-Graves' hyperthyroidism. Its long-term administration (*e.g.,* in bipolar disease) can lead to hypothyroidism (in 34-52% of cases) and goiter; in this situation T_4 preparations must be administered [9]. This may induce cardiac arrhythmias and other cardiac lesions, diabetes insipidus, diarrhea, ataxia and tremor. It has a narrow safety margin, so may be employed only for short treatments in endocrinology under regular monitoring of serum lithium levels. It has the important advantage of stimulating hematopoiesis. On the other hand, in association with clozapine, it can induce agranulocytosis (which is to say, it cannot reverse the action of clozapine).

It is known that patients with hyperthyroidism can develop atrial fibrillation. Although relatively rarely associated with thromboembolisms, given that there is blood hypocoagulability in these states, in some cases (depending on the homocysteinemia), irreversible injury or death can occur. Prevention of thromboembolism can be ensured *via anticoagulant therapy*. At present, however, the criteria of their therapeutic introduction are not yet precisely elaborated. However, any patient with atrial fibrillation or with a history of underlying heart disease or thromboembolic complications requires permanent anticoagulation after they reach 50 years of age [10].

Endocrine ophthalmopathy (usually associated with Basedow-Graves' disease or Hashimoto's chronic thyroiditis) may worsen when the treatment of the underlying disease is too insistent, leading to hypothyroidism. Furthermore, radioiodotherapy or surgery may aggravate the disease if not administered previously and after high-dose *glucocorticoid therapy*. Smoking is another aggravating factor to be completely contraindicated. Starting with stage III/b of ophthalmopathy, this condition requires active, aggressive treatment, including glucocorticoids in high doses, with immunosuppressive effects. Contraindications of glucocorticoids (which are not detailed here) must be respected. We note, however, that their administration for short time periods (*e.g.*, on three consecutive days) in extremely large doses (0.5-1 g/day) in intravenous bolus usually does not lead to their well-known (metabolic and other) complications. It is also noteworthy that these heroic treatments are effective only in active phases of endocrine ophthalmopathy. Retrobulbar irradiation can be performed in advanced stages of ophthalmopathy, but is contraindicated in optic neuropathy associated with altered visual field or rapid alteration of visual acuity. Another contraindication is diabetic retinopathy, which may be aggravated.

Treatment with *radioactive iodine* has some absolute contraindications, such as pregnancy, lactation, desire to conceive in the next six to 12 months, and suspected thyroid cancer. Relative contraindications are youth (specific age being dependent on medical school policies), large goiters, presence of compressive phenomena, severe/untreated hyperthyroidism, contamination with iodine and other situations in which the thyroid cannot capture radioactive iodine. The administration of usual doses of iodine preparations for the prophylaxis and treatment of endemic goiter does not usually lead to complications. However, in the case of nodular goiters, which may prove to be autonomous adenomas or other thyroid autonomies, we must be very cautious, avoiding the use of iodine in any form (medicines such as amiodarone, expectorants with iodine, antiseptic substances, iodine-containing radiological contrast agents, *etc*.). In thyroid autonomies, iodine can trigger a hyperthyroidism/iodine-induced thyrotoxicosis. Iodine preparations are contraindicated in florid hyperthyroidism and in Hashimoto's autoimmune lymphocytic thyroiditis. Regarding indications of *iodine-containing preparations,* we must analyze with responsibility the relationship between the benefits and risk of their administration. Thus, in cases of *emergency* (*e.g.*, myocardial infarction requiring a coronary angiography with an iodinated contrast agent), preparations containing iodine can be used, once appropriate measures are taken. First, a brief thyroidological history and clinical investigation (palpation of the thyroid, heart rate appreciation) is required and, in cases of doubt, hormonal determinations should be performed. If, on the basis of these measures, the risk of hyperthyroidism/thyrotoxicosis caused by iodine is found to be low, potassium perchlorate should be administered. The initial doses of potassium perchlorate are 0.5 g at two to four hours before and after introduction of iodized substance, and then continuation of the treatment at a dose of 3×0.3 g/day for between seven and 10 days. If the risk of hyperthyroidism/thyrotoxicosis is high, these drugs should be associated with methimazole (Thyrozol[R]), 20 mg/day for between seven and 10 days. In the case of *overt hyperthyroidism,* if iodine cannot be avoided in any way, the above-mentioned initial treatment with potassium perchlorate should continue, administered in doses of 3×0.3 g/day for 14 days, along with methimazole 40 mg/day for 14 days, subsequently decreasing the dose depending on the patient's condition. If the administration of iodine is not urgent, the time should be taken to perform complete thyroidological investigations and, in cases of hyperfunction, to carry out a proper treatment, which may include ablative therapy (surgery or radioiodine).

A special problem is the administration of *amiodarone* in patients with or without thyroid disorders. Amiodarone is rich in iodine (a 200 mg tablet contains 75 mg of iodine, of which 6 mg is absorbed) and can cause thyroid disorders, including amiodarone-induced hypothyroidism (AIH) or thyrotoxicosis (hyperthyroidism [AIT type I], especially in patients with preexisting thyroid diseases, or destructive thyroiditis [AIT type II]). In iodine-induced hyperthyroidism (including amiodarone), thioamides must be associated with perchlorates and often even lithium carbonate (although the latter has several side effects). If the iodine preparations (including amiodarone) cause a toxic thyroiditis, antiphlogistic treatment is required with adequate doses of corticosteroids (*e.g.*, prednisone or methylprednisolone – Medrol[R]). Mixed forms (hyperthyroidism with thyroiditis, in about 25% of cases) require both antithyroid and antiphlogistic treatments. Discontinuation of amiodarone is not necessary in hypothyroidism (AIH), which just requires T_4 treatment, but is recommended in hyperthyroidism (AIT type I). AIT type II (destructive thyroiditis) is a self-limiting disease and continuing amiodarone is suitable as it does not pose serious danger. However, this is a controversial issue. This form may rarely present recurrence under amiodarone, which can be easily treated. We have no data on whether the glucocorticoids shorten the time within which euthyroidism is achieved. After restoration of euthyroidism due to interruption of amiodarone, this drug is reintroduced. Recommendations regarding prior thyroidal treatment are controversial [11].

Iatrogenic Thyrotoxicosis clinically resembles the above-mentioned exogenous thyrotoxicosis, but is caused by unfounded medical indication of thyroid hormone preparations. In highly differentiated thyroid cancer treatment, the physician should administer high doses of thyroid hormone for substitution and suppression of endogenous TSH. The manifestations of hyperthyroidism at different ages and physiological states also raise the possibility of iatrogenic pathology. Thus, hyperthyroidism in pregnant women often manifests itself through *hyperemesis gravidarum,* not being diagnosed as an endocrine entity and thereby failing to receive adequate treatment. It is preferable that, in hyperthyroidism during pregnancy, propylthiouracil (Propycil[R]) is initially administered as this fixes to proteins to a greater extent, crossing the placental barrier less than other usual antithyroid drugs. This is recommended for use during lactation, too, for similar reasons. However, propylthiouracil can also induce hepatotoxicity. Therefore, it is only recommended in the first three months of pregnancy, switching after this point to methimazole administration (methimazole is not recommended in the first trimester, due to its rarely encountered teratogenic effect). However, methimazole can be used throughout the whole pregnancy if propylthiouracil allergy or a poor clinical response to it is present [12]. Another problem frequently encountered in hyperthyroidism is its difficult recognition in *elderly patients*, often appearing as an unusual, apathetic form (*"apathetic" hyperthyroidism*), or as thyroid autonomy. In some cases, cardiac arrhythmias (*e.g., atrial fibrillation*) treated with antiarrhythmics without results over a long period indicate hyperthyroid/thyrotoxic origin (induced, for example, by thyroid adenoma). Treatment of this condition, then, leads to cessation of atrial fibrillation.

In the case of *thyrotoxicosis factitia,* when the patient takes thyroid hormone preparations unadvised by physician (*e.g.,* for slimming purposes), medication cessation leads with time to euthyroidism. Exogenous thyrotoxicosis of the *"hamburger"* type, induced by excessive consumption of foods containing animal thyroid, is rare and reversible.

Surgery – in addition to its net benefits, thyroidectomy presents certain dangers and disadvantages. Operative lethality is low (0.1-0.5%) but exists. Its frequent cause is the realization of intervention in a thyrotoxic state in a patient not properly prepared for operation. This leads to the result that the *euthyroid state* is a sine qua non condition of thyroid surgery (excepting the thyrotoxic storm in advanced stages, with impaired patient consciousness and the possibility of patient death, in which case "Frühoperation" can – under certain conditions – be performed). In all other florid forms of hyperthyroidism, surgical interventions are contraindicated. Other contraindications are increased surgical risk (elderly patient, cardiovascular disease and other serious diseases), progressive ophthalmopathy, little or no goiter, and post-thyroidectomy relapse of hyperthyroidism. The most common post-surgery complications are recurrent paresis (1-5%), hypoparathyroidism (0.5-3%), hypothyroidism (10-40%, increasing with time) and worsening ophthalmopathy. Their occurrence depends on the extent of resection and the experience of the surgeon. In elderly patients, intercurrent and thromboembolic complications may occur.

Hypothyroidism

Hypothyroidism in newborns is not manifested clinically in 95% of cases, imposing mandatory screening (by performing TSH at the age of four or five days and, if necessary, also T_4). Not recognizing the diagnosis leads to lack of adequate treatment, and the occurrence of CNS injuries and other complications can have lifelong effects (which may be termed "partial cretinism"). Given that, besides permanent congenital hypothyroidism (not common, occurring with an incidence of 1/4000 births), there are *transitional and subclinical* forms, and that numerous geographic areas are deficient in iodine, the lack of adequate treatment sometimes affects a fairly large number of infants and children. Another category of people at risk of hypothyroidism is pregnant women. Not recognizing hypothyroidism in such patients represents a double danger: for the fetus (primarily regarding the normal development of the CNS) and the pregnant woman. The scope of this paper does not permit detailing the serious repercussions of hypothyroidism for both – we simply stress that the sharp increase of iodine needs during pregnancy imposes prophylaxis and treatment of goiter and hypothyroidism not only on pregnant women living in endemic iodine-deficient areas, but also on all pregnant women [13]. The supply of iodine in adequate doses must be realized even in the presence of autoimmune thyroiditis (doses of 150 μg iodine/day are safe). When, before and during pregnancy, goiter coexists with hypothyroidism (frequently in a subclinical form), the administration of thyroid hormones is also necessary. Postpartum thyroiditis, which appears in the first year after delivery, is essentially an autoimmune thyroiditis. It requires treatment with T_4 preparations only when hypothyroidism develops (in about 54% of cases).

The treatment of hypothyroidism in adults, especially in *elderly patients,* requires some precautions to be observed. Older patients and those suffering from *cardiovascular diseases* should be treated first with medicines for these conditions (primarily with beta blockers, antihypertensive drugs, *etc.*) and only subsequently can thyroid hormones be introduced, starting with low doses (*e.g.,* T_4 12.5-25 mg/day) and gradually increasing. Contraindications of thyroid hormones must be respected, the primary and absolute contraindication being *myocardial infarction.* However, thyroid hormones can cause arrhythmias, angina or even myocardial infarction, cerebral circulation disorders and worsening high blood pressure, so they should be administered with caution in patients with heart diseases, and only under the shield of appropriate medication.

In postmenopausal women chronically overtreated with T_4, *osteoporosis* can develop. This can be prevented by regular monitoring and maintenance of normal serum TSH levels in patients receiving long-term replacement therapy [12].

We have already mentioned issues that may arise during the treatment of *Hashimoto's autoimmune* chronic lymphocytic *thyroiditis.* If treatment is not monitored at the appropriate intervals, complications can occur easily, both in terms of *hypo-* and *hyperthyroidism (thyrotoxicosis)*. The disease has a natural evolutionary tendency to hypothyroidism. Not infrequently, however, it is associated with Basedow-Graves' disease (hashitoxicosis), to be treated with antithyroid agents. These drugs – if the patient is not monitored, usually every six weeks – can promote iatrogenic hypothyroidism. The disease itself presents an undulant development and cannot manage its hyper- and hypothyroid phases – only regular follow-up can do so.

The administration of *immunomodulatory medications* or preparations (*e.g.*, interferon-alpha, *etc*.), for any purposes, can aggravate autoimmune thyroid diseases and Hashimoto's thyroiditis. *Interferon-alpha,* used most frequently for the treatment of chronic hepatitis C virus infection, can activate or induce a preexistent autoimmune thyroiditis, leading to hypothyroidism (often) or thyrotoxicosis (rarely) in about 40% of patients. It exerts both an immunostimulatory effect and a direct deleterious effect on the thyroid gland [9, 14]. At the same time, the hepatitis C virus may also contribute to these lesions.

Bexarotene (Targretin[R]), approved since 1999 as a second-line treatment for late-stage cutaneous T-cell lymphomas, is a vitamin A (retinol)-derivative and RXR-ligand. It provokes central hypothyroidism, reducing the transcription of thyrotropin-releasing hormone (TRH) and TSH-gene. Bexarotene also affects the gene expression of deiodinases 1 and 2, as well as the peripheral clearance of thyroxine [9].

In the majority of cases, *thyroid carcinomas* undergo *total thyroidectomy*. A single *exception* is *papillary microcarcinomas* of diameter less than 1 cm, without metastasis. According to some authors, this exception must fulfill other criteria, too: the patient must be without familial history, unexposed to earlier radiation, and the carcinoma must have developed before the patient reached 35 years of age. This group represents very low-risk patients and only a lobectomy or subtotal thyroidectomy is performed. Apart from this very low-risk group, in highly differentiated carcinomas thyroidectomy is followed by radioiodotherapy, after which the patient receives treatment with thyroid hormones, in substitutive and TSH-suppressive doses. When, if the thyroidectomy is not taken, a free interval of four to six weeks it taken to allow the increase of TSH to about 30 mIU/L, or in this period thyroid hormones or iodine are administered, the efficacy of radioiodine treatment is compromised. This free interval, characterized by postoperative hypothyroidism, is not well supported by some patients. To avoid this inconvenience, it is possible to eliminate the free interval, using recombinant TSH preparations [15]. This resolution, which has been available for a relatively long time, is still very expensive. In the last phase of the treatment of highly differentiated thyroid carcinomas (*e.g.*, suppression of TSH with thyroid hormones) the physician often must use high doses of T_4 (or T_3) preparations, inducing *iatrogenic thyrotoxicosis*. These overdoses are frequently administered to postmenopausal women, increasing the development or aggravation of osteoporosis. At the same time, such overdoses can induce atrial fibrillation. In the final administration, more precise and differential indications regarding the TSH levels appear, which must be maintained, and the duration of treatment is also shortened, reducing the side effects of the TSH-suppressive treatment.

Tyrosine kinase inhibitors (*e.g.*, sunitinib, sorafenib, motesanib, vandetanib, axitinib, *etc.*), used in the treatment of hematologic and solid tumors including thyroid carcinomas, influence thyroid hormone synthesis, can induce destructive hypothyroidism and reduce VEGF-related neoangiogenesis [9].

IATROGENIC PATHOLOGY OF PARATHYROID GLANDS

In *asymptomatic primary hyperparathyroidism,* diagnosis may be difficult due to the lack of clinical symptoms. It is also difficult to recognize and treat the *hypercalcemic crises* induced by *hyperparathyroidism*. These may, in turn, be caused by *other disorders,* such as an overdose of vitamin D preparations (especially those containing modern metabolites with increased activity) or malignant diseases, such as solid tumors (the most common being breast carcinoma) and hematologic malignancies (multiple myeloma, lymphoma, lymphosarcoma, reticulosis), amongst other less common causes that cannot be discussed here. Hypercalcemic crisis, induced by hyperparathyroidism, does not respond to glucocorticoids (which can influence its other forms), requiring instead significant volumes of chloride sodium infusions, furosemide, bisphosphonates (pamidronate injection, *e.g.*, Aredia^R), calcitonin and sometimes mithramycin or plicamycin, or even hemodialysis.

It is also important to note that, in the diagnosis of *parathyroid carcinoma,* fine needle aspiration (FNA) must be avoided because it, unlike highly differentiated thyroid carcinomas, can spread following this intervention. Similarly, vigorous attempts should be made to remove the tumor en bloc [16].

IATROGENIC PATHOLOGY OF ADRENAL GLANDS

The therapeutic problems related to *Cushing's disease* and *syndrome* were discussed earlier, with reference to the hypothalamic-pituitary axis. The side effects of adrenolytic and adrenostatic drugs used in the conservative treatment of Cushing's syndrome cannot be detailed here due to the scope of the study.

Regarding the diagnosis of primary *hypermineralocorticoidism,* especially *primary hyperaldosteronism*, it must be stressed that often hypokalemia does not accompany this disorder, historically considered characteristic, which could contribute to diagnostic errors. Long-term treatment with glucocorticoids should be performed in *congenital adrenogenital syndromes*, so the use of the smallest possible doses that can inhibit hypersecretion of ACTH, characteristic in these states, is recommended. *Adrenal incidentalomas* present problems both for diagnosis and treatment. For practical guidance, we should note the need for surgery when the tumor secretes active hormones, suggests malignancy (*e.g.*, increased secretion) or if its diameter exceeds 3 cm.

In the treatment of *Addison's disease,* a common mistake is to recommend a low-salt diet and other restrictions necessary when corticosteroids are administered in high doses, for pharmacodynamic purposes. In Addison's disease, these corticosteroids are used in relatively low, substitutive doses (*e.g.,* 15-25 mg hydrocortison/day, cortisone acetate in higher doses, or prednisolone 5 mg/day), and the regime should thus be rich in salt and without any metabolic restrictions. The daily glucocorticoid doses must be distributed in two or three parts (with about two thirds taken in the morning), corresponding to the normal biorhythm of cortisol secretion, and must be individualized, mainly based on clinical status (the hormonal results are strongly influenced by the treatments). The other therapeutic problem is the supply of adequate cortisolemia throughout the day. In current practice, in a significant number of cases, the glucocorticoid preparations are *overdosed* (exceeding 7.5 mg/day of prednisolone, or a corresponding dose), so they can induce side effects such as weight gain, obesity, osteoporosis, *etc*. (Table **15-1**). To reduce these complications, *slow-release glucocorticoid preparations* can be used, establishing a more circadian-based serum cortisol profile. In particular, glucose metabolism is improved in patients with concomitant DM [17].

The combined use of other medications can influence the effect of glucocorticoids. Barbiturates, phenytoin, primidone, carbamazepine, rifampicin, rifapentine, ethosuximide and pioglitazone accelerate their hepatic metabolism *via* induction of the enzyme CYP3A4, diminishing the effect of glucocorticoids. By contrast, drugs that impair their metabolism by inhibition of CYP3A4 (fluoxetine, itraconazole, diltiazem, cimetidine, ritonavir, aprepitant, *etc*.) enhance the effects of glucocorticoids. There are also drugs, such as estrogens and mitotane, that increase corticosteroid-binding globulin (CBG) levels and falsely elevate the cortisol serum value [18].

When glucocorticoids alone cannot compensate adrenal insufficiency they must be combined with *mineralocorticoid* preparations (fludrocortisone, such as Astonin^{R}, Florinef^{R}, in doses of 0.05-0.2 mg/day, divided into two equal doses, taken in the morning and evening).

The possibility arises of supplementation of *dehydroepiandrosterone (DHEA)* regarding vitality and libido, especially in postmenopausal women, if all other replacement therapy is adequate. DHEA is used in doses of 25-50 mg/day. A trial of two to three months is usually sufficient to explore any possible benefits [3, 18].

In cases of intercurrent infections, injuries, surgery, childbirth and other overstressing conditions, the dose of glucocorticoids should not be decreased (in terms of their use for pharmacodynamic purposes) – on the contrary, it is necessary to increase the dose to between two and four times the baseline.

Acute adrenal insufficiency, caused by sepsis in infants and young children (Waterhouse-Friderichsen syndrome) and characterized by malaise, high fever and shock, is often not recognized by physicians. Ceasing the administration of higher glucocorticoid doses, used for pharmacodynamic purposes in children and adults, can also precipitate acute adrenal insufficiency. This complication being now more well known, higher therapeutic doses of glucocorticoids are usually withdrawn slowly, and this gradual reduction can be associated with stimulation by ACTH.

Table 15-1. Major side effects and contraindications of systemic glucocorticoids.

Side effects	Mechanisms	Contraindications
Na^+ and water retention, edema, hypertension	Through mineralocorticoid receptors, only after "classic" preparations, or due to very high levels of cortisol	Edema, hypertension (or: adequate treatment)
Exogenous Cushing's syndrome (obesity, hypertension, *etc.*)	After prolonged high-dose therapy, imitating endogenous hypercortisolism	Cushing's syndrome
Osteoporosis	After prolonged high-dose therapy, primarily; Wnt signaling	Osteoporosis (or: adequate treatment)
Myopathy	Direct catabolism of skeletal muscle	Myopathies
Avascular necrosis of femoral head	Damage in venous endothelial cells, bone infarction (?)	Avascular necrosis of femoral head
Hyperlipidemia	As part of metabolic syndrome	Dyslipidemia
Hyperglycemia, rarely steroid diabetes mellitus	Increased gluconeogenesis and hepatic glucose production	DM (or: adaptation of its medication)
Ischemic heart disease, heart failure, hypercoagulability	Increased risk and aggravation of these conditions through obesity, hypertension and other components of metabolic syndrome	Coronary heart disease, heart failure, hypercoagulability
Psychiatric disorders	Alterations of mood, memory deficits, even psychosis (following long-term use)	Psychoses (or: adequate therapy)

(Table 15-1) contd.....

Side effects	Mechanisms	Contraindications
Gastrointestinal disorders	Gastritis, peptic ulcers, hemorrhage (in part due to concomitant use of NSAID)	Peptic ulcers (or: adequate treatment)
Ophthalmological disorders	Glaucoma, due to increased intraocular pressure; cataracts	Glaucoma, cataracts
Immunosuppression	Following high doses, TBC and other infections can be reactivated	Immunodeficiency, which aggravates infections
Adrenal failure (evident following stress)	Through feedback suppression of ACTH	To avoid infections, surgery and stress
Menstrual disorders and anovulation	Through nonspecific gonadotropin suppression, or hyperprolactinemia	Irregular cycles (or: normalization of irregular cycles)
Growth failure, delayed puberty	Decreased GH- and IGF-I-secretion, GH-resistance, inhibition of growth plate, suppression of gonadotropins	Children (or: treatment with rhGH and gonadotropins)
Congenital malformations (disputed)	Small risk following the use in the first trimester of inhaled preparations	Pregnancy (with precaution)

Pheochromocytoma can go undiscovered when the characteristic catecholaminergic crisis (with hypertension) or hypotensive crisis (due to hypersecretion of dopamine, or sometimes epinephrine) is present, or are not manifested in changes to the patient's blood pressure (as in the case of some large tumors, when the secreted catecholamines do not reach general circulation). Catecholaminergic crisis can be triggered by many mechanical and chemical factors, including medicines such as glucagon, tyramine (contained in cheeses and red wine), metoclopramid, opioids, naloxone, tricyclic antidepressants, beta blockers, general anesthetic and contrast agents. The conservative treatment of pheochromocytoma mainly comprises long-term administration of α-adrenolytics, such as phenoxybenzamine. This binds irreversibly to the α-adrenergic receptors, thereby exerting a strong and durable hypotensive effect. Phenoxybenzamine has some side effects, too, including orthostatic hypotension, tachycardia, headache, diplopia, nasal congestion and ejaculation disorders. It is very important that α-adrenolytics be used firstly in the treatment of pheochromocytoma, as nonselective ($\beta 1+\beta 2$) beta blockers can be administered only after α-adrenolytics. This statement is based on the fact that beta blockers without alpha blocking can induce vasoconstriction and consecutive hypertension (as well as hypertensive crisis), as only these effects of endogen epinephrine persists (losing the β_2-adrenoreceptor stimulated vasodilatory actions) [2].

IATROGENIC PATHOLOGY OF GONADS

Of the sexual steroids, we will only here discuss the iatrogenic pathology related to androgenic drugs, the rest of these steroids (including oral contraceptives) being discussed in Chapters 10 and 11.

Androgenic steroids may promote worsening of benign prostatic hyperplasia (BPH) and prostate carcinomas, and are contraindicated in these states. Another contraindication is breast carcinomas occurring in men. Some androgens, like α-alkylated testosterone derivatives, can cause serious liver lesions (including adenomas and adenocarcinomas). Of the *antiandrogens, flutamide* should be mentioned in particular as, in addition to hepatotoxicity, it also has another disadvantage: when used in the treatment of prostatic carcinoma, it can, after some time, behave like an androgenic agonist, exacerbating the patient's condition (in this case it must be substituted with a derivative).

5-phosphodiesterase inhibitors used in the treatment of male impotence, such as sildenafil (Viagra^R), tadalafil (Cialis^R) and vardenafil (Levitra^R), cannot be administered simultaneously with *nitrates* or other drugs that work by stimulating NO formation, because these combinations can induce hypotension, collapse and other acute cardiovascular complications. Phosphodiesterase (PDE) inhibitors should not be used in patients taking alpha blockers due to an increased risk of hypotension. They are also contraindicated when *heart failure* is at an advanced stage, and physical effort relating to intercourse would be dangerous for the patient. The most common side effects of PDE-inhibitors are headache, facial flushing, nasal congestion, dyspepsia and, rarely, priapism. Vardenafil and sildenafil may also cause visual difficulty relating to discrimination of colors (blue and green) and bluish tones in vision. In a small number of patients, a non-arteritic ischemic optic neuropathy (NAION), in which blood flow to the optic nerve is blocked, is reported. If patients experience decreased or sudden loss of vision, they should report to a physician immediately [19]. PDE-inhibitors cannot be administered to patients with *psychotic disorders* or under *treatment with antipsychotics or antidepressants*. Recent data show that sildenafil may elevate melanoma risk [20, 21].

Apomorphine (Uprima^R), used to treat erectile dysfunctions, can cause nausea and vomiting, stimulating the vomiting center of the bulb.

Only limited data support the aphrodisiac effect of *yohimbine,* a selective presynaptic α_2-adrenergic inhibitor, so it is rarely used. The side effects of this drug are nausea, vomiting, irritability, headache, anxiety, tachycardia and hypertension (due to increasing norepinephrine release) [19].

Alprostadil is a prostaglandin E_1 analog that leads to smooth muscle relaxation and rapid arterial inflow in corpora cavernosa. It is available as an intracavernosal injection (Caverject^R) or as a transurethral suppository (medicated urethral system for erection, MUSE^{R}). Side effects include pain upon injection, bleeding or bruising at the injection site, fibrosis and priapism. In sickle cell diseases, patients taking anticoagulants, or those who have bleeding disorders, the risk of priapism and bleeding is increased [19].

Some cases of *cryptorchidism* (caused by congenital hypogonadotropic hypogonadism) can also be treated with GnRH analogs [22], but only when their pulsating administration by a pump is possible. Otherwise, in chronic administration, they exert an inhibitory effect on the gonadotropin secretion, used in the treatment of gonadotropin-dependent precocious puberty, prostate cancer and endometriosis [23]. *Cancerization* of the cryptorchid testicle is a very serious complication, such that if cryptorchidism cannot be resolved by conservative or surgical (orchidopexy) treatment, its removal is necessary.

Regarding the conservative treatment of *polycystic ovarian syndrome*, the biguanide *metformin* is most often used, especially in obese women with insulin-resistance (Table **15-2**). Besides decreasing appetite and thereby reducing weight, it reduces insulin-resistance and hyperinsulinism (as it is an insulin sensitizer, like thiazolidinedione), ameliorating the metabolic syndrome present in a significant number of patients with polycystic ovarian syndrome. A great deal of recent evidence shows that metformin exerts antitumoral effects on many tumors, not only in diabetic patients, but also in non-diabetics (Table **15-2**).

Table 15-2. The mechanism of action and the side effects of metformin.

Mechanism of action	**Side effects**
Decrease of appetite	Nausea, vomiting, abdominal pain, diarrhea or constipation
Weight reduction	Side effects may be attenuated by gradually increasing the dosage
Reduction of insulin-resistance (IR) and hyperinsulinism	Gastrointestinal side effects may be reduced by administering after meals
Improving lipid levels	Side effects can be reduced by ensuring the daily dose does not exceed 2-2.5 g
Decrease of cardiovascular complications	Administration must cease in pregnancy, but its use in early pregnancy does not justify an interruption
Direct and indirect antitumoral effects: - Activation of adenosine monophosphate-activated protein kinase (AMPK) induces (through down-regulation) reduction of mammalian TOR-complex 1 (mTORC1), an mTOR signalization complex, and increases liver kinase B1 (LKB-1) - Inhibition of the IGF-I/Akt (PKB) pathway and stopping of the p53-mediated cell cycle - AMPK-independent (*e.g.*, IR reduction)	

CONFLICT OF INTEREST

The authors confirm that this chapter content has no conflict of interest.

ACKNOWLEDGEMENTS

Declared none.

REFERENCES

[1] Robinson AG, Verbalis JG. Williams Textbook of Endocrinology. Elsevier-Saunders, Philadelphia 2011; pp. 308-14.

[2] Kun IZ, Szanto Zs. Acromegalia. Prolactinomák és egyéb hyperprolactinaemiás állapotok. Cushing-kór. Thyreotrop adenomák. Gonadotrop és klinikailag nem-funkcionáló hypophysis-adenomák. Phaeochromocytoma In: Kun IZ, Szanto Zs, Eds. Neuroendocrinologia. Erdélyi Múzeum-Egyesület Kiadó, Kolozsvár 2012; pp. 170-472.

[3] Racz K. Leövey A, Nagy VE, Paragh Gy, Racz K. Prolactinoma és hyperprolactinaemiás állapotok. Az endokrin és anyagcsere-betegségek gyakorlati kézikönyve. Medicina Budapest Hungary 2011; pp. 71-328.

[4] Petersenn F. Medical therapy with pasireotide. In: Lamberts SW, Ed. Handbook of Cushing's Disease. Bristol, UK: BioScientifica 2011; pp. 139-49.

[5] Pivonello R, De Leo M, Cozzolino A. Medical therapy with dopamine receptor analogues. In: Lamberts SW, Ed. Handbook of Cushing's Disease. Bristol, UK: BioScientifica 2011; pp. 125-36.

[6] Castinetti F, Brue T. Medical therapy with ketoconazole and mifepristone. In: Lamberts SW, Ed. Handbook of Cushing's Disease. Bristol, UK: BioScientifica 2011; pp. 95-107.

[7] Toth M. Nelson-szindróma. In: Leovey A, Nagy VE, Paragh Gy, Racz K, Eds. Az endokrin és anyagcsere-betegségek gyakorlati kézikönyve. Medicina, Budapest, Hungary 2011; pp. 115-6.

[8] Beck-Peccoz P, Persani L. Thyrotropinomas. In: Hay ID, Wass JA, Eds. Clinical Endocrine Oncology. 2nd ed. Oxford: Blackwell Publishing 2008; pp. 268-73. [http://dx.doi.org/10.1002/9781444300222.ch33]

[9] Orgiazzi J. The thyroid as a victim. Iatrogenicity of non-iodinated drugs. Acta Endocrinol (Bucur) 2014; 10: 41-2.

[10] Davies TF, Larsen PR. Williams Textbook of Endocrinology. 11th ed. Elsevier-Saunders, Philadelphia 2008; p. 334.

[11] Wiersinga W. Amiodarone and thyroid. Acta Endocrinol (Bucur) 2014; 10: 39-41.

[12] Cooper DS. The Thyroid Gland. In: Gardner DG, Shoback D, Eds. Greenspan's Basic & Clinical Endocrinology. McGraw-Hill Companies: Lange 2011.

[13] Kun I. Patologia iatrogenă în endocrinologie. In: Jung J, Ed. Patologie iatrogenă. Târgu Mureş, Romania: University Press 2006; pp. 97-107.

[14] Duncea I, Georgescu C. Interferon α-induced autoimmune thyroid disease in chronic viral hepatitis C: case report and review of literature. Acta Endocrinol (Bucur) 2011; 7: 25.

[15] Schlumberger M, Ricard M, De Pouvourville G, Pacini F. How the availability of recombinant human TSH has changed the management of patients who have thyroid cancer. Nat Clin Pract Endocrinol Metab 2007; 3(9): 641-50. [http://dx.doi.org/10.1038/ncpendmet0594] [PMID: 17710085]

[16] Bringhurst FR, Dernay MB, Kronenberg HM. Williams Textbook of Endocrinology. 11th ed. Elsevier-Saunders: Philadelphia 2008; p. 1232.

[17] Johannsson G, Nilsson AG, Bergthorsdottir R, *et al.* Improved cortisol exposure-time profile and outcome in patients with adrenal insufficiency: a prospective randomized trial of a novel hydrocortisone dual-release formulation. J Clin Endocrinol Metab 2012; 97(2): 473-81. [http://dx.doi.org/10.1210/jc.2011-1926] [PMID: 22112807]

[18] Grossman AB. The diagnosis and management of central hypoadrenalism. J Clin Endocrinol Metab 2010; 95(11): 4855-63. [http://dx.doi.org/10.1210/jc.2010-0982] [PMID: 20719838]

[19] Liday C, Heyneman C. Erectile dysfunction. In: Chisholm-Burns MA, Wells BG, Schwinghammer TL, Eds. Pharmacotherapy Principles and Practice. NY Chicago, San Francisco: McGraw Hill Medical 2008; pp. 784-6.

[20] Li WQ, Qureshi AA, Robinson KC, Han J. Sildenafil use and increased risk of incident melanoma in US men: a prospective cohort study. JAMA Intern Med 2014; 174(6): 964-70. [http://dx.doi.org/10.1001/jamainternmed.2014.594] [PMID: 24710960]

[21] Grichnik JM. Sildenafil may elevate melanoma risk. Dermatol Ther (Heidelb) 2014; 27(5): 313. [http://dx.doi.org/10.1111/dth.12162] [PMID: 25285874]

[22] Boehm U, Bouloux PM, Dattani MT. European Consensus Statement on congenital hypogonadotropic hypogonadism - pathogenesis, diagnosis and treatment. Nat Rev Endocrinol 2015; 11: 547-64. [PMID: 26194704]

CHAPTER 16

Iatrogenic Pathology in Anesthesiology and Intensive Care

Leonard Azamfirei* and **Iudita Badea**

Department of Intensive Care, University of Medicine and Pharmacy, Tirgu-Mures, Romania

Abstract: The iatrogenic pathology occurring in anesthesiology and intensive care is a consequence of errors made due to ignorance (the incapacity to identify suddenly appearing pathological situations), negligence (deficiencies in applying correct medical conduct) or clinical misjudgment. In the field of anesthesiology, this type of pathology comprises complications in pre-anesthetic, anesthetic and post-anesthetic periods, the consequences of pharmacological effects of the administered anesthetic drugs, technical complications related to airway security, anesthetic machine functioning and monitoring equipment, the anesthetic technique utilized and the differing reactivity of patients to the chosen anesthetic procedure. In intensive care, regarding critical care patients with multiple organ dysfunctions, the main source of iatrogenesis is represented by invasive maneuvers (mechanical ventilation techniques, monitoring, vascular approaches). To all these are added complications related to administered drugs, artificial nutrition, volemic therapy and the high risk of infection.

Keywords: Anesthetic drugs, Artificial nutrition, Fluid therapy, General anesthesia, Infection, Intensive care, Loco-regional anesthesia, Maneuvers, Mechanical ventilation, Oxygen therapy.

INTRODUCTION

Iatrogenic complications appearing in the ICU are defined as adverse effects or pathological situations that occur independently of the underlying disease. In the USA, it is estimated that 4% of hospitalized patients in ICUs experience iatrogenic complications and 14% of such complications contribute to death [1].

These complications can be fatal (being primarily responsible for patient death), life-threatening (requiring intensive care measures such as mechanical ventilation, hemodialysis, vasopressors and thoracotomy) or moderate (requiring routine monitoring and management) [2].

* **Corresponding author Leonard Azamfirei:** Department of Intensive Care, University of Medicine and Pharmacy, Tirgu-Mures, Romania; Tel/Fax: 0040-744-828224; E-mail: leonard.azamfirei@umftgm.ro

There are three main ***types of errors*** that can induce iatrogenic pathology in the ICU [3]:

- *Ignorance* – failure to recognize an unusual pathological situation, which can lead to a failure to provide the appropriate treatment.
- *Negligence* – failure to comply with universally accepted standards (*e.g.*, noncompliance with aseptic measures, failure to ask about allergies).
- *Erroneous judgment* – exaggerated optimism, unjustified designation of emergency status, "fashion" therapy, perfectionism, abstention, insufficient deliberation, *etc.*

The relationship between drugs (Table **16-1**) or medical procedures (Table **16-2**) and pathological situations can be definite (certain consequence of intervention), probable (likely consequence of intervention), possible (intervention-related), conditional (patient-related) or uncertain (not meeting any of these conditions) [4]:

Table 16-1. Drug-related iatrogenic lesions occurring in the ICU.

Type of drug	Disorders
Diuretics	Hypokalemia, hyperkalemia
NSAIDs	Gastrointestinal bleeding
Oral anticoagulants	Bleeding
Fluids	Fluid overload
Antibiotics	Hepatitis, allergies
Anesthetics	Respiratory failure, cardiac failure
ACEs	Acute renal failure, dehydration
Miscellaneous	Coma, metabolic disorders

Table 16-2. Medical procedure-related iatrogenic diseases occurring in the ICU.

Type of procedure	Type of disorder
Cardiac catheterization	Arrhythmia
Central venous catheterization	Bacteremia, pneumothorax
Peripheral venous catheterization	Bacteremia
Urinary tract catheterization	Infection
Radiocontrast infusion	Acute renal failure
Radiotherapy	Enteritis, leukemia

COMPLICATIONS OF GENERAL ANESTHESIA

During the patient's premedication and general anesthesia, various complications can be drug-induced or can be caused by technical malfunctions in equipment and unexpected reactions of the patient's body.

Side Effects of Drugs Used in General Anesthesia

Drugs Used in Premedication

Benzodiazepines (diazepam), barbiturates and opioids can produce respiratory depression, especially in elderly patients [5]. Minor neuroleptics (promethazine) can induce hypotension, xerostomia, skin reactions, esophageal sphincter hypotonia, *etc.* [6].

Intravenous Anesthetics

Thiopental can produce cough, hiccups, laryngospasm, bronchospasm, allergic reactions, respiratory depression, tachycardia and vasodilation. Perivascular extravasation can be followed by severe tissue injuries. Unintentional intraarterial injection leads to the formation of thiopental microcrystals in arterioles, followed by platelet aggregation and risk of thromboembolism.

Etomidate can induce cough, hiccups, laryngospasm, bronchospasm and adrenal suppression. Venous thrombosis is more common in this case than following use of other agents [7].

Propofol induces hypotension (20% of patients), transient apnea and allergic reactions. The rapid growth of microorganisms can also be a consequence [8].

Droperidol exerts cholinergic and sympatholytic effects and produces extrapyramidal motor symptoms, but does not induce respiratory depression. Dysphoria can also be noted.

Ketamine produces hypersalivation, hypotension, tachycardia, restlessness and transient apnea. It can also induce vivid dreams, increased intracranial pressure and allergic reactions.

Fentanyl causes respiratory depression and severe chest wall rigidity, and increases the tone of the sphincter of Oddi.

In patients treated with monoamine oxidase inhibitors, ***pethidine*** can cause serious complications, potentially fatal, ranging from hypotension and respiratory depression to hypertension and hyperpyrexia, seizures and coma.

Morphine depresses the respiratory centers [9].

Rapid injection of ***alfentanil*** with another vagal stimulation maneuver (laryngoscopy) or administration of a neuromuscular blocking agent with vagotonic effect (succinylcholine) may produce extreme bradycardia and asystolia [10].

Inhaled Anesthetics – Effects On Specific Organs

Cerebrovascular Disorders include progressive depression of cortex functions, basal ganglia and cerebellum, and sensitive motor spinal nerves, vasomotor and respiratory centers. The annihilation of central inhibitory effects leads to exacerbation of excitatory reactions.

The main ***myocardial effects*** relate to depressed myocardial contractility *via* enflurane, halothane and isoflurane, in descending order. Cardiac output decreases proportionately to the depth of anesthesia. Patients with dystrophic myotonia present a higher susceptibility to anesthetics-related cardiovascular injuries.

Respiratory Disorders refer to decreased frequency and amplitude of spontaneous breathing, drops in functional residual capacity (FRC) and modification of the ventilation/perfusion ratio.

Renal Effects result from decreasing the renal blood flow and glomerular filtration rate and increasing the ADH release that induces oliguria.

Other Effects: volatile anesthetics, except nitrous oxide, are proven triggers in the occurrence of malignant hyperthermia.

Inhaled Anesthetics – Specific Drug-Related Effects

Nitrous Oxide may produce increased intracranial pressure and bone marrow suppression. Nitrogen accumulation produces distension of hollow organs ("the effect of dark space") and increases the risk of gaseous embolism. At the end of the anesthetic period, when the partial pressure of oxygen decreases in the pulmonary alveoli for about 10 minutes, nitrogen-induced diffusion hypoxia can be noted. By activating methylcobalamin, nitrous oxide stimulates myelin and DNA synthesis. The effects can include spontaneous abortions, congenital anomalies, megaloblastic anemia and agranulocytosis. Prolonged exposure to nitrous oxide can be followed by degeneration of the lateral horns of the spinal cord and subsequent peripheral sensory or motor polyneuropathy.

Halothane predisposes the patient to arrhythmias, breathing centers depression, bronchodilation, cerebral perfusion and intracranial pressure increase, and uterine smooth muscle relaxation. Immune mediated halothane hepatitis, which is characterized by extensive hepatic necrosis, occurs in 1/10,000-35,000 adult patients. One third of patients present unexplained fever associated with eosinophilia, skin reactions and arthralgia. The mortality rate is about 20-50%. The risk of hepatitis is higher in patients receiving multiple anesthesia with halothane, the latter appearing 30 days before the appearance of hepatitis. Although halothane decreases portal blood flow and increased hepatic artery flow, it can accentuate the severity of a preexisting hepatic injury [11]

Enflurane can cause hypotension and reflex tachycardia. In deep anesthesia, electroencephalic changes characteristic of seizures can be noted [12]. ***Isoflurane*** produces hypotension, respiratory depression, bronchodilation, increased intracranial pressure and, infrequently, coronary vasodilation [13]. ***Desflurane*** increases intracranial pressure and is irritating to the upper airways. Arterial hypertension and tachycardia can also occur [14]. ***Sevoflurane*** increases intracranial pressure but does not produce seizures [15].

Neuromuscular Blocking Agents

The depolarizing neuromuscular blocker ***succinylcholine*** can produce muscle fasciculation and pain, transient ocular hypertension, sinus bradycardia, rhabdomyolysis, hyperkalemia and myoglobinuria. In newborns and infants up to eight weeks of age, fulminant pulmonary edema can occur. Succinylcholine is a trigger for malignant hyperthermia. In patients with burns, suxamethonium can induce a massive release of potassium from skeletal muscles, potentially resulting in cardiac arrest [16].

Nondepolarizing Neuromuscular Blockers such as vecuronium, pancuronium, and alcuronium, exert sympathomimetic and vagolytic effects. They have unpredictable effects in myasthenia gravis. Up to 75% of intraoperative anaphylactic reactions are caused by muscle relaxants, due to their potential to stimulate the release of histamine. In patients with a damaged BBB, intracranial pressure will rise [17 - 19].

Technical Complications of General Anesthesia

Technical Malfunctions in Equipment and the Anesthetic Circuit

These malfunctions are usually produced by inadequate oxygen/anesthetic gases intake, with hypoxia and hyperventilation (accidental disconnections, incorrect setting of ventilation parameters, incorrect introduction of the anesthetic circuit, decalibrated vaporizers) being the main consequences. The clinical effects are cyanosis, tachycardia and abnormal ECG, followed by bradycardia and hypotension [20].

Incorrect Positioning of the Patient on the Operating Table

The main consequences are atelectasis (by intrabronchial placing of the intubation cannula), peripheral nerve injuries (due to vicious position of limbs or hyperextension with nerve plexus elongation) and ocular lesions (corneal abrasion).

Patient-Related Complications

Bronchial Aspiration of Gastric Content – gastric content is especially aspirated in the upper airways during the induction phase. It is a silent aspiration that is difficult to detect, but becomes obvious when the gastric content is aspirate through the intubation cannula. It is considered that about 25 ml of gastric acid is enough to induce acute pulmonary inflammation. The main predisposing factors are gastric hypersecretion and high gastric pressure (full stomach, acute abdomen, pregnancy, obesity, ileus). The main consequences are surfactant degradation, pulmonary edema, atelectasis, hypoxia, Mendelson's syndrome (autodigestion of pulmonary parenchyma by acid gastric secretion), ARDS, pneumonia and formation of pulmonary abscesses [21].

Laryngospasm (Glottis Spasm), Bronchospasm – the predisposing factors are catarrh, smoking, superficial anesthesia and repeated intubation attempts [22]. Ventilation attempts with positive pressure increase pressure in the airways and cause the appearance of pneumothorax through barotrauma. This is manifested as subcutaneous emphysema, pneumomediastinum or pneumopericardium [23].

Pneumothorax can be a consequence of blebs rupture or high intrathoracic pressure.

Pulmonary Interstitial Emphysema and Air Embolism are caused by the increased pressure of gases in the anesthesia machine. The mechanism comprises the occurrence of septal tearing and the air and gases reaching the lung parenchyma, inducing interstitial emphysema. In patients with pulmonary vein injuries, air embolism can result. Air embolism can also be induced by pneumoperitoneum with CO_2 during laparoscopic surgery.

Acute Pulmonary Edema usually occurs *via* the association of myocardial dysfunction with intraoperative fluid overload [24].

Anaphylactic Reactions During Surgery can be triggered by any drug or substance used during anesthesia [25].

Hypertensive Crises usually occur in patients with hypertension when premedication is not appropriate or perioperative analgesia is insufficient. It can induce hypertensive encephalopathy, cardiac failure and cerebral and renal complications.

Arterial Hypotension can occur during the induction of anesthesia or intraoperatively, through bleeding or uncompensated losses (decreased preload), decreasing afterload or myocardial depression [26].

Intraoperative Myocardial Infarction depends on the preexisting coronary distress level, the type of surgery and the degree of volume replacement. It occurs most commonly on the third to fifth day after surgery [27].

Malignant Hyperthermia is the result of massive calcium release from sarcoplasmic reticulum in skeletal muscle fibers, which produces powerful muscle contractions and hyperthermia. The main clinical features are tachycardia, tachypnea, muscle rigidity, hyperthermia, abnormal ECG and arrhythmias [28].

Laryngotracheal Decubitus Ulcers are late consequences of long-term endotracheal intubation as a result of the mechanical effect (compression) of the tube inserted into the airways [29].

Other Complications include arterial hypotension, cardiac arrhythmias, prolonged respiratory depression, epistaxis produced by the nasogastric tube, *etc.*

COMPLICATIONS OF LOCO-REGIONAL ANESTHESIA

Local Anesthetics-Related Complications

Overdose – local toxic effect is very rare. Subarachnoid administration in high doses (usually accidentally, during alleged epidural administration or prolonged Trendelenburg positioning) produces prolonged blockage of nerve conduction with subsequent emergence of total motor block. Subsequently, the rising anesthesia level reaches the respiratory muscles. A properly executed epidural administration can also induce motor block through diffusion of the local anesthetic into the subarachnoid space.

Systemic toxicity is usually the consequence of accidental intravenous administration of the anesthetic drug. In early phases, the main affected systems are the central nervous (restlessness, delirium, tonic-clonic seizures) and cardiovascular systems (tachycardia, hypertension, skin erythema). The late consequences are coma, apnea and cardiovascular disorders (bradycardia, decreased myocardial contractility, dysrhythmia, vasodilatation, thready pulse, cardiocirculatory arrest, *etc.*). Overdosed prilocaine causes methemoglobinemia [30].

Arterial hypotension appears *via* the lowering of peripheral vascular resistance, especially following subarachnoid anesthesia [31].

Anaphylactic Allergic Reactions are rare complications of local anesthesia, occurring more frequently following administration of the amino ester class of anesthetics [32].

Complications Due to Anesthesia Technique

An improper anesthesia technique can induce peripheral nerve injury (paresthesias, paralyses) [33] or spinal artery syndrome (total or partial occlusion of the artery of Adamkiewicz) with subsequent paraplegia.

Based on the type of anesthesia, the following specific complications may occur [34]:

- ***Intercostal Anesthesia:*** pneumothorax and accidental intravenous or epidural injection.
- ***Spinal Anesthesia:*** intraspinal hematoma (compression), acute bacterial meningitis, chronic adhesive meningitis, spinal nerve traumatic injuries, spinal cord lesions, bone/ligament injuries and post-dural puncture headache (due to the leakage of cephalorachidian fluid through the opening of the puncture area).
- ***Epidural Anesthesia:*** accidental puncture of dura, epidural hematoma, arterial hypotension, acute systemic toxicity (especially of the cardiovascular system), total spinal anesthesia.

COMPLICATIONS OF INTENSIVE CARE

Complications Associated with Mechanical Ventilation

Controlled mechanical ventilation may cause complications *via* the following:

• ***<u>Increased Intrapulmonary Pressure</u>*** – controlled mechanical ventilation can induce acute dilation of the lungs (acute emphysema), interstitial emphysema followed by mediastinal and subcutaneous emphysema, pulmonary refraction with pneumothorax or air embolism. Air embolism occurs as a result of ventilation pushing into the pulmonary veins, and subsequently into the great systemic arteries (meningeal, cerebral, coronary arteries, *etc*.). The main symptoms of air embolism are cerebral petechiae, presence of air bubbles in the meningeal and retinal arteries, and marble appearance of the skin and tongue [35].

• ***<u>Decreased Venous Return</u>*** – controlled mechanical ventilation can produce generalized venous stasis.

• ***External Contamination*** – controlled mechanical ventilation can increase the risk of respiratory infection [36].

• ***Mechanical Effect*** – in long-term intubation or tracheostomy, cannula may cause ulcerative lesions of the tracheal wall with improper healing, or the formation of granulomas with subsequent tracheal stenosis or tracheopathia [37].

Complications of oxygen therapy

Prolonged inhalation of pure oxygen (100%) produces the following effects:

• ***Pulmonary Changes*** – injuries progress from tracheobronchial irritation to extravasation of plasma proteins, formation of hyaline membranes, dystelectasis and progressive interstitial fibrosis [38]. The mechanism of oxygen's toxic effect is based on the ozone effect against the alveolar capillary endothelium. Oxygen free radicals, arachidonic acid and other mediators of the inflammatory process are involved [39]. The toxic effect of oxygen explains the occurrence of Wilson-Mikity syndrome in newborns who undergo prolonged oxygen therapy. This syndrome is characterized by dyspnea, recurrent cyanosis, diffuse pulmonary fibrosis and chronic cor pulmonale.

• ***Ocular Changes*** – in adults, retinal vasoconstriction is a reversible process without clinical consequences. In premature infants, pure oxygen produces retrolental fibroplasia characterized by edema, retinal hemorrhages, retinal gliosis and vessels neoformation. Clinically, a gray-white mass can be seen in the anterior vitreous followed, infrequently, by definitive blindness.

• ***Neurological Effects*** – the main signs of such effects are seizures that can mimic a grand mal epileptic crisis. These symptoms disappear following discontinuation of oxygen therapy.

Complications of Maneuvers Used in Intensive Care

The central venous access can involve the following complications [40 - 43]: catheter-induced infection and sepsis, thrombophlebitis or thrombosis, air embolism, catheter embolism (due to its inadequate fixation or the accidentally sectioning of the catheter tip), aberrant tracks on other veins routes, pneumothorax (after subclavicular approach of the subclavian vein), arterial puncture with local hematoma (*e.g.,* carotid injury during puncture of the internal jugular vein), nerve damage (vagus or phrenic nerve). Injuries of the stellate ganglion or the cervical plexus can induce the Claude Bernard-Horner syndrome.

Side Effects of Drugs used in Intensive Care

One of the specific ADR is the propylene glycol intoxication that is induced, in ventilated patients, by benzodiazepines (lorazepam, diazepam). The sedative/anxiolytic agents are also dissoluted in propylene glycol. The main clinical effects are the hyperosmolarity, hemolysis, cardiac arrhythmias, agitation, seizures, and coma. This intoxication may mimic an inflammatory syndrome characterized by acidosis, hypotension and multiple organ dysfunction [44].

Heparin-induced thrombocytopenia syndrome can also occur in the ICUs due to the formation of abnormal antibodies that activate platelets. It can induce various forms of thromboembolism [45].

Neurological Complications in Intensive Care

ICU-Acquired Delirium is often underdiagnosed and can occur in two forms: hyperactive or hypoactive. It is caused by dementia, sedatives and strong analgesics, prolonged immobilization and changes to the patient's circadian rhythm.

ICU-Acquired Weakness represents an alteration of neuromuscular function that impacts ventilator weaning and patient mobility. It is especially linked to prolonged duration of mechanical ventilation (at least seven days), but also to the use of corticosteroids [46].

Relaxants-Induced Neuropathy is related to nondepolarizing muscle relaxants and is reversible in weeks/months.

Complications Related to Artificial Nutrition

Dysmetabolic Complications

Malnutrition can emerge in critical patients receiving only 50-80% of their energy and nutritional requirements, despite existing enteral/parenteral nutrition formulas. It increases the number of days of required mechanical ventilation, especially in patients with body mass indices below 25. The risk of death is increased in patients with a deficit of 1200 kcal/day [47].

Propofol-Related Infusion Syndrome is a serious complication evidenced by rhabdomyolysis, acute kidney injury and cardiac failure, acidosis, hepatomegaly, hyperlipidemia and high serum values of lactate and creatine kinase. It occurs as a result of propofol-induced damage to the mitochondrial respiratory chain. The main risk factors are over 48 hours of propofol therapy with a dose of more than 4 mg/kg/h, low intake of carbohydrates, and increased intake of exogenous corticosteroids and catecholamines [48]. Propofol-induced hypertriglyceridemia occurs in patients with alterations in lipid metabolism or those with an excess of serum lipids [49].

Enteral Nutrition

During artificial enteral nutrition, gastroesophageal reflux can be followed by aspiration of gastric contents into the airways, leading to aspiration pneumonia. Irritations or erosions of the pharyngeal or esophageal mucosa can occur following long-term catheter maintenance. The risk of erosions is lower for silicone or polyurethane catheters. Diarrhea appears in 10-20% of cases and can be associated with cramping, abdominal distension, bloating, flatulence, nausea, vomiting and gurgling. It is caused by inadequate food formula, inanition, hypoalbuminemia, antibiotherapy, impaired pancreatic function, malabsorption, enteritis, lactose intolerance or contamination of food formulas. Glucose intolerance may be manifested by hyperglycemia, hyperosmolarity, nonketotic dehydration and even coma. It is caused by temporary insulin-resistance or preexisting DM. Hyponatremia is the consequence of intestinal or dilution losses and is treated with diuretics, lost sodium replacement and dilution losses control. Hypernatremia occurs following dehydration or in patients with diabetes insipidus. Hypokalemia results from the administration of diuretics, dilution, insulin excess or intestinal losses [50, 51].

Parenteral Nutrition

Total parenteral nutrition can induce intestinal atrophy and is a risk factor for cholecystitis. Intestinal atrophy is the consequence of changes in the intestinal mucosa, appearing a few days following cessation of enteral feeding. The altered mucosal barrier causes penetration of microorganisms into systemic circulation. Noncalculous cholecystitis is caused by biliary stasis, due to the absence of cholecystokinin-induced gallbladder contractions [52, 53].

Post-Transfusion Complications

Metabolic Complications include Hyperkalemia, Hypocalcemia and Acidosis

Immune-Mediated Complications (immediate hemolytic reactions) are the result of ABO incompatibility. The mechanism is based on the recipient's IgG and IgM antibodies' attack on the donor red blood cells. It induces hemolysis, erythrocyte agglutination and DIC. Clinically, it presents a sudden onset. In the first two to three hours post-transfusion, the patient can present chills, fever, tachycardia, dyspnea, chest pain, nausea, vomiting, hypotension, hemoglobinuria, signs of anaphylactic shock, congestive heart failure, oliguria and anuria. Angioedema, pulmonary edema, urticaria, tubulonephrosis, obstructive necrosis through hemoglobinuria and disseminated microthrombosis are characteristic. During general anesthesia, the symptoms are usually masked and attenuated [54, 55].

Late Hemolytic Reaction is due to a subgroup incompatibility. Increasing the antibodies of the Rh, Kidd, E and D systems induce lysis of the donor erythrocytes, especially in the monocyte-macrophage system of the recipient. Clinically, this reaction occurs one to two weeks or months following transfusion and is characterized by fever, anemia, jaundice and renal failure. Hepatic and splenic hemosiderosis are characteristic.

Nonhemolytic Febrile Reactions occur as a result of formation of cytotoxic or agglutination antibodies. They attack the lymphocytes, granulocytes and plasma cells of the donor. The clinical features vary from mild forms, manifesting as fever, tachycardia and dyspnea, to severe forms that include anaphylactic reactions.

Allergic Reactions induce urticaria, nausea, vomiting, abdominal cramps, diarrhea and vascular instability. ARDS and shock can be associated. Angioedema, urticaria, skin erythema and shock organs are seen in severe forms [56].

Infections are relatively rare. However, bacterial infections with Pseudomonas, Citrobacter freundii, Escherichia coli and other Gram-negative bacteria have been reported. Fever, vomiting, diarrhea, abdominal cramps and infrequent septic shock are the main clinical features [57]. Viral contamination involves cytomegalovirus, hepatitis B and C, HIV and HTLV-1 viruses. Contamination with prions can cause Creutzfeldt-Jakob disease [58].

Massive Transfusion Syndrome relating to thrombocytopenia and microvascular bleedings occurs by diluting the blood of the recipient. The donor blood is preserved without an adequate number of functional platelets.

Acute Lung Injury (ALI) is produced by the antileukocytes antibodies of the donor plasma, which agglutinate the pulmonary recipient's leukocytes. Clinically, this condition can mimic noncardiogenic acute pulmonary edema [59].

Other Post-Transfusion Complications are hemodynamic overload with subsequent cardiac failure and, more rarely, hypothermia, coagulation disorders, impaired oxygen affinity for hemoglobin and air embolism.

Complications Of Fluid Therapy

Infusion solutions are crystalloids (glucose, saline, Ringer's solution, hypertonic salt solution, sodium bicarbonate) or colloids (albumin, hydroxyethyl starch, dextrans and gelatin derivatives).

Crystalloid Solutions can cause hyperkalemia and lactic acidosis (Ringer's solution), hypernatremia, increased production of carbon dioxide (sodium bicarbonate). Large volumes of crystalloids (over 3.5 l) determine hyperhydration and can cause a colloid osmotic pressure drop, peripheral edema, pulmonary edema and volume expansion of short physiological duration (23-28 mmHg) [60].

Colloid Solutions may cause allergic reactions (dextrans, gelatin derivatives) and use in excess can produce dilution coagulopathy. Allergic reactions to dextran occur in 0.02% of users [61].

CONFLICT OF INTEREST

The authors confirm that this chapter content has no conflict of interest.

ACKNOWLEDGEMENTS

Declared none.

REFERENCES

[1] Abdellatif S, Ksouri H, Ben Hamida A, *et al.* Iatrogenic complications in the ICU: a prospective study during 10 months. Crit Care 2003; 7: 247.
[http://dx.doi.org/10.1186/cc2136]

[2] Darchy B, Le Mière E, Figuérédo B, Bavoux E, Domart Y. Iatrogenic diseases as a reason for admission to the intensive care unit: incidence, causes, and consequences. Arch Intern Med 1999; 159(1): 71-8.
[http://dx.doi.org/10.1001/archinte.159.1.71] [PMID: 9892333]

[3] Couch NP, Tilney NL, Rayner AA, Moore FD. The high cost of low-frequency events: the anatomy and economics of surgical mishaps. N Engl J Med 1981; 304(11): 634-7.
[http://dx.doi.org/10.1056/NEJM198103123041103] [PMID: 7453740]

[4] Karch FE, Lasagna L. Adverse drug reactions. A critical review. JAMA 1975; 234(12): 1236-41.
[http://dx.doi.org/10.1001/jama.1975.03260250028021] [PMID: 1242749]

[5] Taittonen M, Kirvelä O, Aantaa R, Kanto J. Cardiovascular and metabolic responses to clonidine and midazolam premedication. Eur J Anaesthesiol 1997; 14(2): 190-6.
[http://dx.doi.org/10.1097/00003643-199703000-00012] [PMID: 9088819]

[6] Gin T. Hypnotic and sedative drugs anything new on the horizon? Curr Opin Anaesthesiol 2013; 26(4): 409-13.
[PMID: 23820101]

[7] Mayer M, Doenicke A, Nebauer AE, Hepting L. [Propofol and etomidate-Lipuro for induction of general anesthesia. Hemodynamics, vascular compatibility, subjective findings and postoperative nausea]. Anaesthesist 1996; 45(11): 1082-4.
[http://dx.doi.org/10.1007/s001010050343] [PMID: 9012304]

[8] Moneret-Vautrin DA, Mertes PM. Anaphylaxis to general anesthetics. Chem Immunol Allergy 2010; 95: 180-9.

[http://dx.doi.org/10.1159/000315951] [PMID: 20519890]

[9] Devlin JW, Mallow-Corbett S, Riker RR. Adverse drug events associated with the use of analgesics, sedatives, and antipsychotics in the intensive care unit. Crit Care Med 2010; 38(6) (Suppl.): S231-43. [http://dx.doi.org/10.1097/CCM.0b013e3181de125a] [PMID: 20502176]

[10] Barnes BJ, Hollands JM. Drug-induced arrhythmias. Crit Care Med 2010; 38(6) (Suppl.): S188-97. [http://dx.doi.org/10.1097/CCM.0b013e3181de112a] [PMID: 20502173]

[11] Landoni G, Bignami E, Oliviero F, Zangrillo A. Halogenated anaesthetics and cardiac protection in cardiac and non-cardiac anaesthesia. Ann Card Anaesth 2009; 12(1): 4-9. [http://dx.doi.org/10.4103/0971-9784.45006] [PMID: 19136748]

[12] Rörtgen D, Kloos J, Fries M, *et al.* Comparison of early cognitive function and recovery after desflurane or sevoflurane anaesthesia in the elderly: a double-blinded randomized controlled trial. Br J Anaesth 2010; 104(2): 167-74. [http://dx.doi.org/10.1093/bja/aep369] [PMID: 20042477]

[13] Canet J, Roigé J, Bandrés R, Campos JM, Chiveli MA, Campbell J. [Comparison of the effect of desflurane with isoflurane in patients over 65 years of age: multicenter study]. Rev Esp Anestesiol Reanim 1998; 45(7): 280-4. [PMID: 9780764]

[14] Marana E, Russo A, Colicci S, *et al.* Desflurane *versus* sevoflurane: a comparison on stress response. Minerva Anestesiol 2013; 79(1): 7-14. [PMID: 23090102]

[15] Sakai EM, Connolly LA, Klauck JA. Inhalation anesthesiology and volatile liquid anesthetics: focus on isoflurane, desflurane, and sevoflurane. Pharmacotherapy 2005; 25(12): 1773-88. [http://dx.doi.org/10.1592/phco.2005.25.12.1773] [PMID: 16305297]

[16] Baur CP, Schlecht R, Jurkat-Rott K, Georgieff M, Lehmann-Horn F. [Anesthesia in neuromuscular disorders. Part 1: introduction]. Anasthesiol Intensivmed Notfallmed Schmerzther 2002; 37(2): 77-83. [http://dx.doi.org/10.1055/s-2002-20392] [PMID: 11865384]

[17] Soukup J, Doenicke A, Hoernecke R, Vorhammer B, Seebauer A, Moss J. [Cardiovascular effects after bolus administration of cisatracurium. A comparison with vecuronium]. Anaesthesist 1996; 45(11): 1024-9. [PMID: 9012296]

[18] Raft J, Chenot ED, Longrois D, Meistelman C. [Analysis of neuromuscular blocking drugs and sugammadex expenses, one year after its introduction into routine clinical practice]. Ann Fr Anesth Reanim 2011; 30(10): 758-9. [http://dx.doi.org/10.1016/j.annfar.2011.06.013] [PMID: 21820269]

[19] Warr J, Thiboutot Z, Rose L, Mehta S, Burry LD. Current therapeutic uses, pharmacology, and clinical considerations of neuromuscular blocking agents for critically ill adults. Ann Pharmacother 2011; 45(9): 1116-26. [http://dx.doi.org/10.1345/aph.1Q004] [PMID: 21828347]

[20] Crossingham GV, Sice PJ, Roberts MJ, Lam WH, Gale TC. Development of workplace-based assessments of non-technical skills in anaesthesia. Anaesthesia 2012; 67(2): 158-64. [http://dx.doi.org/10.1111/j.1365-2044.2011.06977.x] [PMID: 22251107]

[21] Levichev EA, Nedashkovskiĭ EV. [Prevention of regurgitation and aspiration during emergency care of patients under general anesthesia]. Anesteziol Reanimatol 2008; 4(4): 8-12. [PMID: 18819388]

[22] Hobaika AB, Lorentz MN. [Laryngospasm]. Rev Bras Anestesiol 2009; 59(4): 487-95. [http://dx.doi.org/10.1590/S0034-70942009000400012] [PMID: 19669024]

[23] Rampersad S, Elwood T. Risk factors for laryngospasm. Paediatr Anaesth 2009; 19(1): 59-60. [http://dx.doi.org/10.1111/j.1460-9592.2008.02809.x] [PMID: 19076513]

[24] Kilpatrick B, Slinger P. Lung protective strategies in anaesthesia. Br J Anaesth 2010; 105 (Suppl. 1): i108-16.
[http://dx.doi.org/10.1093/bja/aeq299] [PMID: 21148650]

[25] Ebo DG, Fisher MM, Hagendorens MM, Bridts CH, Stevens WJ. Anaphylaxis during anaesthesia: diagnostic approach. Allergy 2007; 62(5): 471-87.
[http://dx.doi.org/10.1111/j.1398-9995.2007.01347.x] [PMID: 17441788]

[26] Rooke GA. Cardiovascular aging and anesthetic implications. J Cardiothorac Vasc Anesth 2003; 17(4): 512-23.
[http://dx.doi.org/10.1016/S1053-0770(03)00161-7] [PMID: 12968244]

[27] Biboulet P, Aubas P, Dubourdieu J, Rubenovitch J, Capdevila X, dAthis F. Fatal and non fatal cardiac arrests related to anesthesia. Can J Anaesth 2001; 48(4): 326-32.
[http://dx.doi.org/10.1007/BF03014958] [PMID: 11339772]

[28] Schuster F, Moegele S, Johannsen S, Roewer N. Malignant hyperthermia in the intensive care setting. Crit Care 2014; 18(2): 411.
[http://dx.doi.org/10.1186/cc13744] [PMID: 24602556]

[29] Bouattour K, Prost-Lapeyre A, Hauw-Berlemont C, Diehl JL, Guérot E. [A post-intubation tracheal rupture in intensive care unit]. Ann Fr Anesth Reanim 2014; 33(11): 590-2.
[http://dx.doi.org/10.1016/j.annfar.2014.09.005] [PMID: 25450732]

[30] Mercado P, Weinberg GL, Brockow K. Local anesthetic systemic toxicity: prevention and treatment. Anesthesiol Clin 2011; 29(2): 233-42.
[http://dx.doi.org/10.1016/j.anclin.2011.04.007] [PMID: 21620340]

[31] Dogan Z, Bakan M, Idin K, Esen A, Uslu FB, Ozturk E. Total spinal block after lumbar plexus block: a case report. Braz J Anesthesiol 2014; 64(2): 121-3.
[http://dx.doi.org/10.1016/j.bjane.2013.03.002] [PMID: 24794455]

[32] Ring J, Franz R, Brockow K. Anaphylactic reactions to local anesthetics. Chem Immunol Allergy 2010; 95: 190-200.
[http://dx.doi.org/10.1159/000315952] [PMID: 20519891]

[33] Mulroy MF, Weller RS, Liguori GA. A checklist for performing regional nerve blocks. Reg Anesth Pain Med 2014; 39(3): 195-9.
[http://dx.doi.org/10.1097/AAP.0000000000000075] [PMID: 24718017]

[34] Doherty H, Hameed S, Ahmed I, Russell IF. Post-dural puncture headache and posterior reversible encephalopathy syndrome: a misdiagnosis or co-presentation? Int J Obstet Anesth 2014; 23(3): 279-82.
[http://dx.doi.org/10.1016/j.ijoa.2014.02.003] [PMID: 24768557]

[35] Futier E, Godet T, Millot A, Constantin JM, Jaber S. Mechanical ventilation in abdominal surgery. Ann Fr Anesth Reanim 2014; 33(7-8): 472-5.
[http://dx.doi.org/10.1016/j.annfar.2014.07.007] [PMID: 25153670]

[36] Bobik P, Siemiątkowski A. [Ventilator-associated pneumonia and other infections]. Pneumonol Alergol Pol 2014; 82(5): 472-80.
[http://dx.doi.org/10.5603/PiAP.2014.0062] [PMID: 25133817]

[37] Terragni P, Faggiano C, Martin EL, Ranieri VM. Tracheostomy in mechanical ventilation. Semin Respir Crit Care Med 2014; 35(4): 482-91.
[http://dx.doi.org/10.1055/s-0034-1383862] [PMID: 25111644]

[38] De Jong A, Futier E, Millot A, *et al.* How to preoxygenate in operative room: healthy subjects and situations at risk. Ann Fr Anesth Reanim 2014; 33(7-8): 457-61.
[http://dx.doi.org/10.1016/j.annfar.2014.08.001] [PMID: 25168301]

[39] Lumb AB, Walton LJ. Perioperative oxygen toxicity. Anesthesiol Clin 2012; 30(4): 591-605.

[http://dx.doi.org/10.1016/j.anclin.2012.07.009] [PMID: 23089497]

[40] Miguelena D, Pardo R, Morón-Duarte LS. [Central venous catheter-related complications in critically ill children]. Rev Salud Publica (Bogota) 2013; 15(6): 916-28. [PMID: 25124354]

[41] Lebeaux D, Joly D, Zahar JR. [Long-term central venous catheter-related infections]. Rev Prat 2014; 64(5): 626-33. [PMID: 24923045]

[42] New KA, Webster J, Marsh NM, Hewer B. Intravascular device use, management, documentation and complications: a point prevalence survey. Aust Health Rev 2014; 38(3): 345-9. [http://dx.doi.org/10.1071/AH13111] [PMID: 24869909]

[43] Bowdle A. Vascular complications of central venous catheter placement: evidence-based methods for prevention and treatment. J Cardiothorac Vasc Anesth 2014; 28(2): 358-68. [http://dx.doi.org/10.1053/j.jvca.2013.02.027] [PMID: 24008166]

[44] Wilson KC, Reardon C, Theodore AC, Farber HW. Propylene glycol toxicity: a severe iatrogenic illness in ICU patients receiving IV benzodiazepines: a case series and prospective, observational pilot study. Chest 2005; 128(3): 1674-81. [http://dx.doi.org/10.1378/chest.128.3.1674] [PMID: 16162774]

[45] Baglin TP. Heparin induced thrombocytopenia thrombosis (HIT/T) syndrome: diagnosis and treatment. J Clin Pathol 2001; 54(4): 272-4. [http://dx.doi.org/10.1136/jcp.54.4.272] [PMID: 11304842]

[46] Vasilevskis EE, Ely EW, Speroff T, Pun BT, Boehm L, Dittus RS. Reducing iatrogenic risks: ICU-acquired delirium and weakness crossing the quality chasm. Chest 2010; 138(5): 1224-33. [http://dx.doi.org/10.1378/chest.10-0466] [PMID: 21051398]

[47] Faisy C, Lerolle N, Dachraoui F, *et al.* Impact of energy deficit calculated by a predictive method on outcome in medical patients requiring prolonged acute mechanical ventilation. Br J Nutr 2009; 101(7): 1079-87. [http://dx.doi.org/10.1017/S0007114508055669] [PMID: 18778528]

[48] Imam TH. Propofol-related infusion syndrome: role of propofol in medical complications of sedated critical care patients. Perm J 2013; 17(2): 85-7. [http://dx.doi.org/10.7812/TPP/12-114] [PMID: 23704851]

[49] Barr J. Propofol: a new drug for sedation in the intensive care unit. Int Anesthesiol Clin 1995; 33(1): 131-54. [http://dx.doi.org/10.1097/00004311-199500000-00008] [PMID: 7635554]

[50] Choi EY, Park DA, Park J. Calorie intake of enteral nutrition and clinical outcomes in acutely critically ill patients: a meta-analysis of randomized controlled trials. J Parenter Enteral Nutr 2015; 39(3): 291-300. [http://dx.doi.org/10.1177/0148607114544322] [PMID: 25078609]

[51] Saran D, Brody RA, Stankorb SM, Parrott SJ, Heyland DK. Gastric *vs* Small Bowel Feeding in Critically Ill Neurologically Injured Patients: Results of a Multicenter Observational Study. J Parenter Enteral Nutr 2015; 39(8): 910-6. [http://dx.doi.org/10.1177/0148607114540003] [PMID: 24947058]

[52] Olveira G, Tapia MJ, Ocón J, *et al.* Parenteral nutrition-associated hyperglycemia in non-critically ill inpatients increases the risk of in-hospital mortality (multicenter study). Diabetes Care 2013; 36(5): 1061-6. [http://dx.doi.org/10.2337/dc12-1379] [PMID: 23223407]

[53] Thibault R, Pichard C. Parenteral nutrition. World Rev Nutr Diet 2013; 105: 59-68. [http://dx.doi.org/10.1159/000341269] [PMID: 23075587]

[54] Osterman JL, Arora S. Blood product transfusions and reactions. Emerg Med Clin North Am 2014,

32(3): 727-38.
[http://dx.doi.org/10.1016/j.emc.2014.04.012] [PMID: 25060259]

[55] Vucelić D, Savić N, Dordević R, Dokić M, Vavić N, Velimirović I. [Acute hemolytic transfusion reaction]. Acta Chir Iugosl 2002; 49(1): 61-7.
[http://dx.doi.org/10.2298/ACI0201061V] [PMID: 12587485]

[56] Domen RE, Hoeltge GA. Allergic transfusion reactions: an evaluation of 273 consecutive reactions. Arch Pathol Lab Med 2003; 127(3): 316-20.
[PMID: 12653575]

[57] Le Niger C, Dalbies F, Narbonne V, *et al.* [Transfusion-transmitted bacterial infection of a apheresis platelet concentrate with *Streptococcus gallolyticus*: Analysis of one case]. Transfus Clin Biol 2014; 21(3): 107-10.
[http://dx.doi.org/10.1016/j.tracli.2014.05.001] [PMID: 24934685]

[58] Liu Y, Zeng P, Wang J, *et al.* Hepatitis B virus infection in a cohort of HIV infected blood donors and AIDS patients in Sichuan, China. J Transl Med 2014; 12: 164.
[http://dx.doi.org/10.1186/1479-5876-12-164] [PMID: 24923206]

[59] Chung YT, Wu YC, Chen YH. Postoperative pulmonary edema, transfusion-related?a case report. Acta Anaesthesiol Sin 2003; 41(1): 43-6.
[PMID: 12747347]

[60] Bartels K, Thiele RH, Gan TJ. Rational fluid management in todays ICU practice. Crit Care 2013; 17 (Suppl. 1): S6.
[http://dx.doi.org/10.1186/cc12771] [PMID: 23514431]

[61] Hiltebrand LB, Kimberger O, Arnberger M, Brandt S, Kurz A, Sigurdsson GH. Crystalloids *versus* colloids for goal-directed fluid therapy in major surgery. Crit Care 2009; 13(2): R40.
[http://dx.doi.org/10.1186/cc7761] [PMID: 19302713]

CHAPTER 17

Iatrogenic Pathology in Surgery

Tivadar Jr. Bara[*], **Bogdan Andrei Suciu** and **Tivadar Bara**

Department of Surgery, University of Medicine and Pharmacy, Tirgu-Mures, Romania

Abstract: Surgical intervention remains a trauma for patients even given modern techniques and the use of highly specialized instruments. Any surgical maneuver can cause injuries and complications. The severity of such injuries is determined by the disease itself, the patient's comorbidities and the surgeon's experience. In this chapter, we present the iatrogenic complications arising following major surgeries performed openly or laparoscopically. In the first section, general complications, such as hemorrhage, fever, ileus and abscesses, are presented. Next, organ-related complications occurring during laparotomy, drainage of the abdominal cavity or abdominal wall reconstruction are described in detail. We then turn to the specific intra- and postoperative complications of various organs' surgical treatment due to erroneous surgery indications, vascular lesions and lesions of the neighboring organs. We describe complications in the surgery of the mediastinum, thoracic and abdominal cavity and describe the particularities of thyroid, lung, esophagus, stomach, small intestine, appendix, colon, pancreas, hepatobiliary tract and hernia surgery and postoperative parietal defects. Complications occurring as a result of laparoscopic intervention, erroneous indications or complications in performing pneumoperitoneum during insertion of the trocars are also presented. Finally, we consider the specific iatrogenic complications arising during minimally invasive bile, hiatal hernia, cardiac achalasia, spleen and morbid obesity (gastric sleeve and gastroplication) surgery.

Keywords: Abscess, Chylothorax, Duodenal stump insufficiency, Fistula, Hematoma of the scrotum, Hemoperitoneum, Hemopneumothorax, Mediastinitis, Pancreas, Peritonitis, Suture dehiscence.

INTRODUCTION

The severity of surgery-related injuries is directly influenced by the type of disease, the patient's comorbidities and the surgeon's experience. Unexpected complications may manifest after surgery, which can spoil the patient's prognosis and endanger his life. The surgeon thus faces a new pathology, which is often difficult to diagnose or treat because it is caused by the original disease or the surgical procedure used during treatment.

[*] **Corresponding author Tivadar Jr. Bara:** Department of Surgery, University of Medicine and Pharmacy, Tirgu-Mures, Romania; Tel/Fax: 0040-744-848456; E-mail: barativadar@yahoo.com

Simona Gurzu & Ioan Jung (Eds.)

GENERAL COMPLICATIONS

The purpose of the atraumatic, tissue-friendly surgical technique is to minimize tissue damage, preserve vascular and nervous integrity, and prevent additional injury. Thus, we can ensure optimal tissue regeneration and reduce the rate of intra- or postoperative complications.

Fever of unknown origin, pain, infections, anastomotic insufficiency and wound dehiscence appearing after surgery is often caused by nonuse of *atraumatic techniques*. The requirements for the application of atraumatic surgical techniques are: expertise in the field of surgical anatomy, biomechanics and physiology of wound healing, and an excellent knowledge of the application of special surgical tools used during surgery. These techniques prevail, especially, during tissue dissection, when blood-free anatomic target areas are created by dividing the tissues. In order to prevent complications, correct hemostasis and knowledge of the advantages and disadvantages of the preparation techniques, as well as their proper application, are required (sharp, dull, electrical, ultrasonic, *etc.*).

To remove the blood, whey and tissue fragments created in the surgical area, it may be necessary to use *drainage*. This, however, is not a substitution for atraumatic technique. The rate of drainage-related complications depends on the quality, size, location and timing of surgical tube use.

The *quality of suture* is also an aspect of the atraumatic technique, most trauma being caused by the inadequate use of surgical needles. Nowadays, the use of atraumatic needles is more common, yet the diameter of the needle, its profile (round, triangular) and thickness, as well as the quality of the thread (monofilament, multifilament, absorbable, *etc.*) are all important considerations. The *suture method* also affects the quality of the atraumatic technique. Knots in suturing with dense stitches cause tissue ischemia and necrosis.

Aggressive surgical maneuvers induce tissue trauma with further functional or morphological damage [1].

SURGERY OF THE MEDIASTINAL CAVITY

In this section, we will present the lesions related to surgery of the esophagus and thyroid gland.

Iatrogenic Lesions in Surgery of the Esophagus

Surgery of the Esophageal Diverticula

Diverticulectomy is indicated in symptomatic cases (dysphagia, regurgitation) and not for incidentally identified pulsating diverticula. Surgery is also indicated in associated inflammation, hemorrhages and chronically aspirated food remnants with aspirated pneumonia or lung fistulae. Reflux disease can be resolved with anti-reflux surgery.

Complications of such surgery can be related to the *surgical technique* and relate to recurrence as a result of clogging the diverticulum or incomplete myotomy. Sutures applied to close the diverticulum's aperture may cause stenosis, which can induce increased pressure and, in turn, lead to suture dehiscence.

Intraoperative Injuries include the following main lesions: hemorrhages (injuries of the common carotid artery, inferior thyroid artery or jugular vein), injuries of the recurrent laryngeal nerve (with postoperative hoarseness) and perforation of surrounding organs (esophagus, stomach, spleen, liver, pleura, lung).

Postoperative Injuries include fistulae (especially for Zenker's diverticulum), dehiscence of the epiphrenic diverticulum (with life-threatening mediastinitis displayed with dyspnea, fever, retrosternal pain, pleural and mediastinal fluid accumulation), stenosis (with dysphagia) and diverticulum recurrence (errors in surgical technique) [1 - 4].

Surgery of Malignant Tumors of the Esophagus

Incorrect Surgical Indication for esophagectomy can be the result of weak investigation of the patient. Improper preoperative assessment of metastatic status is a relatively common error, esophagectomy not being recommended in advanced stages, when the tumor infiltrates the respiratory tract, recurrent laryngeal nerve, lung or thyroid, even in the presence of liver or distant metastases. For example, in one of our cases, we intended to remove a diaphragmatic tumor reported preoperatively in a CT scan. Intraoperatively, a huge tumor of the middle third esophagus with infiltration of the trachea carina was identified, changing the operative protocol. The patient died 12 days after the surgery. This case attests to the necessity of attentive evaluation of the patient and choice of surgical procedure based on the tumor stage and localization, the patient's status and comorbidities, as well as the surgeon's experience and skill.

There is no consensus on the radical surgical treatment for malignant tumors of the esophagus. For subtotal esophagectomy, three principles should be respected: transhiatal method (Orringer), transthoracic block dissection (Skinner), and "two fielded" lymph node dissection (Akiyama) [1, 5].

Errors Regarding the Surgical Technique are mainly related to the surgeon's experience. For potentially curative tumors, oncologic radicalism and preserving esophageal function should be the main objectives, taking into account the patient's status and comorbidities. To preserve functionality, a Roux loop constructed from the jejunum is ideal, however such a loop long enough to replace the whole esophagus is not possible. Replacement of the esophagus with stomach "tube" is effective. However, during the replacement, in some cases, we discover that its length is still not enough. Functionality is then better preserved using a retrosternally built gastric tube. The risk of duodenal gastroesophageal reflux is decreased, but the risk of dehiscence increases. The use of a colon tube is associated with a higher rate of postoperative complications [1, 6].

Intraoperative injuries during esophagectomy without thoracotomy comprise a large spectrum of lesions, including the following main complications: injury or perforation of the abdominal esophagus (with mediastinitis, gastritis or purulent complications), injury of the left hepatic lobe (during preparation of the abdominal esophagus), injury of the spleen (during preparation of the "gastric tube"), injury of the pancreas (during removal of adherences between the stomach and pancreas), injury of the stomach (during preparation of the "gastric tube"), vascular lesions (with hematoma formation or gastric wall ischemia), injuries of the recurrent laryngeal nerve, injury of the trachea or pleura (risk of pneumo- or hemothorax) and cardiac arrhythmia (during transhiatal preparation of the esophagus) [6 - 8].

Intraoperative Injuries during Esophagectomy with Thoracotomy include the following complications: pleural or pulmonary injuries (during removal of the pleural adherences), hemorrhages (lesions of the intercostal vessels, such as vena azygos, or of the aortic branches) and injuries of the thoracic duct (risk of chylothorax), trachea and bronchi [6 - 8].

Postoperative Complications are relatively common and primarily involve cervical, intrathoracic or pyloric suture dehiscence (with fistulae formation, dyspnea, thoracic pain, tachycardia, fever, hydrothorax) and necrosis of the organ that was intraoperatively injured [1, 7].

Gastric dilatation can be caused by incomplete pyloromyotomy. In these cases, gastric secretions are expelled through the nasogastric tube or by the patient vomiting. Lack of gastric emptying can be identified through radiology with contrast agents [6].

Several other complications can be associated. Swallowing disorders are more common in cervical anastomosis. Injury of the recurrent laryngeal nerve can lead to recurrent aspiration pneumonia. Chylo-, hemo- or pneumothorax can be consequences of injuries to the thoracic duct or pleura. Postoperative esophageal reflux, anastomotic stenosis (especially in retrosternal cervical esophagogastrectomy), internal hernia and mechanical ileus on the hiatus of the dilated esophagus can also occur as postoperative complications [1].

Iatrogenic Lesions in Surgery of the Thyroid Gland

Preoperative Errors

Incorrect surgical indication is still considered to be based on the histological tumor type, although adapting the operative technique and extent of the surgery (partial *versus* total thyroidectomy) based on this differentiation is not endorsed by all surgeons.

Partial Thyroidectomy is considered a method of conservative surgery and includes lobectomy, hemithyroidectomy, subtotal thyroidectomy, total istmo-lobectomy on the lesion side and subtotal contralateral lobectomy. The arguments for partial thyroidectomy relate to the following: lack of multicentric clinical significance, low percentage of relapses in the remaining lobe or tissue (under 5%), possibility of iodine sterilization of the remnant tissue, low rate of postoperative morbidity, and less aggressive substitution therapy.

Total Thyroidectomy is indicated for multicentric tumors (30-80% of papillary carcinomas) to decrease the risk of recurrence (the rate is 4.7-24% after conservative excisions). The arguments against total thyroidectomy relate to the intraoperative risk of damage to the surrounding structures (parathyroid gland and nerves), postoperative functional dysfunctions and the necessity of hormone substitution. The arguments for total thyroidectomy relate to the following: minimal risk of loco-regional recurrences and distant metastases, no risk of secondary tumor of the remnant tissue (postirradiation), proper monitoring of relapses by determining the thyroglobulin level and correct iodine capture. If the survival rate in thyroid cancer after total thyroidectomy does not seem superior to more conservative approaches, it must be noted that disease-free survival appears significantly prolonged.

For thyroid tumors over 1.5 cm in size, total thyroidectomy followed by radioiodine therapy and substitution is usually indicated. Conservative methods should only be applied following an accurate preoperative assessment based on the prognostic score, complemented by the intraoperative assessment of an experienced surgeon. In recent times, in cases of preoperatively suspected thyroid cancer confirmed by fine needle biopsy and reconfirmed intraoperatively on frozen sections, most surgeons have agreed to perform total thyroidectomies. This is also the surgery technique used for medullary carcinomas. Partial thyroidectomy is usually performed in minimally invasive follicular carcinomas and intraparenchymal encapsulated papillary carcinomas less than 1 cm in size, and also in children and teenagers [9 - 11].

Intraoperative Complications

Hemorrhages are the most common complications occurring during thyroid surgery. Venous injuries (internal jugular vein, anterior jugular vein, thyroid veins) can occur during cervical lymphadenectomy and can be complicated by gas embolism. Immediate compression is necessary. The most common arterial structures that can be damaged are the thyroid vascular pedicles, the superior thyroid artery (which can slip from the sealant forceps) and inferior thyroid artery (usually associated with injury of the recurrent nerve).

Lesions of the Recurrent Nerves occur in 2% of cases, the rate of injury being based on the surgeon's experience and the tumor characteristics. In most cases, the injury occurs during preparation of the inferior thyroid pedicle, which should be as close to the thyroid capsule as possible. To avoid its lesion in thyroid cancer, thyroidectomy is performed after preparation of the recurrent nerve. The clinical consequences are recurrent unilateral or bilateral palsy with voice changes, phonation disorders, swallowing disorders and hoarseness. The bilateral damage can also cause respiratory failure and tracheostomy is sometimes necessary [7].

Postoperative Complications

Hematomas can compress the trachea and esophagus and sometimes evacuation, sealant or Redon drainage is necessary.

Respiratory Disorders occur due to bilateral injuries of the recurrent nerves, tracheal compression by hematoma, laryngeal edema, tracheitis or tracheomalacia.

Postoperative Hypoparathyroidism is caused by surgical removal of the parathyroid glands. It is clinically manifested by paresthesia, numbness, tingling, muscle cramps and tetany seizures. Following total thyroidectomy, with or without parathyroid autotransplantation, hypocalcemia occurs in one third of cases, persisting for more than three months in only 2% of cases, calcium supplementation being necessary.

Pneumothorax is the result of pleural injuries during surgical removal of a retrosternal goiter.

Perforation of the Esophagus and/or Trachea predisposes the patient to fistulae formation.

Thoracic Duct Injury is a rare complication that occurs during left cervical lymphadenectomy and is manifested by lymphorrhagia.

Other Local Complications include swelling of the skin flap, wound suppuration, adherence of the skin flap to the trachea, and movement of the flap with swallowing [7, 12].

Iatrogenic Lesions in Lung Surgery

Thoracic surgery is associated with high rates of mortality and morbidity. Lobectomy has a mortality rate of 3%, rising to 4.5% for double lobectomy and 6-10% for pneumectomy [13].

Intraoperative Complications

Intraoperative incidents in thoracic surgery include incidents of anesthesia and intraoperative injuries (injuries of the chest wall, heart and great vessels, thoracic duct, diaphragm and esophagus).

Incidents of Anesthesia

These incidents primarily occur during tracheal intubation and relate to lesions of the mouth (tongue, teeth and lips), larynx, pharynx and vocal cords. Difficult intubation can be followed by arterial desaturation and gastric reflux, further followed by aspiration pneumonia. Endobronchial intubation can also be difficult and often requires intraoperative bronchoscopy. Furthermore, during general anesthesia, pulmonary ventilation disorders can be associated with cardiac dysfunctions, such as arrhythmias, rhythm disturbances and acute myocardial infarction.

Intraoperative Injuries

Chest Wall Injuries comprise rib fractures, which are the most common, followed by intercostal vessel and intercostal muscle injuries. Rib fractures usually do not require immobilization or osteosynthesis. Intercostal vessel injuries require prompt recognition and appropriate homeostasis. Otherwise, severe bleeding occurs in the early postoperative period, and surgical reintervention can be necessary. Intercostal muscle injuries can be avoided by practicing thoracotomy on the upper edge of the lower rib.

Heart and Large Vessels Injuries should be recognized and treated promptly, as they are followed by severe bleeding. Small injuries of the heart can be resolved with simple suturing, but severe injuries often require extracorporeal circulation. The most common injury involves the left atrium, which can occur during preparation of the pulmonary veins. If heart injuries are extended, they can also involve the coronary arteries. The latter are difficult to recognize and myocardial infarction can occur during surgical intervention. Such incidents can be resolved by aortocoronary bypass.

Large vessel injuries are often secondary to intrathoracic surgery-induced dissection. The vessels of the lungs (artery and veins) can be affected. If the intrapleural approach is difficult, a pericardial window should instead be performed. During left thoracotomy, the thoracic aorta is most vulnerable to trauma, but the left carotid common artery and left subclavial artery are also vulnerable. During right thoracotomy, the superior cava vein, brachiocephalic vein, azygos vein and brachiocephalic trunk can also be injured. Usually, these injuries are followed by severe and even life-threatening bleeding that must be promptly recognized and treated.

Pericardium Injuries can occur during left thoracotomy. Small pericardial lesions do not require surgical treatment, being well tolerated. Serious injuries usually occur during right thoracotomy, and can be followed by the torsion of the great vessels and heart.

Lung Injuries can occur during thoracotomy, especially in patients with pleural adhesions. These lesions should be quickly recognized and sutured as they are followed by air leaks, leading to postoperative lung atelectasis and pneumothorax.

Injuries of the Upper Airways refer to lesions of the trachea and bronchial tree. Tracheal lesions should be recognized and treated promptly, and simple suturing is usually not sufficient. Protective patches, such as heterologous bovine pericardium, are usually necessary [14]. Small bronchial tree lesions can be resolved *via* simple suture and the suture line can be protected with an intercostal muscle pedicle, pleural pedicle, pericardial fat or greater omentum flap. For large lesions, resection of the adjacent lung parenchyma should be performed. The aim of this resection is to prevent the occurrence of postoperative bronchial fistulae. Failure to obtain pulmonary inflation following thoracic surgery can be due to a large volume of bronchial liquid. However, this liquid can be removed through bronchoscopy, suction and lavage.

Esophageal Injuries primarily involve the thoracic esophagus. The lesions are more common during right than left thoracotomy. Small lesions can be resolved by simple suturing, but large injuries usually require partial resection of the esophagus to prevent further esophageal fistulae.

Injuries of the Thoracic Duct can occur during thoracotomies performed on both sides, but most often on the left side. The potential for postoperative chylothorax is resolved by introducing octreotide one week before surgery [15].

Injuries of the Diaphragm can be resolved by simple suturing, but larger injuries can require diaphragm reconstruction, with heterologous patch or diaphragm reinsertion. These injuries should be recognized in early stages to avoid the occurrence of respiratory insufficiency or diaphragmatic hernia.

Injuries of the Phrenic Nerve primarily occur in patients with pleural adhesions [16].

Postoperative Complications

Postoperative complications can be divided into two categories according to the time of onset: early (local and systemic) and delayed (local only).

Early Postoperative Complications

Systemic complications of thoracic surgery are the same as those associated with general surgery and include cardiovascular lesions (arrhythmia, conduction disorders, acute myocardial infarction, stroke, thrombophlebitis, pulmonary embolism, acute urinary retention, *etc.*).

Early local complications primarily refer to serious complications, such as hemothorax and risk of hemorrhagic shock. Surgical intervention and homeostasis are imposed if external drainage collects more than 1000 milliliters overall, or 200 milliliters of blood/hour for four to six hours [17].

Persistent air leaks are the most common postoperative complication of pulmonary resections that determines prolonged hospitalization [18]. Pneumothorax occurs in cases of ineffective external pleural drainage or significant air leakage. In such cases, the condition is resolved by treating the cause of the pneumothorax. Subcutaneous or mediastinal emphysema is usually secondary to ineffective pleural drainage. Postoperative atelectasis is attributable to a large volume of endobronchial liquid. This can be removed by bronchoscopy, suction and lavage.

Acute respiratory failure usually requires mechanical ventilation and/or respiratory support and orotracheal intubation. It should be accompanied by identification and proper treatment of its leading cause. Following lung resection, bronchial fistulae occur in 6-10% of cases [19]. This can be resolved by performing passive lavage of the pleural cavity, pleural drainage and insertion of local antiseptic solutions. ARDS can emerge in patients who require prolonged respiratory support or mechanical ventilation.

Late Local Complications

The persistence of pleural effusion or empyema may demand pleural decortication. Following pneumectomy, approximately 2-15% of patients present empyema, with a mortality rate of 10%.

Late bronchial stump fistulae can occur after radiotherapy, and can require surgical treatment.

Bronchial stump granuloma can occur after pneumectomy or lobectomy and usually demand surgical repair [20, 21].

Specific Complications after Lung Transplantation

Besides the specific surgical complications of thoracic surgery, some specific postoperative complications can be associated with lung transplantation. The most common early postoperative complications relate to bronchial anastomosis and include stenosis or anastomotic fistulae. In the late postoperative period, bronchial stenosis is common [22].

Other complications involve acute and chronic rejection. The risk of acute rejection is present until the first postoperatively day. The rate of acute rejection is about 70-80%, despite correct immunosuppressive treatment [23]. The most common signs of acute rejection are fever, hypoxemia, worsening of lung function and infiltrates on the chest X-ray [16].

The clinical signs of chronic rejection (bronchiolitis obliterans) include dyspnea and signs of obstruction on spirometry. These signs are present in 60% of recipients who survive for at least five years postoperatively and are associated with poor survival rates [24].

Due to high doses of immunosuppressives and exposure of the transplanted lung to environmental factors, the incidence of the post-transplant infectious diseases (bacterial, viral and fungal) is quite high [25]. The most common infection is pneumonia, occurring in 33-66% of recipients [26].

SURGERY OF THE ABDOMINAL CAVITY

In this section, we will present lesions related to the surgery of the stomach, colon, appendix, liver, bile ducts and pancreas.

Complications Related to Tissue Trauma

Tearing the mesentery can cause temporary loss of nerve function (neurapraxia) which leads to motility disorders. Aggressive maneuvers can cause subcapsular hematoma or tears on the liver or spleen, mesenteric or subserosal hematomas and even luminal openings. In cases of malignant tumors, aggressive manipulation can lead to a spread of tumor cells (implantation metastasis), and therefore the principle of "no touch isolation" should be respected. Other clinical manifestations of tissue trauma include the following lesions [1, 7]:

- ***Hemorrhage*** demands hemostasis, which is often time-consuming, difficult, partial, can occur postoperatively and requires reintervention. Injuries of the splenic hilum or its lower pole can call for splenectomy.
- ***Subileus and Paralytic Ileus*** can be the consequence of intestine and mesentery traction, peritonitis or peritoneal irritation.
- ***Intra-Abdominal Abscess*** can be caused by encapsulated seroma, hematoma or intestinal contents, which are consequences of trauma.

Vomiting, Hiccups and Fever

Vomiting, hiccups and fever are common surgery-related complications whose exact mechanisms should be clarified [7].

Vomiting is most common following abdominal interventions. Intestinal tears, gastrointestinal resection and drugs used for anesthetic purposes may be involved in its etiology. Vomiting may occur pre-, intra- and postoperatively. It can be an early or delayed postoperative complication. Prolonged vomiting can be related to surgery (peritonitis, ileus) or metabolic disorders.

Hiccups are involuntary convulsive contractions of the diaphragm. They can intensify pain and cause insomnia. The pathomechanism is based on four main causes: barbiturates used in anesthesia, traction of the supramesocolic organs (during incomplete general anesthesia), irritation of the phrenic nerve (due to the drain tube under the pouch, blood accumulation or abscess) and acute gastric dilatation (associated with flatulence, ileus, peritonitis, *etc.*).

Fever can be a sign of purulent inflammations, such as abdominal wall phlegmon, abscesses, enterocolitis, *etc.*

Postoperative Ileus

In patients undergoing complex abdominal surgery (long-term interventions, especially for colorectal lesions), postoperative ileus can be a life-threatening lesion. The pathomechanism is based on the postsurgical sympathomimetic-adrenergic reaction. It induces decreasing levels of digestive enzymes and intestinal motilities. Dysfunctions of intestinal absorption lead to hypokalemia, intensification of the tone of the sphincter and increase of the volume of intestinal gases. The patient experiences abdominal pain and distension. At palpation, the abdomen is rigid, sensitive to touch, without bowel movements. Abdominal X-ray exam shows hydroaeric shadows. Details regarding this lesion will be presented below in the section on surgery of the abdominal cavity [7].

Laparotomy-Related Lesions

Laparotomy refers to the transection of abdominal wall tissue during surgery. It is intended to assure intraoperative accessibility, flexibility (allowing extension in any direction during surgery) and security (maintaining the integrity and functionality of the vascular and nervous structures of the abdominal wall).

The correctly performed laparotomy should be based on the following principles: provision of optimal penetration and exploration of the organ or surgical area; causing minimal damage to the abdominal wall; allowing extension, if necessary; permitting easy, functional and resistant wound closure; causing little damage to the resistance of the abdominal wall; and leaving an aesthetic scar after surgery.

Midline laparotomies are easy to perform and reconstruct, yet they do not always ensure the most optimal exploration of the target organ. In the case of the liver or pancreas, especially for obese patients, bilateral subcostal or subcostal laparotomy (Lecler's incision) ensures more effective exploration. Subcostal, transverse laparotomies are time-consuming during penetration and reconstruction. Not only the muscle but also the nerves are damaged and, following surgery, dermal hypo- or anesthesia and low muscle tonus can emerge. Nowadays the "great surgeon, great incision" principle is no longer valid. In the optimal exploration process, in addition to the incision, the laparotomy itself, the patient's position on the surgical table and the correct use of the exploration spatula and isolation fields all play key roles. The main complications of laparotomy include the following [1, 7]:

- ***Liver Injuries*** are more common following midline laparotomy. The left lobe is usually damaged and the extent of injury depends on the surgical tool. In the case of scalpel use, tissue injuries are deeper and more prone to bleeding as compared to the use of an electric knife.
- ***Splenic Injury*** primarily occurs following left subcostal laparotomies. Injury to the spleen may be superficial, with only the capsule being damaged, or deep, often demanding a splenectomy.
- ***Omentum Injury*** manifests as hemorrhage. Additional injuries, such as lesions of the small intestine, can be associated.
- ***Injuries of the GI Tract*** primarily relate to the small intestine, stomach or

colon. Scalpel-related injuries are usually linear and easy to control. In some cases, luminal opening can be associated, leading to infection or suture failure. These injuries can be prevented by lifting the abdominal wall. After the opening of the peritoneum, the abdominal wall is lifted with two fingers, allowing for incision between the fingers. Injuries caused by electric knife use are wider and more linear, and it is extremely important to notice and immediately treat them, as necrosis may induce an intestinal fistula. In the case of relaparotomies, damage to the intra-abdominal organs may be partial or complete, and may be extended if the serosa is damaged on a larger surface or even the whole intestinal wall. The injury is not linear and suture failure may result.

Complications following closure of the abdominal wall are relatively common and include the following five lesions:

1. ***Wound Hematoma*** can occur in patients with hepatic disorders or coagulopathies, or users of anticoagulants. In some cases, it is caused by cough or incorrect hemostasis. The wound is swollen, its periphery is discolored, ecchymosis can be associated and the patient's complaints include painful pressure. Protrusion of the abdominal wall, wound leakage and/or suppuration can be associated.
2. ***Wound Suppuration*** can be caused by superinfection with pathogens, inadequate immunity and vascular disorders (vasculitis, ischemia, collagen disorders). Wound infection prophylaxis includes the following principles: respect for asepsis and antisepsis; prevention of hematoma and/or seroma formation; use of Redon drainage; and prophylactic pre- and intraoperative antibiotherapy. Wound treatment involves reopening, cleaning and removing the infected tissue. Adequate blood flow to the wound periphery is assured by pressure relief through a sparse suture or incision.
3. ***Thread Suppuration/Granuloma*** is a delayed wound complication occurring after use of nonabsorbable multifilament threads. It can be complicated by postoperative abdominal wall defects.
4. ***Wound Dehiscence*** can be classified as partial or total, superficial or deep dehiscence. The deep tissues are first affected, the skin being implicated in the final steps. It can be complicated by evisceration (usually between five and 10 days following surgery). The risk of postoperative dehiscence is influenced by the following local and general factors: incision location (more common after midline laparotomy), improper healing (associated hematoma, seroma, suppuration), inadequate surgical technique and/or suturing material, high intra-abdominal pressure (ascites, cough, distension), associated comorbidities (DM, uremia, jaundice, hypoproteinemia, anemia, obesity) and specific medications (steroids, chemotherapeutics, immunosuppressive agents).

5. ***Postoperative Abdominal Wall Defects*** occur in more than 10% of patients undergoing laparotomy. The risk of defects is influenced by the factors outlined regarding the genesis of wound dehiscence.

Hernia Surgery and Postoperative Defects of the Abdominal Wall

Incorrect Surgical Indication refers to the optimal time of the procedure, which depends on the associated comorbidities [1].

Errors Regarding Surgical Technique are difficult to avoid. Complications are common following suture performed under tension, the rate decreasing to 20-30% for Bassini-type procedures and to 1% for the Lichtenstein technique. Postoperative defects of the abdominal wall are primarily attributable to use of implants/surgical meshes. Post-implant complications are related to the type, structure and composition of the meshes, as well as the type of technique. The mesh can be placed in relation to the layers of the abdominal wall in an onlay, sublay or inlay manner. Most complications occur during placement of the onlay mesh. The most commonly used mesh is the monofilament, unabsorbable, macroporous, prolene mesh; however, its contact with the intestines must be prevented, as it causes erosions. Therefore, prolene mesh cannot be used for inlay techniques. In cases of inlay techniques, double-layered meshes (Dual Mesh, Composix Mesh) are recommended, the visceral side of which prevents the formation of adherences [27].

Intraoperative Complications include the following lesions: opening of a hollow organ (injuries of the small intestine, colon or bladder, and sepsis), reinsertion of an unviable intestinal loop into the abdominal cavity (with further postoperative complications), hemorrhages (injury of the inferior epigastric artery, femoral artery, femoral vein, "corona mortis", referring to the vascular anastomosis between the obturator artery and inferior epigastric artery, testicular artery with further testicular necrosis), injuries of the ductus deferens, and neural damage (causing neurinoma, pain and sensorial dysfunctions) [7].

Postoperative Complications include the following lesions: hematomas (scrotum and abdominal wall hematomas are caused by insufficient hemostasis and predispose the patient to infections), seroma formation (after eventrations and hernias, being caused by long-term preparation; Rendon's drainage can prevent its formation), wound suppuration, local edema (penis, testicles and scrotum can be affected after compression or injury of the spermatic cord), testicular atrophy (after ischemia) or necrosis (caused by the ligation of testicular veins), and evisceration (following postoperative defects of the abdominal wall).

Hernia recurrence can be caused by choosing the wrong mesh size (too small causes shrinkage, too large causes "dead zones" and infections).

Other postoperative complications include respiratory failure (raising the diaphragm when the reconstruction is performed under tension), formation of foreign body granulomas (caused by multifilament threads and meshes), intestinal fistulae and postoperative ileus (caused by intestinal adhesions) [1].

Complications Caused by Abdominal Drainage

Drainage is used to remove the fluid, blood and/or tissue fragments generated during surgery. The surgical drain tube should be flexible, maintain its form, have appropriately sized lumens and be equipped with side holes. If the drain tube is too rigid or hard, it erodes the walls of hollow organs. Drainage through the laparotomy hole causes wound suppuration, therefore the tube should be guided through another aperture.

If the drainage is performed for too long it can lead to ascending infection or intestinal obstruction due to the bowel's adhesion to the drainage tube. To avoid complications, the tube should be removed if the volume of the secretion is less than 50 ml in 24 hours.

During tube insertion, the forceps can cause injuries to the liver, small intestine, colon or bladder. In one of our cases, the drainage tube was mobilized, migrated through the inguinal region into the Douglas pouch and perforated the external iliac artery. On the fourth postoperative day, a significant hemorrhage occurred after the drainage tube was shortened and hemostasis was necessary. To avoid and successfully resolve such complications, the drainage tube should be inserted and controlled by the operating surgeon [1, 7, 28, 29].

Errors and Complications in Laparoscopic Surgery

Laparoscopic surgery is preferred in clinical practice due to its shorter surgery time as compared to traditional open surgery, minimal invasiveness, minimal trauma and lower rates of complications [1].

Preoperative Errors

Incorrect surgical indications can lead to necessary transformation of the laparoscopic technique into open surgery. This especially occurs in patients with associated morbidities, such as cardiorespiratory diseases.

Intraoperative Complications

Pneumoperitoneum-Related Complications especially include injuries to organs/structures such as the omentum, small intestine, transverse colon and, rarely, the liver. In cases of suspected organ damage, extensive exploration is mandatory. Other consequences include air accumulation in the round ligament and major omentum, usually without clinical complaints. However, these consequences can nevertheless be avoided with careful insertion of the Veress needle, lifting of the abdominal wall and attentive checking of specific parameters (the needle's interoperability and the pressure of the insufflators). Moreover, the pneumoperitoneum should be gradually induced and, in patients with previous surgeries, the pneumoperitoneum can be performed *via* open surgery [1].

Complications Caused by Trocars are more severe and especially relate to the hemoperitoneum, the optical trocar being "blindly" inserted after creating the pneumoperitoneum, most often along the linea alba above the omphalocele. However, hemorrhages at the level of the optical trocars are rare, being the result of vascular injuries (epigastric arteries, umbilical veins and, very rarely, large abdominal vessels). They can be prevented by checking the trocar's placement after translumination. After finishing the procedure, besides optical inspection, all trocars should be removed and, in case of hemorrhage, hemostasis should be performed.

Injuries of the abdominal wall can have an appearance similar to a hernia. They can occur after using trocars with closure larger than 10 mm. They can be prevented by inserting the trocar diagonally through the layers of the abdominal wall, or by closing the large closures. Trocar-induced damage can also involve the liver, omentum, spleen, colon, small intestine and stomach, which are inflated during intubation. Nonrecognition of these lesions can demand reintervention [1].

Preparation-Related Complications depend on the technique that is used and the organ that is removed [1, 7, 30]:

Laparoscopic cholecystectomy can be associated with hemorrhages (most often in the liver, due to injury of the cystic artery or right hepatic artery), bile leakage (injury of the gallbladder), injuries of the cystic duct or extrahepatic biliary tracts, bilirrhagia and postoperative jaundice (clipping of the biliary tracts).

Laparoscopic surgery of hiatal hernia can be associated with hemorrhages (esophageal rupture during preparation of the greater curvature or rupture of the spleen or liver), organs/structures damage (esophagus, vagus nerve, intestine) and pneumothorax/pneumomediastinum (pleural lesions).

Technical errors can occur during reconstruction of the hiatus (the diaphragm being too tight, inducing dysphagia, or too loose, a feature that can be prevented by correct suture placement and the insertion of a 34-36 cm width probe into the stomach during reconstruction) or during creation of the stomach "muff". A "muff" that is too tight causes dysphagia, whereas a "muff" that is too loose or inadequately fixed to the esophagus can lead to the stomach telescoping into the mediastinal cavity. This "muff" complication can be prevented by using adequate technique – with the preparation of the greater curvature, the "muff" must fit smoothly around the esophagus, as it is to be fixed with a suture to the esophagus, so its length should be about 2 cm and during its creation the Fouche probe should be inserted into the stomach.

Laparoscopic surgery of achalasia can be associated, during preparation, with hemorrhages (from the periesophageal/pericardial arteries, arteries of the abdominal wall or hepatic injuries). Perforation of the esophagus or stomach can occur during myotomy (with tools) or during the insertion of probes. It requires treatment and covering with Dor fundoplication, which prevents postoperative complications. Lesions of the distal esophagus cannot be recognized during surgery, but gradual postoperative perforation with mediastinitis can occur. This is why fundoplication is necessary during laparoscopic correction of achalasia. Injury of the pleura can cause pneumothorax, whereas incomplete myotomy can cause postoperative dysphagia.

Laparoscopic splenectomy can be complicated by hemorrhages (from the arteries of the omentum or gastrocolic ligament, spleen arteries or spleen parenchyma). In severe hemorrhage, conversion to open surgery might be necessary. Spleen lesions, which can occur during preparation or in cases of large spleen removal, can cause splenosis or idiopathic thrombocytopenic purpura (ITP). Accessory spleen incidentally identified intraoperatively should be removed to avoid postoperative functional complications.

Laparoscopic hernioplasty can be associated with intraoperative hemorrhages (injury of the inferior epigastric arteries and veins, or external iliac artery and veins), intestinal injuries with fistulae (caused by diathermic tools or mesh erosion), injury of the bladder (requiring conversion), nerve damage (by the clasps used for fixation of the mesh during the TAPP technique; this can be prevented by not applying a clasp to the inguinal ligament), seroma or hematoma formation, injury of the spermatic cord, subcutaneous emphysema of the scrotum (during gas insufflations), peritonitis, orchiepididymitis, *etc.*

Complications during Laparoscopic Surgery of Morbid Obesity

Minimally invasive techniques have allowed increasing numbers of patients to undergo laparoscopic therapy for morbid obesity. The methods used can be restrictive, malabsorptive or mixed. Restrictive methods decrease the reservoir function of the stomach and include gastric banding, longitudinal gastrectomy, sleeve gastrectomy and gastroplication. Malabsorptive methods include the jejunoileal bypass, biliopancreatic diversion and duodenal switch. Mixed methods used both above-mentioned classes of technique (*e.g.,* Roux-Y gastric bypass). Restrictive methods are preferred as they are easier and faster for the surgeon to perform, as compared to the malabsorptive methods, and the rate of complications is lower. Use of gastric banding has been abandoned due to the increased risk of foreign body reactions.

General Complications

Hemorrhages primarily occur from the veins of the gastrocolic ligament, spleen vessels or incision surface following transection of the stomach. During gastric preparation, the vascularity can be damaged and, rarely, the spleen can be ruptured. Hemostasis is necessary in such cases. During construction of the stomach "tube" and after applying Endo-GIA, bleeding from the gastric vessels and resection surface can occur. Covering the resection surface with a biodegradable material (Peri-Strips Dry) is necessary, alternatively applying suture with continual stitches, usually using absorbable thread. Bleeding of the resection surface constitutes the majority of postoperative bleedings (intraperitoneally or intraluminally, with melena).

Transection of the esophagus is a very rare complication that primarily occurs during the Endo-GIA longitudinal gastrectomy. It can be prevented by using an adequate technique. A 34-36 cm diameter Faucher tube can be inserted into the stomach to appreciate the stomach "tube" diameter and prevent esophageal transection [31, 32].

Suture dehiscence is the most severe complication, with a 5% occurrence rate. Its occurrence is accompanied by fever, tachycardia and tachypnea, and can be diagnosed using imagistic methods and contrast agents. Peritonitis and hemodynamic instability are signs of severe dehiscence that demands reintervention [33].

Abscess can be the consequence of superinfection of released fluid or blood, but also of suture dehiscence.

Stenosis of the stomach "tube" rarely occurs during the early postoperative period (being caused by mucosal edema), and is more commonly a delayed complication that involves the angular incision area. The main clinical symptom is vomiting [33].

Malnutrition occurs due to disorders of gastric absorption of vitamin B12, iron and other microelements [33].

Complications of Laparoscopic Gastroplication

Laparoscopic gastroplication is a restrictive method used in minimally invasive treatment of morbid obesity. The most widespread method is the plication of the gastric greater curvature, but plication of the frontal wall is also used. The aim of this technique is to infuse the greater curvature towards the lumen, after skeletonization with double- or triple-layered suture, decreasing the gastric lumen. It seems to cause fewer complications (1%) than the other resection methods, is less expensive and presents similar postoperative results [34, 35].

Nausea, vomiting and sialorrhea usually decrease before stopping three to five days after bowel movement recovery. It can persist in patients with high pressure in the stomach's lumen, being more common after three-row gastroplication [34, 35].

Stenosis of the stomach "tube" can be indicated by nausea and vomiting, and is more common after three-row gastroplication, when the stomach's lumen is tightened too forcefully. It can be prevented by inserting a 34-36 cm Faucher probe into the stomach during the procedure. Gastric stenosis can be caused by stomach kinking, angulation along the sutures or protrusion of the abdominal wall between two sutures that are placed too far from each other. It occurs most commonly in the stomach's fundus due to decrease visibility [34, 35].

Gastroparesis can be caused by seroma or fluid accumulation between the sutures. It can be prevented by using the correct suturing technique. Three-row plicature is rarely advised. Two days after surgery, before removing the probe, a gastric emptying test with gastrografin and even endoscopy is necessary to check the gastric wall functionality [34, 35].

Gastric fistulae can be formed along the suture both intra- and postoperatively. This is a rare complication that occurs most commonly at the gastric fundus. The gastroplication begins 2 cm from the cardia at the stomach fundus, where visibility is low, the suture penetrates too deeply into the wall of the abdomen and is transfixed. However, the sutures can be verified during the intraoperative phase. After finishing gastroplication, the Faucher probe is removed and a 16 cm stomach probe is inserted by the anesthesiologist, through which 100 ml of methylene blue solution is introduced into the stomach, to check for fistulae formation. The clinical symptoms are intensive abdominal pain, fever and tachycardia.

Postoperative perforation can be caused by excessive pressure in the stomach. For example, in one of our patients, stomach pain, fever, tachycardia and tachypnea emerged four days after surgery. The patient declared that he had consumed excessive amounts of potato and lentil pottage eight hours before the onset of symptoms. Relaparoscopy was performed. Gastric wall prolapse at the gastric fundus and a 2 cm perforation were identified. One layer closing of the perforation was performed and the patient survived without complications. This case highlights the necessity of informing the patient about the required postoperative diet and amount of food to be taken. The diet should contain 800 kilocalories, 25-50 ml per meal, with gradually augmentation [34, 35].

Gastric dilatation and postoperative increasing of body weight are usually patient-related complications. In our patients, body weight increases were associated with gastric dilatation at between eight and 10 months after surgery, when the patients returned to their previous lifestyle, consuming excessive amounts of food. During laparoscopic reintervention in one patient, we detected a broader stomach and three sutures of gastroplication were performed. However, postoperative education is mandatory [34, 35].

IATROGENIC LESIONS IN GASTRIC SURGERY

Surgery of the Peptic Ulcer

Nowadays, the indication of surgery for treating gastroduodenal ulcers has been significantly lowered by the availability of medicines such as histamine-H2 receptor antagonists, proton pump inhibitors (PPIs) and antibiotics used for *Helicobacter pylori* eradication. Surgical therapy is used in cases of complications such as perforations, stenosis and severe bleeding. The surgical-related complications depend on the associated lesions.

Surgery of the Peptic Ulcer with Associated Hemorrhage is especially centralized on bleeding control that can be endoscopically obtained in 80-90% of cases. However, in cases where endoscopic hemostasis fails or bleeding reoccurs, open gastric suture or gastrectomy is necessary. The surgery indications should take into account the following parameters: the patient's age, general status, comorbidities, ulcer location and intensity of the hemorrhage. The suture of the ulcer should be performed by an experienced surgeon. However, in giant ulcers penetrating into the pancreas or liver, ulcer suture is only a temporary intervention, and gastrectomy is recommended [1, 7].

An important therapeutic issue is the differential diagnosis of peptic ulcers and vascular malformations, such as gastric angiodysplasia or Dieulafoy's lesion (abnormally large and tortuous vessels in gastric submucosa, without caliber loss, protruding through a small mucosal defect). In these patients, associated vascular lesions can cause recurrent bleeding and fistulae formation, a life-threatening sepsis being sometimes associated. In our hospital, we have encountered some cases of gastric vascular malformations in which fulminant hematemesis masqueraded as a tumor or peptic ulcer. In one of these cases, endoscopic suture was followed by open laparotomy suture. The bleeding did not stop and gastrectomy was necessary. However, the patient died of septic shock. A section of the gastric wall revealed intramural hematoma with large tortuous vessels under the microscope (Fig. **17-1**) [36, 37]. In another case, a young female was diagnosed with early gastric cancer, which was endoscopically resected, but recurrent bleeding called for partial gastrectomy. No tumor was identified but multifocal gastric angiodysplasia was found under the microscope. In the remnant stomach and duodenum, a fistula reoccurred and death was the ultimate result. In the final case relevant to this section, a patient with previously diagnosed myocardial and intestinal infarctions presented with acute abdominal pain and emergency laparotomy revealed segmental necrosis with perforation of the gastric wall from the smaller curvature. Longitudinal gastric wall resection was performed and angiodysplasia was also identified.

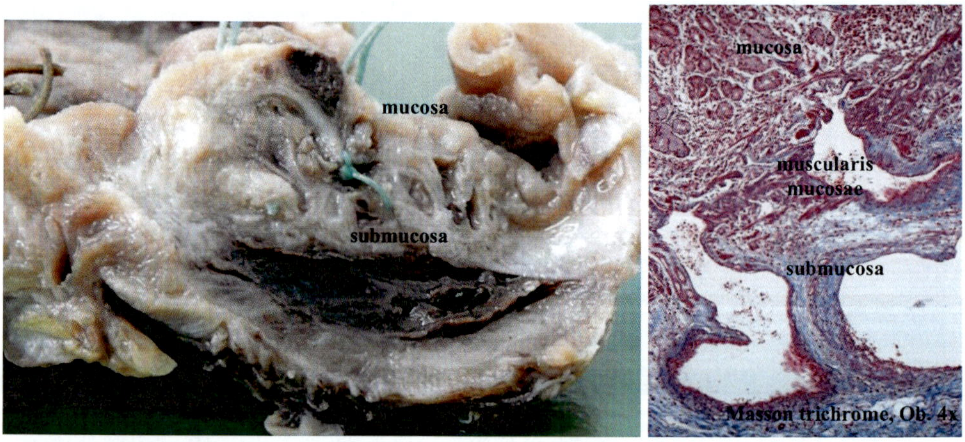

Fig. (17-1). Gastric vascular malformation characterized by intramural hematoma (left) and large intramucosal tortuous vessels that cross the muscularis mucosae (right), predisposing the patient to mucosal bleeding (courtesy of Prof. Simona Gurzu).

Surgery of the Perforated Peptic Ulcer is associated with minimal errors, this lesion being usually recognized early and treated through open laparoscopy. However, in some cases, a perforated ulcer can masquerade as an associated benign or malignant lesion. For example, in one of our more challenging cases, a young patient presented with sharp pain in the epigastrium, muscular defense in the right iliac fossa and leukocytosis (14500/microliter). Appendectomy was performed using McBurney's incision. The appendix was perforated and pseudomembranes were identified on the cecum wall. After surgery, the patient presented intensified abdominal pain, muscular defense and worsening general status. Re-exploration of the abdominal cavity through midline laparotomy revealed a prepyloric ulcer perforated in the omental bursa. This ulcer was sutured, abdominal lavage was applied and no postoperative complications were associated.

To exclude a malignancy, in patients with large perforated ulcers, gastric excision should be performed, whereas intraoperative biopsy and suture are recommended for small perforated and hemorrhagic ulcers. If excision or biopsy cannot be performed during surgery, gastroscopic biopsy should be indicated after recovery [1].

Gastrectomy or truncal vagotomy with pyloroplasty is today rarely performed in patients with perforated duodenal ulcer. Ulcer suture with infrequent omentum Graham patch is usually indicated [38, 39].

Ulcer suture can be followed by a large spectrum of postoperative complications, including reperforation (due to suturing that is too tight or too close to the periphery of the perforation), duodenal stenosis (due to suturing that is too far from the periphery of the perforation, taking too much out of the duodenal wall), remnant undiagnosed malignancy, delayed gastric emptying (remnant pyloric stenosis) and postoperative subphrenic abscess (inadequate lavage/drainage) [1, 7].

Truncal vagotomy can be followed by recurring ulcer (due to incomplete vagotomy), lack of truncal transection, or injuries/perforation of the pleura or esophageal/gastric wall (during preparation of the vagal trunks). During preparation of the anterior vagal trunk, removal of the gastric tube is recommended, as it may otherwise be confused with the vagal trunk, leading to esophageal injuries. Proximal selective vagotomy can be associated with lack of denervation of the abdominal esophagus or delayed gastric emptying/ gastroparesis (injury of the nerve of Laterjet). Other associated complications are hemorrhages, spleen injuries caused by excessive pull of the stomach (for superficial or capsular lesions, hemostasis may be performed *via* TachoSil and splenectomy may be necessary for deep hematomas), gastric dilatation with/without aspiration pneumonia, diarrhea (direct effect of vagotomy), hiccups, mediastinitis, *etc.* [1, 7].

Pyloroplasty can be associated with false pylorectomy (the duodenum is opened instead of the pylorus) or large pyloroplasty, with subsequent risk of wound dehiscence [7].

Gastrectomy can be associated with a risk of postoperative wound bleeding, suture dehiscence, peritonitis, subphrenic abscess, sepsis, infection of the abdominal wall and nonfunctional pyloroplasty (delayed gastric emptying).

Intraoperative Hemorrhages primarily occur during the preparation of the stomach and duodenum (injuries of the left and right gastroepiploic artery, left gastric artery, gastroduodenal artery and short gastric artery). Lesions of the common hepatic artery can occur during surgery of giant ulcers of the lesser curvature. The vessels of the transverse mesocolon (arteries and middle colic vein) can be damaged during preparation of the gastric posterior wall. These lesions are minimal but can induce ischemia, requiring segmental colectomy.

Postoperative Hemorrhages can be an indicator of unrecognized intraoperative vascular damage and suggest a need for reintervention. For example, in one of our cases, partial gastrectomy was performed for a perforated peptic ulcer. After surgery and closure of the abdominal wall, an excessive amount of arterial blood was continuously released through the subhepatic drainage tube. Re-exploration identified the source of bleeding as the inadequate ligature of the left gastric artery. Hemostasis was performed, without other postoperative complications. Anastomotic hemorrhages can lead to the release of fresh blood through the nasogastric tube. Conservative hemostasis should be performed, but reintervention with hemostasis in the suture line is sometimes necessary.

During gastrectomy, the following organs can be injured: pancreas (leading to pancreatitis, fistulae and suture dehiscence), spleen, liver and colon (very rarely, during preparation of the greater curvature). Intraoperative spleen lesions are caused by intensive pulling of the stomach, or injury *via* abdominal spatula. Hemoperitoneum can be associated. In some cases, splenectomy is necessary.

Intraoperative injuries of the bile ducts occur in large ulcers penetrating the hilum of the liver or pancreas. The common bile duct (CBD) may be injured during the preparation of the duodenum, or tilting of the duodenal stump. This injury can result from a lack of continuity, hematoma or ligature of the common bile duct, which manifests as bile leaking. Failure to identify the injury leads to postoperative biliary peritonitis or mechanical icterus. Injuries of the papilla of Vater occur in patients with highly localized papilla or overprepared duodenum. Disinsertion of the papilla is a serious lesion that is difficult to treat.

Incorrect reconstruction of the gastrointestinal tract can be followed by suture dehiscence, internal hernia, recurrent ulcer, peritonitis, *etc*. Vomiting, fever and leukocytosis are usually associated.

Postoperative ileus is a severe, life-threatening lesion that can be caused by internal postoperative hernia, peritonitis and intestinal adhesions [1, 7].

Surgery of Gastric Tumors

Preoperative Errors

Incorrect Surgical Indication for gastrectomy can be the result of weak investigation of the patient and lack of or improperly performed biopsy. For example, gastric wall rigidity can be induced by a tumor, but gastric ulcers or pancreatitis can also be associated with increased resistance of the gastric wall. Moreover, a diagnosis of lymphoma established upon biopsy can be an indicator of non-surgical therapy [1].

Incorrect Preoperative Tumor Stage refers to improper evaluation of the metastatic status. For example, hepatic metastases should be attentively differentiated from hemangiomas or cystic nontumor lesions upon CT or MRI scan. Hemangiomas present as hypoattenuated masses upon ultrasonographic examination, and, in contrast CT scans, progressive iodophilia from the periphery to the center, from the arterial through the venous/delayed phase, are seen, with the specific feature of "tongues of fire". The metastatic nodules are primarily subcapsularly located (Fig. **17-2**), whereas cystic benign lesions involve the inside parenchyma [40, 41].

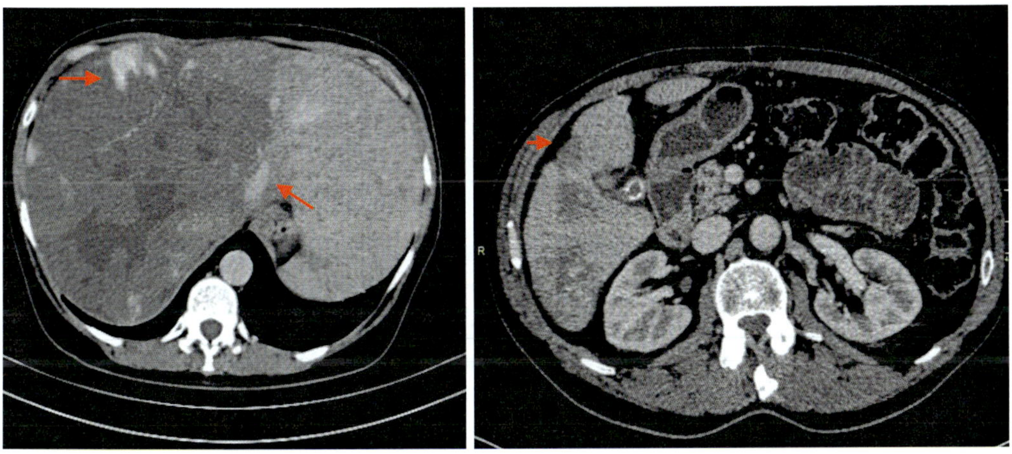

Fig. (17-2). Upon contrast CT scan examination, hepatic hemangioma displays a progressive iodophilia from the periphery to centrum (left) *versus* capsular retraction in liver metastases (right).

For example, in one of our cases, endoscopic examination revealed a large antral carcinoma that was histologically confirmed. The abdominal CT scan indicated a

2.5 cm metastatic nodule in the second segment of the liver, and the patient was declared as inoperable (the hematocrit was 24%). However, due to obstructive symptoms, surgery was nevertheless initiated and the supposed hepatic liver was found to be a hemangioma. The patient is still alive. This case highlights the necessity of very attentive differentiation of liver metastases. In difficult cases, suspected hepatic metastasis or peritoneal carcinomatosis can be certified through laparoscopic biopsies.

Intraoperative Errors

Incorrect Assessment of Unresectability primarily depends on the surgeon's experience. For example, suprapancreatic adherence as a result of lymph nodes metastases around the celiac trunk, or tumor penetration into the pancreas, does not signify unresectability if R_0 resection can be performed [1].

Incorrect Achievement of Radical Tumor Resection can be caused by failure to respect oncologic principles. Based on international guidelines, the upper edge of the resectomy should be performed at 6-8 cm distance from the tumor, and the lower edge at 2-3 cm from the pylorus. For radical resection of a gastric tumor, subtotal, total and superior polar gastrectomy, as well as total esophagogastrectomy, are recommended. To obtain a complete R_0 resection, the small and large omentum should also be removed.

The Japanese Gastric Cancer Association (JGCA) recommends assessment of the upper edge of the resection based on the T stage: for the T2 stage, this edge should be from 3 cm (for macroscopic Bormann's type 1, 2) to 5 cm (for macroscopic Bormann's type 3, 4 and for tumors with esophageal involvement) from the tumor, whereas, for the T1 stage, a distance of 2 cm is proposed [42 - 44].

JGCA also recommends quick histological analysis of the resection's edge for R_0 resection in order to guarantee the free resection margin. Based on this intraoperative assessment, they categorize the curative treatment of gastric cancer as standard, non-standard or extensive. For standard gastrectomy, two thirds of the stomach are removed and D_2 lymphadenectomy is performed. For non-standard gastrectomy, subtotal gastrectomy (below two thirds) and D1 lymphadenectomy is executed. Extensive surgery includes gastrectomy, resection of other organs, hepatic metastasectomy and extended lymphadenectomy (more than D_2 resection). Gastrectomy is classified as total, distal, pylorus-preserving, proximal or segmental. For early gastric cancer, laparoscopic segmental gastrectomy or endoscopic resection is indicated [42 - 45].

In cases of mandatory radical resection, R_0 can be obtained only with great difficulty. For example, in advanced tumors of the cardia, esophagectomy is difficult to obtain without thoracotomy. It is also challenging to preserve the spleen or perform splenectomy. Non-extended lymph node resection, especially in advanced cases, can cause tumor relapse. JGCA advises that the extension of lymphadenectomy be based on T stage: D_1 lymphadenectomy is recommended for T_1a cases (that do not match the criteria for endoscopic resection) and T_1bN_0 tumors, D_2 lymphadenectomy is used for T_2-T_4 resectable or cT_1N+ tumors, as well as in all cases in which lymph node metastases are suspected, while extension beyond D_2 is reserved for advanced stages with potential curative gastrectomy [42 - 44].

Incorrect Reconstruction can be followed by several postoperative complications. For example, in patients undergoing distal gastrectomy, performing Billroth-I gastroduodenostomy can result in taut anastomosis, suture dehiscence and/or recurrence. Some types of reconstruction (esophagoduodenostomy, esophagojejunostomy with omega loop and Braun anastomosis, esophagoduodenostomy with short Roux loop) can cause biliary reflux. Malnutrition can be a consequence of a Roux-Y loop that is too long. Suture material-related complications relate, for example, to monofilament-induced foreign body granuloma [1].

Other Intraoperative Complications include the following lesions: hemorrhages (following lymphadenectomy or lesions of the capsule of the spleen), drainage-related complications and co-injuries of other organs/structures, such as the CBD, portal vein, common and proper hepatic artery, pancreas and colon [1].

Postoperative Errors

Early Postoperative Complications include the following lesions: hemorrhages (suture dehiscence, intraoperative vascular injuries, spleen rupture), pancreatic fistulae (occurring after resection of the pancreatic tail and potentially leading to left subphrenic abscess), postoperative pancreatitis (as a result of intraoperative pancreas resection or postoperative shock), bile leakage (due to liver or bile ducts injuries), suture dehiscence (associated with fever, pain, dyspnea and leukocytosis, and potentially inducing life-threatening septic shock), duodenal stump insufficiency (a rare complication in which duodenum and pancreas fluids flow through the drainage tube, inducing skin irritation around the drainage tube), abscesses formation (subphrenic, intraperitoneal), mechanical ileus (as a result of visceral adherences or adherences around the drainage tube if it is left in for too long) and lymphorrhagia (following extended lymphadenectomy) [1].

Late Postoperative Complications include the following main lesions: alkaline reflux esophagitis (caused by errors in reconstruction, presenting with retrosternal burning sensation and ingestion difficulties), anemia (absence of the intrinsic factor) and anastomotic stenosis [1].

IATROGENIC LESIONS IN SURGERY OF THE SMALL INTESTINE

In most cases, emergency surgery is performed for mechanical ileus. Errors can involve the indication of the surgery and a longer obstruction period, associated with a higher risk of intestinal necrosis.

Intraoperative Complications can be associated with improper intestinal preparation or surgery technique. Incorrect surgical preparation, without equalization of fluid and electrolyte balance, is an error. Even a few hours, small intestinal ileus can cause hypovolemia which affects the circulatory, respiratory and renal systems. Hypotonia, anuria and high serum levels of urea and creatinine delay surgical intervention. The short but intensive preoperative preparation is important, as is monitoring of the central venal pressure and the amount of urine. An important aspect of preoperative preparation is the insertion of the nasogastric tube. This helps to monitor the amount and quality of the fluid and decompresses the stomach to prevent accidental aspiration.

Surgical incision should also be attentively planned. Midline laparotomy is primarily used. In cases of laparotomy performed along a previous incision, the colon, small intestine and omentum can be injured, resulting in further adhesions formation. For example, in one of our cases, a patient treated for abdominal trauma was transferred to our clinic, four days after surgery, with suspected suture dehiscence. Perforation of the small intestine was confirmed and sutured. However, symptoms of paralytic ileus and peritonitis later appeared. Upon reintervention, resuture was necessary, the second perforation being induced by adherences along the incision line.

Intraoperative hemorrhages are the result of injuries to the mesenteric veins and can induce hematoma formation in the mesenteric tissue.

During surgery, the small intestine must be fully checked, from the duodenojejunal flexure to the Bauhin valve, in order to exclude co-injuries, distally located adhesions or synchronous tumors that can cause postoperative complications and demand reintervention. At the same time, it is necessary to take into account the fact that the small intestine can be easily perforated and abdominal wall purulent inflammation can also be associated. This is why intestinal checking for decompression should be avoided.

Postoperative Complications primarily refer to anastomotic insufficiency. The risk of this lesion is greater following radiotherapy, cortisone use and obstruction of the mesenteric arteries, but technical errors, dense suturing-induced ischemia and inadequately chosen stapler can also increase this risk. The most common complications are fistulae formation, peritonitis and septic shock.

A challenging issue relates to the postoperative ileus. Distinguishing paralytic from mechanical ileus is difficult, and mistaken reintervention for a paralytic ileus is a serious error with potentially life-threatening complications. Knowledge of the symptoms, physical examination (intensive peristalsis and vomiting in mechanical ileus *versus* absence of bowel sounds in paralytic ileus) and native radiography are necessary for a correct diagnosis. Moreover, the upper small intestinal ileus is not associated with abdominal distension, but convulsive pain is present and large amounts of fluid flow through the nasogastric tube. Contrast radiology with liquid agents can help to establish the diagnosis as it indicates the location of the obstruction. Postoperative ileus is also difficult to distinguish from postoperative paralytic state or Ogilvie syndrome. Adhesions appear from the second postoperative day and can induce a slowly but gradually developing mechanic ileus. The main consequences of postoperative ileus are septic shock, adhesions formation, perivisceritis, internal hernia and even postoperative shock and death.

Postoperative complications of the abdominal wall include wound suppuration, wound dehiscence, foreign body granuloma formation and myositis ossificans [1, 46].

IATROGENIC LESIONS IN SURGERY OF THE COLORECTAL SEGMENTS AND APPENDIX

Surgery of the Colon and Rectum

Preoperative Errors

Incorrect Surgical Indications for colectomy include the tumor location, preoperative stage and improver evaluation of the patient's status [1].

Incorrect Patient Preparation refers to several aspects, including preoperative antibiotic prophylaxis. On the day of the surgery, it is necessary to administer antibiotics to maintain the integrity of colonic flora. Moreover, cleaning of the colon is especially indicated in associated stenosis. In highly contaminated colons, Hartmann's procedure or colostomy might be necessary [1].

Intraoperative Complications

Surgical Technique-Related Complications can depend on the type of technique and the surgeon's experience. For example, right hemicolectomy is not mandatory to include in resection of the transverse colon – tumors on the distal sigmoid and upper rectum can be removed using Dixon's procedure (anterior resection of the rectosigmoid colon), whereas tumors of the lower rectum can be excised through abdominoperineal rectum extirpation [47, 48].

Intraoperative Hemorrhages can be the result of injuries of the pericolonic or presacral blood vessels during preparation, with further formation of a hematoma in the mesocolon. During preparation of the splenic flexure, the lower pole of the spleen can be damaged, especially in obese patients. This injury is primarily superficial (subcapsular hematoma) and can be followed by hematoma or adherences formation. Deep intraparenchymatous hematomas can require splenectomy. However, it is important to examine the left subphrenic region and the origin of the blood accumulation after the preparation of the splenic flexure [1, 7].

Errors Related to the Extension of Resection relate to functional disorders or the necessity of extension in cases of vascular injury-related colonic ischemia. Unnecessary large resections can be performed for benign tumors in patients if they are not correct investigated or if a biopsy is not preoperatively performed [1, 7].

Ureteral Injuries can involve partial or complete perforation. Oral administration with tea of methylene blue solution aids identification of such potential injuries (blue drainage fluid) that can predispose the patient to fistulae formation. Blue mucus excreted through the drainage tube can confirm the necessity of an abdominal CT scan using contrast agents. Unilateral ureteral injuries can occur after right or left hemicolectomy, whereas bilateral injuries can be complications of Dixon's procedure or abdominoperineal rectum extirpation [1, 7].

Injuries of the Gallbladder and Biliary Ducts occur especially in patients with previous cholecystectomy and presence of adherences between the hepatic flexure of the colon and the gallbladder. Debulking can induce injuries and colonic rupture can be followed by peritonitis and septic shock. Because damage to the gallbladder leads to biliary flow, examination of the integrity of the biliary tracts should be performed after removing the gallbladder [1].

Hepatic Injuries can be complications of surgical removal of tumors located on the hepatic flexure or transverse colon, especially in associated adherences. Injury to the liver caused by abdominal spatula can also occur [1].

Injuries of the Stomach refer to lesions of the greater curvature of the stomach or its blood vessels (gastroepiploic artery or veins) during preparation of the stomach for removal of tumors located on the transverse colon [1].

Duodenal Injuries can occur after right hemicolectomy, during the mobilization of the hepatic colic flexure, especially in cases of duodenal infiltration. Treating a duodenal injury is a serious task for a surgeon, the risk of postoperative complications being quite high [1].

Injuries of the Terminal Ileus and/or Colon can occur during the preparation of the terminal ileus or hemicolectomy, respectively. In cases of intraoperative lesions, resection extension is required. Damage to the colon primarily occurs during the linear mobilization of the splenic flexure, especially in cases of forceful pulling. However, injuries can also occur during skeletonization. The main consequence is increased risk of postoperative infections [7].

Injuries of the Pelvic Organs primarily occur in cases of adherences between the sigmoid colon and ovary, uterus or bladder. The risk is even higher in females with previous gynecological surgeries. These injuries can also emerge during preparation of the rectum (lesions of the vagina or bladder). In males, prostatic lesions can be followed by hemorrhages or fistulae formation [1, 47, 48].

Anastomotic Complications primarily refer to taut anastomosis and suture dehiscence. Taut anastomosis is the result of manual, multilayered suturing, or the use of an inadequate stapler. However, multilayered sutures only provide "false security", as stenosis leads to increased pressure, which causes suture dehiscence [1, 48].

Extension of Surgical Removal should be based on the tumor characteristics, the number of adherences, the patient's age and status, comorbidities and postoperative quality of life (as large surgery can increase the risk of complications). The most difficult intraoperative decisions relate to the involvement of the following organs or structures: loops of the small intestine, ureters, uterus, ovaries, bladder, arteries and nerves [1].

Postoperative Complications

Duodenal Suture Dehiscence can be identified through oral administration of a small dosage of tea containing methylene blue. In patients with dehiscence, a blue colored secretion will appear in the drainage fluid. The treatment can be conservative or surgical, depending on the quantity of the secretion and the symptoms (*e.g.,* peritonitis).

Unidentified Ureteral Injury can lead to the formation of a urinary phlegmon. The symptoms and signs are fever, leukocytosis and the absence of bowel movements. Moreover, a large quantity of urine-scented fluid is excreted through the drainage tube. Orally administered methylene blue will be eliminated in the blue drainage fluid/urine. Ligation of the ureter can cause obstruction, which can be confirmed *via* a CT scan using contrast agents or urography [7].

Postoperative Hemorrhages can be detected by blood release through the drainage tube. Reintervention is chosen based on bleeding severity. Blood can accumulate in the abdominal cavity (right/left subphrenic area, Douglas pouch, abdominal cavity), leading to superinfection and abscesses formation, and demanding reintervention. Rectorrhagia can be an indicator of bleeding from the suture line. In other cases, intraluminal hematoma can induce mechanical ileus [1, 7].

Anastomotic Insufficiency is a dreaded complication of colon surgery. Its occurrence is determined by general (biological condition of the patient) and local factors, of which the most important is the technique of the anastomosis. It can be partial or total, with local (abdominal pain, meteorism, suppuration of the surgical wound, fecal excretion through the drainage tube or stercoral fistula) or systemic symptoms. Its occurrence on the third to fifth postoperative day is an indicator of a technical error, comorbidities (malnutrition, other malignant tumors, DM) or some drug administration (chemotherapeutics, immunosuppressive drugs and NSAIDs). Suture dehiscence, which forms after the eighth to 12th postoperative day, is usually caused by ischemia, taut anastomosis or a too tightly sutured anastomosis [1, 7].

Gastric Emptying Dysfunction should be suspected in patients who present early postoperative vomiting or release of a large quantity of gastric secretion through the nasogastric tube. This complication can occur after resection of the transverse colon or extended left hemicolectomy. In these cases, the colocolic anastomosis or colorectal anastomosis can be constricted by the duodenal flexure, causing ileus and further gastric complications. After left hemicolectomy, to prevent complications, the transverse colon should lead to the rectum through a transmesenteric or retroperitoneal route, followed by colorectal anastomosis [1, 48, 49].

Complications of Colostomy and Ileostomy

Colostomy and ileostomy involve the creation of a stoma on a segment of the colon or the terminal ileus. Such a stoma can be temporary or permanent. In the case of permanent stomas, distally situated colic, rectal and anal parts are completely removed. The stoma can also be made permanent by bringing the transected intestine's oral end to the surface of the skin, allowing the intestinal contents to excrete through it. This can be performed in a lateral manner, when the loops of the colon or ileus are pulled out to the surface of the skin. This loop constitutes the ileostomy or colostomy. The stoma is an infirmity for the patient, a psychological burden that is difficult to handle, and therefore it is necessary to explain the circumstances to the patient and seek their consent.

Errors during Stoma Creation can relate to its location (it should be situated 4-6 cm from the laparotomic wound). Stomas created at the level of the surgical intrusion can cause wound suppuration and dehiscence, and can demand reintervention. In associated high-pressure contexts, the exteriorized intestinal segment can slip back or its vascularization can be damaged, inducing necrosis.

Suturing the intestinal segment to the peritoneum and skin aids proper healing and security. In cases of partial suturing or lack of suturing, small intestinal loops can wedge in or the extracted intestine segment can slip back.

Another important point regards the aspect of the stoma after its creation. It is important to ensure that the intestinal segment is easily brought to the surface of the skin. Usually, when creating the opening, it is an accepted principle that the stoma allows the easy insertion of the surgeon's two fingers [1].

Postoperative Complications include the following lesions: retraction of the intestine's loop (with early stercoral peritonitis or pyostercoral phlegmon and late stenosis of the loop), hemorrhages (from the blood vessels supplying the intestine's loop or from the surface of the transected loop), loop necrosis, peristomal skin irritation, peristomal abscess (due to incorrect joining of the skin and mucosa, suture stitching through the intestinal wall, loop retraction or superinfection of the peristomal hematoma), peristomal evisceration (due to a large stoma opening or the loops not being fixed to the layers of the abdominal wall, or cases of suppuration of suture dehiscence), stoma stenosis, prolapse of the mucosa and peristomal hernia [1, 7].

Surgery of the Appendix

Incorrect Surgical Indication for appendectomy primarily relates to improper preoperative examination and the surgeon's lack of experience.

Incorrect Surgical Preparation is rarely encountered, acute appendicitis usually not requiring specific preparations. Associated comorbidities or disorders of the fluid and electrolyte balance should be attentively corrected. For antibiotic prophylaxis, a single dose of metronidazole is usually administered in our clinic, and wide-spectrum cephalosporin is added for patients with peritonitis.

Intraoperative Complications during open or laparoscopic appendectomy mainly refer to incorrect penetration. The placement and size of the incision can cause difficulty in terms of location and preparation of the appendix. Associated peritonitis can cause postoperative complications, and relaparotomy can be necessary. Penetration performed without adequate exploration can cause technical difficulties and intestinal injuries with other late complications. The small intestine and cecum are primarily affected.

Intraoperative hemorrhages from the meso-appendix can be caused by injury to the appendicular artery or slipping of the ligature. Hemostasis is usually difficult, in which case the incision should be expanded and the cecum sometimes excised. Purulent inflammations, such as peritonitis, can be caused by rupture of the appendix. Injury of the muscles of the abdominal wall can also occur intraoperatively.

Postoperative Complications include the following lesions: hemorrhages (*e.g.*, hemoperitoneum), abscesses (Douglas abscess, internal abscesses, appendix stump abscess), fistulae, mechanical ileus (caused by peritonitis or adhesions), superinfection of the surgical wound (injury of the gangrenous or phlegmonous appendix) and late consequences of injuries to the abdominal wall (hematoma formation, wound suppuration, abdominal wall abscess, incisional hernia) [1, 7].

IATROGENIC LESIONS IN SURGERY OF THE LIVER, GALLBLADDER, BILIARY TRACT AND PANCREAS

Surgery of the Liver

Liver Cysts, Echinococcosis

Incorrect Surgical Indication for hepatic cysts can occur as a result of their confusion with metastases, though this is rare in the era of development of medical imaging technology. Echinococcosis is usually treated with antiparasitic drugs (mebendazole), and only large cysts (greater than 5 cm) and cysts unresponsive to medicinal treatment indicate resection. However, laparoscopic excision of echinococcosis liver cysts can be performed once parasite spreading is prevented. Punction is insufficient, as the cavity of the cyst can refill in time. Percutaneous drainage is part of the procedure, with emptying of the contents and resection of the wall being performed *via* fenestration and pericystectomy. Percutaneous drainage can be performed and sclerotherapy is required [1, 50].

Intraoperative Complications include the following lesions: scattering of the cyst's contents (with risk of peritoneal hydatidosis; to avoid this risk, aspiration of the cyst's contents and neutralization with hypertonic solution can be performed), hemorrhages (rupture of the hepatic parenchyma during fenestration or pericystectomy), bile leakagc, burning (historically backfires in cases where neutralization with alcohol is followed by electric knife resection) and remnant cysts (in multiple lesions).

Postoperative Complications include the following lesions: hemorrhage, bile leakage (due to undetected intraoperative injuries of the biliary tracts and veins), superinfection and abscesses formation (due to insufficient fenestration or resection of the pericyst).

Primary Liver Tumors

Incorrect Preoperative Estimation of Resectability can induce several intraoperative complications. For primary tumors, 30% of the liver parenchyma should remain intact (with 1-2 cm free margins), this requirement rising to 40% in patients with liver cirrhosis [1, 51].

Intraoperative Complications primarily refer to hemorrhages (injuries of the portal vein, inferior cava vein, hepatic vein, hepatic artery), perforation of the CBD and injuries of the diaphragm (during the transection of the falciform ligament or tumors with adherences) [1].

Postoperative Complications include the following lesions: hemorrhages, bile leakage (resection of the small biliary ducts) and functional disorders.

Surgery of the Gallbladder and Biliary Tracts

Incorrect Surgical Indication is difficult to estimate in an era of cholecystectomy as a daily surgical intervention. However, although malignant transformation of cholecystitis is a known possibility, there are still physicians who indicate antibiotherapy as an acute process, and patients known to have gallbladder stones for 10-15 years admitted with gangrenous cholecystitis and histologically confirmed gallbladder carcinoma. In one of our cases, cholelithiasis was diagnosed during pregnancy, inducing biliary pancreatitis during lactation. These cases are not easy to manage. In elderly patients with severe comorbidities and no significant complaints, surgical intervention is not always indicated.

Differential diagnosis of cholecystitis from peptic ulcer, right colon tumor, early pancreatic head tumor and cardiovascular diseases should be very attentively assessed. For example, a patient with cholelithiasis and severe retrosternal pain was transferred to our dcpartment and laparoscopic cholecystectomy was performed. At three hours after surgery, sudden death occurred as a result of a preoperatively unidentified dissection of the thoracic aorta. In another case, the patient died a short time after surgery, and rupture of a preoperatively unidentified aneurysm of the thoracic aorta was found upon autopsy. For cases involving cholecystitis, the cardiologist must offer their opinion and consent for surgery. Moreover, complaints that persist after cholecystectomy demand further examination.

In patients with cholecystitis, bile tract stones and jaundice, preoperative ERCP and sphincterotomy must be performed, followed by laparoscopic cholecystectomy. During laparoscopic cholecystectomy, if choledocholithiasis is suspected, the surgeon can confirm it with a transcystic cholangiogram and remove it, or can decide to perform postoperative ERCP. The surgeon's task is to choose the treatment with the lowest risk factor for the patient.

The contraindications of laparoscopic cholecystectomy are advanced pregnancy, gallbladder carcinoma and severe comorbidities, such as decompensated hepatic cirrhosis and cardiorespiratory lesions [1, 7].

Intraoperative Complications during Open Cholecystectomy primarily include injuries of the bile ducts and/or biliary tract that can occur during preparation (due to intensive pulling of the cystic duct, ligation of the cystic artery or in patients with gangrenous or scleroatrophic cholecystitis). Biliary injuries (common or right hepatic duct) are more common in retrograde than antegrade cholecystectomy. Injuries of the liver parenchyma can occur during the preparation of the gallbladder or due to the use of a stomach spatula.

Hemorrhages can result from vascular injuries during preparation (cystic artery, right hepatic artery) or originate from the gallbladder bed (in gangrenous cholecystitis). Monopolar electrocautery is not advised as it can damage the wall of the CBD.

Other intraoperative complications include the following lesions: spread of infection (in patients with empyema), duodenal injuries (during gallbladder preparation), gallstone ileus, fistulae formation (cholecystoduodenal, cholecystocholic, cholecystocholedochal), injuries of the colon (in cases involving adherences between the gallbladder, colon, duodenum and great omentum) and incorrect placement of Kehr's tube (with further postoperative complications) [1, 7].

Postoperative Complications Following Open Cholecystectomy include the following lesions: wound infection, suture/wound dehiscence, fistulae, biliary peritonitis, bilirrhagia, angiocholitis (after choledochoduodenostomy) and mechanical jaundice (due to injuries of the biliary tracts, ligation or the presence of stone remnants in the CBD). A nonfunctional Kehr's tube can induce angiocholitis, biliary fistulae, septic gall retention or tube rupture [7].

Intraoperative Complications during Laparoscopic Cholecystectomy are rare, being primarily related to trocar misplacement. Intraoperative hemorrhage can arise from rupture of the liver during forceful gallbladder exertion, injury of the gallbladder bed during gallbladder preparation or injury of the cystic artery or right hepatic artery. Bilirrhagia can be a consequence of gallbladder injuries during exertion with pliers. Injury of the cystic duct or biliary ducts, forced dissection/preparation, close preparation of the CBD and infection spreading can also occur.

Biliary tract rupture and severe hemorrhages require the conversion of laparoscopy into open surgery. Failure to recognizing bile duct perforation can cause postoperative bilirrhagia, peritonitis and jaundice. Rare injuries include lesions of the duodenum, colon, diaphragm, stomach, small intestine and colon [1, 7].

Postoperative Complications Following Laparoscopic Cholecystectomy are rare and primarily involve postoperative hemorrhage (as a result of an unrecognizing intraoperatively vascular injury) and peritonitis (intraoperative duodenum or colon injury, or biliary peritonitis caused by injury of the biliary ducts).

Bilirrhagia can be a consequence of injuries of the CBD. Early small quantities spontaneously cease, but reintervention with clipping of the damaged area is necessary for early large quantities. Late bile leakage is usually caused by cystic or primary biliary tract necrosis.

Early jaundice can be a consequence of clipping of the extrahepatic biliary ducts, whereas late jaundice can be caused by angiocholitis or remnant biliary tract stones [1, 7].

Surgery of the Pancreas

Preoperative Errors

Incorrect surgical indications primarily refer to the optimal time for surgery. For example, in patients with acute pancreatitis, it is advised to avoid surgical intervention in the first 14 days. Moreover, premature and unnecessary surgeries increase postoperative morbidity and mortality risk. Surgical intervention is indicated for biliary pancreatitis, infected pancreatic necrosis, complications of pancreatitis and sterile pancreatic necrosis if the patient's status does not improve after conservative treatment.

In patients with chronic pancreatitis, the main aim is to manage its complications. In many cases, chronic pancreatitis can be distinguished from malignant tumors only during intraoperative exploration. However, while it is considered an error to treat a benign lesion with radical surgery, as this exposes the patient to high risk, it is also considered a mistake to treat a malignant lesion with noncurative surgery.

To avoid these inconveniences, a correct preoperative assessment should be based on modern medical imaging methods, such as ultrasound, CT, ERCP, endoscopic ultrasound examination and magnetic resonance cholangiopancreatography (MRCP), and also on needle biopsy. However, in some cases, distinguishing between benign and malignant tumors represents a diagnostic difficulty. Distinguishing pancreatic cystitis from malignant cystic mucinous neoplasms or chronic pancreatitis is also challenging. In these cases, it is necessary to perform biopsies from the cyst wall and also from the surrounding parenchyma and, in noneloquent cases, open surgery should be preferred over laparoscopic removal of the tumor. In one of our representative cases, a patient with non-Hodgkin's lymphoma presented with a 2 cm cystic lesion in the tail of the pancreas associated with enlarged lymph nodes in the splenic hilum identified at CT scan. Due to severe splenomegaly, the hematologist transferred the patient for splenectomy. Open splenectomy with resection of the pancreatic tail, without intraoperative histological examination, was performed. The histopathological diagnosis was invasive ductal carcinoma of the pancreatic tail with invasion of the proximal resection margin. The lymph nodes assessment confirmed the non-Hodgkin's lymphoma. Reintervention was necessary (subtotal pancreatectomy) and the patient is still alive. This case highlights the necessity of taking synchronous tumors into account. Moreover, remnant postoperative complaints demand supplementary investigation. In another case, laparoscopic excision of a cystic encapsulated lesion of the pancreatic tail, without a solid component reported at CT scan, was performed, and a benign cystic lesion was diagnosed under the microscope. A few weeks later, the patient presented with complaints that indicated cholecystitis. The CT scan also identified a solid infiltrating component in the remnant pancreas. Laparoscopic cholecystectomy was performed as the patient refused open surgery. This case highlights the necessity of extensive preoperative investigation of the cystic pancreatic lesions that can be associated, in many cases, with an invasive component.

Before unresectability is determined, correct assessment of the CT-MRI is mandatory. In patients with tumors that infiltrate the superior mesenteric vein, partial or segmental vein resection can be performed by experienced surgeons. Invasion of the superior mesenteric artery is frequently considered unresectable.

However, in some cases, resection of the superior mesenteric artery and celiac artery can be performed along with the tumor [1, 7, 52 - 54].

Intraoperative Complications

These complications can be related to incorrect preoperative preparation. Intraoperative hemorrhage is common in pancreatic surgery and preoperative blood supply is necessary (at a minimum of two units). For patients with mechanical jaundice caused by pancreatic tumors, endoprosthesis should be inserted during ERCP to prevent cholestasis. Correct surgical preparation is the result of proper cooperation between the surgeon and anesthesiologist, the latter being prepared for a lengthy surgery. It is also important to note that pancreatic radical surgeries present a significantly high risk of septic complications. Intraoperatively, it is also mandatory to perform a complete abdominal evaluation, even in extensively investigated patients. The Kocher maneuver of the duodenum and the opening of the bursa omentalis can be necessary for exploration. Intraoperative biopsy can also be performed in suspected cases. The following organs/structures can be injured: small intestine, liver, duodenum, stomach and bile ducts. Such injuries increase the risk of bile leakage, peritonitis and septic shock.

Hemorrhages are the result of vascular injuries, the most commonly damaged vessels being the branches of the portal vein, superior mesenteric artery, splenic vein and artery, and middle colic artery. Ischemia of the transverse colon can be detected during hemostasis and demands segmental colectomy [1, 7].

Postoperative Complications

Hemorrhages can occur as following pancreaticogastrostomy a result of dehiscence of vein ligation, spread of pancreatic necrosis through the vascular wall, or hemorrhage of the pancreatic stump (and can be accompanied by hematemesis).

Pancreatic fistulae are the result of suture dehiscence of the pancreatic stump and can heal spontaneously using sandostatin. Biliary fistulae are caused by the necrosis or insufficient anastomosis of CBD and demand reintervention. Gastrojejunal fistulae are rare, being caused by anastomotic insufficiency. The severe consequences of fistulae are peritonitis and septic shock.

In patients with a thin CBD, choledochojejunostomy is difficult to perform. For proper anastomosis, slowly absorbable monofilament, 4/0 or 6/0 atraumatic sutures and Volcker's drainage are indicated.

Anastomotic suture dehiscence is usually an indicator of the insufficiency of pancreatic anastomosis, as a result of segmental necrosis of the pancreatic stump and postoperative pancreatitis or necrosis.

Postoperative ileus is rare, being caused by expanded preparation during surgery, perivisceritis, septic processes or adhesions around a drainage tube that is kept in for too long.

Other postoperative complications include angiocholitis (caused by the reflux of intestinal contents into the biliary tracts, commonly after choledochojejunostomy) and necrosis of the pancreatic stump (caused by damage to the pancreatic tissue or ducts during preparation or suturing) [1, 7].

CONFLICT OF INTEREST

The authors confirm that this chapter content has no conflict of interest.

ACKNOWLEDGEMENTS

Declared none.

REFERENCES

[1] Olah A, Gaal C. Errors and complications in abdominal surgery. Medicina, Budapest: Hungary 2006.

[2] Rossetti G, Fei L, del Genio G, *et al.* Epiphrenic diverticula mini-invasive surgery: a challenge for expert surgeons personal experience and review of the literature. Scand J Surg 2013; 102(2): 129-35. [http://dx.doi.org/10.1177/1457496913482242] [PMID: 23820690]

[3] Tedesco P, Fisichella PM, Way LW, Patti MG. Cause and treatment of epiphrenic diverticula. Am J Surg 2005; 190(6): 891-4. [http://dx.doi.org/10.1016/j.amjsurg.2005.08.016] [PMID: 16307941]

[4] Varghese TK Jr, Marshall B, Chang AC, Pickens A, Lau CL, Orringer MB. Surgical treatment of epiphrenic diverticula: a 30-year experience. Ann Thorac Surg 2007; 84(6): 1801-9. [http://dx.doi.org/10.1016/j.athoracsur.2007.06.057] [PMID: 18036889]

[5] Avital S, Zundel N, Szomstein S, Rosenthal R. Laparoscopic transhiatal esophagectomy for esophageal cancer. Am J Surg 2005; 190(1): 69-74. [http://dx.doi.org/10.1016/j.amjsurg.2004.12.004] [PMID: 15972176]

[6] Mackenzie DJ, Popplewell PK, Billingsley KG. Care of patients after esophagectomy. Crit Care Nurse 2004; 24(1): 16-29. [PMID: 15007889]

[7] Jung J, Ed. Patologie iatrogena. Tirgu Mures, Romania: University Press 2006.

[8] Katariya K, Harvey JC, Pina E, Beattie EJ. Complications of transhiatal esophagectomy. J Surg Oncol 1994; 57(3): 157-63. [http://dx.doi.org/10.1002/jso.2930570305] [PMID: 7967604]

[9] Bancu S. General surgery of the neck, "Petru Maior. Tirgu-Mures, Romania: University Press 2015.

[10] Alecu L, Bărbulescu M, Ursuţ B, Enciu O, Slavu I, Braga V. Occult thyroid carcinoma in our experience should we reconsider total thyroidectomy for benign thyroid pathology? Chirurgia (Bucur)

2014; 109(2): 191-7.
[PMID: 24742409]

[11] Pacini F, Schlumberger M, Dralle H, Elisei R, Smit JW, Wiersinga W. European thyroid cancer taskforce. European consensus for the management of patients with differential thyroid carcinoma of the follicular epithelium. Eur J Endocrinol 2006; 154: 787-803.
[http://dx.doi.org/10.1530/eje.1.02158] [PMID: 16728537]

[12] Asari R, Passler C, Kaczirek K, Scheuba C, Niederle B. Hypoparathyroidism after total thyroidectomy: a prospective study. Arch Surg 2008; 143(2): 132-7.
[http://dx.doi.org/10.1001/archsurg.2007.55] [PMID: 18283137]

[13] Popescu I, Ed. Tratat de Chirurgie Chirurgie Toracică. Bucuresti Romania: Academiei Romane 2008; vol IV.

[14] Carter JJ, Evans D, Shah P, Ura M. Iatrogenic tracheal rupture: bovine pericardial patch repair without flap reinforcement. Interact Cardiovasc Thorac Surg 2012; 14(4): 502-3.
[http://dx.doi.org/10.1093/icvts/ivr132] [PMID: 22228286]

[15] Ismail NA, Gordon J, Dunning J. The use of octreotide in the treatment of chylothorax following cardiothoracic surgery. Interact Cardiovasc Thorac Surg 2015; 20(6): 848-54.
[http://dx.doi.org/10.1093/icvts/ivv046] [PMID: 25784759]

[16] Sugarbaker JD, Ed. Adult chest surgery. The McGraw-Hill Companies 2009.

[17] Miyahara S, Iwasaki A. Diagnosis and treatment of hemothorax. Kyobu Geka 2015; 68(8): 650-3.
[PMID: 26197910]

[18] Royer AM, Smith JS, Miller A, Spiva M, Holcombe JM, Headrick JR. Safety of outpatient chest tube management of air leaks after pulmonary resection. Am Surg 2015; 81(8): 760-3.
[PMID: 26215236]

[19] Di Maio M, Perrone F, Deschamps C, Rocco G. A meta-analysis of the impact of bronchial stump coverage on the risk of bronchopleural fistula after pneumonectomy. Eur J Cardiothorac Surg 2015; 48(2): 196-200.
[http://dx.doi.org/10.1093/ejcts/ezu381] [PMID: 25342849]

[20] Kuhtin O, Kenanidis T, Haas V, Lampl L, Schulz T. Differential treatment strategy of pleural empyema in a post-pneumonectomy cavity. Pneumologie 2015; 69(8): 463-8.
[PMID: 26258420]

[21] Hu FB, Kou RY, Zou ZQ, *et al.* [Technical improvement of mechanical suture of bronchial stumps in pneumonectomy]. J First Mil Med Univ 2004; 24(10): 1203-4.
[PMID: 15501740]

[22] Cho EN, Haam SJ, Kim SY, Chang YS, Paik HC. Anastomotic airway complications after lung transplantation. Yonsei Med J 2015; 56(5): 1372-8.
[http://dx.doi.org/10.3349/ymj.2015.56.5.1372] [PMID: 26256982]

[23] Baz MA, Layish DT, Govert JA, *et al.* Diagnostic yield of bronchoscopies after isolated lung transplantation. Chest 1996; 110(1): 84-8.
[http://dx.doi.org/10.1378/chest.110.1.84] [PMID: 8681672]

[24] Boehler A, Estenne M. Post-transplant bronchiolitis obliterans. Eur Respir J 2003; 22(6): 1007-18.
[http://dx.doi.org/10.1183/09031936.03.00039103] [PMID: 14680094]

[25] Peghin M, Monforte V, Martin-Gomez MT, *et al.* 10 years of prophylaxis with nebulized liposomal amphotericin B and the changing epidemiology of *Aspergillus spp*. Infection in Lung Transplantation 2016; 29: 51-62.

[26] Speich R, van der Bij W. Epidemiology and management of infections after lung transplantation. Clin Infect Dis 2001; 33 (Suppl. 1): S58-65.
[http://dx.doi.org/10.1086/320906] [PMID: 11389524]

[27] Amid PK, Shulman AG, Lichtenstein IL. The Lichtenstein open tension-free mesh repair of inguinal hernias. Surg Today 1995; 25(7): 619-25. [http://dx.doi.org/10.1007/BF00311436] [PMID: 7549274]

[28] Srivastava P, Srivastava S, Sahu M. Iatrogenic bowel perforation secondary to surgical drain after cholecystectomy: a case report with review of literature. Intern J of Sur 2006; 13: 1-5.

[29] Sahu S, Bahl D, Husain M, Sachan P. Drain erosion into bowel: an unsual complication. Internet J of Surg 2007; 16: 1-5.

[30] Edward F. Complications of laparoscopic inguinal hernia repair. Prevention and Management of Laparoendoscopic Surgical Complications. J Soc Laparoend Surg , 2016 [21 February, 2016]; Available at: http://laparoscopy.blogs.com/prevention_management_3

[31] Meshikhes AW, Al-Saif OH. Iatrogenic oesophageal transection during laparoscopic sleeve gastrectomy. BMJ Case Rep 2014; 2014: bcr2013201260. [http://dx.doi.org/10.1136/bcr-2013-201260] [PMID: 24591379]

[32] Kenneth D, Cruz D, Pathak T. Nayaka. A rare complication of laparoscopic sleeve gastrectomy: Gastro-esophageal transection. IOSR-JDMS 2014; 13: 16-8. [http://dx.doi.org/10.9790/0853-131161618]

[33] Sarkhosh K, Birch DW, Sharma A, Karmali S. Complications associated with laparoscopic sleeve gastrectomy for morbid obesity: a surgeons guide. Can J Surg 2013; 56(5): 347-52. [http://dx.doi.org/10.1503/cjs.033511] [PMID: 24067520]

[34] Talebpour M, Motamedi SM, Talebpour A, Vahidi H, Vahidi H. Twelve year experience of laparoscopic gastric plication in morbid obesity: development of the technique and patient outcomes. Ann Surg Innov Res 2012; 6(1): 7. [http://dx.doi.org/10.1186/1750-1164-6-7] [PMID: 22913751]

[35] Kourkoulos M, Giorgakis E, Kokkinos C, *et al.* Laparoscopic gastric plication for the treatment of morbid obesity: a review. Minim Invasive Surg 2012; 2012: 696348. [http://dx.doi.org/10.1155/2012/696348]

[36] Gurzu S, Copotoiu C, Azamfirei L, Jung I. Caliber persistent artery (Dieulafoys lesion) which is associated with an early-stage gastric stump cancer following distal gastrectomy. J Clin Diagn Res 2013; 7(8): 1717-9. [PMID: 24086889]

[37] Gurzu S, Copotoiu C, Molnar C, Azamfirei L, Jung I. Lethal gastric hemorrhage from a caliber-persistent artery of the antrum - a branch of the right gastric artery. Hippokratia 2014; 18(2): 172-6. [PMID: 25336884]

[38] Hill AG, Fracs MD. , Management of perforated duodenal ulcer. In: Holzheimer RG, Mannick JA, Eds. Surgical treatment Evidence-based and problem-oriented. Zuckschwerdt Munich 2001.

[39] Di Saverio S, Bassi M, Smerieri N, *et al.* Diagnosis and treatment of perforated or bleeding peptic ulcers: 2013 WSES position paper. World J Emerg Surg 2014; 9: 45. [http://dx.doi.org/10.1186/1749-7922-9-45] [PMID: 25114715]

[40] Bara T Jr, Gurzu S, Jung I, Muresan M, Szederjesi J, Bara T. Giant cavernous hepatic hemangioma diagnosed incidentally in a perimenopausal obese female with endometrial adenocarcinoma: A case report. Anticancer Res 2016; 36(2): 769-72. [PMID: 26851037]

[41] Suciu BA, Gurzu S, Marginean L, *et al.* Significant shrinkage of multifocal liver metastases and long-term survival in a patient with rectal cancer, after trans-arterial chemoembolization (TACE). Medicine (Baltimore) 2015; 94: e1848.

[42] Japanese gastric cancer treatment guidelines 2010 (ver. 3). Gastric Cancer 2011; 14(2): 113-23. [http://dx.doi.org/10.1007/s10120-011-0042-4] [PMID: 21573742]

[43] Japanese classification of gastric carcinoma: 3rd English ed. Gastric Cancer 2011; 14(2): 101-12. [http://dx.doi.org/10.1007/s10120-011-0041-5] [PMID: 21573743]

[44] Yada T, Yokoi C, Uemura N. The current state of diagnosis and treatment for early gastric cancer. Diagn Ther Endosc 2013; 2013: 241320. [http://dx.doi.org/10.1155/2013/241320]

[45] Gurzu S, Jung I, Kadar Z. Aberrant metastatic behavior and particular features of early gastric cancer. APMIS 2015; 123(12): 999-1006. [http://dx.doi.org/10.1111/apm.12469] [PMID: 26547366]

[46] Gurzu S, Bara T, Bara T Jr, Jung I. Metaplastic bone formation in the abdominal wallan incidental finding in a patient with gastric cancer. Case report and hypothesis about its histogenesis. Am J Dermatopathol 2013; 35(8): 844-6. [http://dx.doi.org/10.1097/DAD.0b013e318285db5c] [PMID: 24257191]

[47] Philip HG, Santhat N. Principles and practice of surgery for the colon, rectum, and anus. 3rd ed., Informa Healthcare 2007.

[48] Carol EH. Scott-Conner Chassin's Operative Strategy in Colon and Rectal Surgery. Springer 2006.

[49] Ushigome T, Kawahara H, Watanabe K, Yanagisawa S, Kobayashi S, Yanaga K. Colorectal anastomosis using retroperitoneal window after wide colorectal resection. Hepatogastroenterology 2011; 58(112): 1983-4. [http://dx.doi.org/10.5754/hge11273] [PMID: 22024065]

[50] Manterola C, Fernández O, Muñoz S, *et al.* Laparoscopic pericystectomy for liver hydatid cysts. Surg Endosc 2002; 16(3): 521-4. [http://dx.doi.org/10.1007/s00464-001-8125-7] [PMID: 11928040]

[51] Bara T, Bancu S, Gyorgy-Fazakas I, *et al.* Two-step hepatectomy with right portal branch ligature for a right lobe metastasis. Hepatogastroenterology 2008; 55(84): 1071-2. [PMID: 18705330]

[52] Khan AZ, Smith AM, Irving GR, Cameron I, Dehn T. Portal vein resection during pancreaticoduodenectomy for cancer. Ann R Coll Surg Engl 2009; 91(2): 95-9. [http://dx.doi.org/10.1308/rcsann.2009.91.2.95] [PMID: 19317932]

[53] Hackert T, Büchler MW, Werner J. Current state of surgical management of pancreatic cancer. Cancers (Basel) 2011; 3(1): 1253-73. [http://dx.doi.org/10.3390/cancers3011253] [PMID: 24212660]

[54] Torres OJ, Moraes-Junior JM, Fernandes EdeS. [Distal pancreatectomy with en-bloc celiac trunk resection for locally advanced pancreatic body cancer (Appleby procedure): case report]. Arq Bras Cir Dig 2013; 26(2): 151-3. [http://dx.doi.org/10.1590/S0102-67202013000200018] [PMID: 24000032]

CHAPTER 18

Iatrogenic Lesions in Obstetrics and Gynecology

Bela Szabo*

Department of Gynecology, University of Medicine and Pharmacy, Tirgu-Mures, Romania

Abstract: Gynecological surgery is associated with general risks that also occur in general surgery, but specific lesions are frequently encountered. For example, due to the fact that the genital organs are closely related to the organs of the urinary tract, they can easily be injured. These injuries primarily include lesions of the urinary bladder and ureters, but intestinal and nerve damage can also occur. Regarding drugs, dose- and time-dependent effects are controversial. These effects include thromboembolic complications, myocardial infarction, cerebrovascular accidents and even the carcinogenic risk of development of an endometrium or breast cancer.

Keywords: Cancer, Drugs, Gynecological surgery, Gynecology, Hormonal therapy, Intestinal lesions, Menopause, Nerve lesions, Side effects, Urinary tract lesions.

COMPLICATIONS OF SURGICAL INTERVENTIONS

In addition to the risks of general surgery, gynecological surgery has some specific characteristics and risks.

Lesions of the Urinary Tract

Due to the fact that the genital organs are closely related to the urinary tract, the urinary bladder is especially vulnerable to injury during gynecological surgery. It can be damaged in the process of opening the peritoneal cavity if the lower angle of the medial subumbilical incision is adherences between the bladder and the anterior abdominal wall can also cause its injury. The bladder can also be injured during total hysterectomy, as it is necessary to push the bladder down when performing this surgery. Another risk factor is preoperative radiotherapy for pelvic tumors. Although rare, surgical treatment of genital prolapse can also be associated with bladder injuries. These lesions should be sutured during surgical intervention, although minor lesions can heal spontaneously. Undetected lesions can cause uroperitoneum, peritonitis or vesico-vaginal fistulae. In some cases,

* **Corresponding author Bela Szabo:** Department of Gynecology, University of Medicine and Pharmacy, Tirgu-Mures, Romania; Tel: 0040-265-212111; Fax: 0040-372-653250; E-mail: szabobela2006@yahoo.com

Simona Gurzu & Ioan Jung (Eds.)

nonabsorbable suture material can accidentally be passed through the bladder wall and the urothelium during hysterectomy. This can act as a nucleus for the formation of foreign body granulomas or urinary sectioned too close to the symphysis. In patients with previous surgical interventions (*e.g.,* cesarean section), calculi [1].

Lesions of the ureter are not so common but more serious complications. Based on a large body of data, it has been proven that at least one ureter is damaged in every 200 hysterectomies. Moreover, 50% of all iatrogenic ureter injuries occur during gynecological surgery, especially the surgery of cervical cancer (Wertheim's hysterectomy). Minor lesions can go unidentified during surgery and are associated with postoperative complications, such as macroscopic hematuria, ureterovaginal fistulae or urinary leak through the wound during micturition. Postoperative treatment of ureteric lesions is usually performed by urologists [2 - 4].

Intestinal Lesions

These lesions primarily occur during the opening of the peritoneal cavity, being caused by the presence of adhesions between the intestines and anterior abdominal wall in patients with previous laparotomies. They can also occur during laparoscopic interventions, especially during insertion of the trocars. Large bowel injuries are severe complications of laparoscopic surgery that are reported in 0.62-1.6/1000 laparoscopy cases. The treatment involves simple suture or segmental resection of the bowel in large lesions or perforations. Rectal lesions can occur during delivery (expulsion of the presenting part) or during the postpartum period (repair of perineal tears) [5, 6].

Nerve Injuries

These injuries occur in 1.1-1.9% of patients undergoing gynecological interventions. The main causes are malpositioning of the patient, incorrect placement of self-retaining retractors, hematoma formation, direct nerve entrapment and nerve transaction.

Although it is more aesthetic, the transverse Pfannenstiel laparotomy is associated with a greater risk of nerve lesions than median incision. The abdominal wall can potentially lose tone and become flaccid. Damage to the obturator nerve can occur during radical surgery, usually without significant consequences. Lesions of the genitofemoral nerve or ilioinguinal nerve can cause paresthesia of the vulva and inner thighs.

During vaginal surgery, the lower limbs of the patient are immobilized and the knee joints lean on metallic supports. In prolonged interventions or prolonged compression (*e.g.,* if the assistant leans on the knee of the patient), paralysis of the peroneus nerve can arise [7, 8].

ADVERSE DRUG REACTIONS IN OBSTETRICS AND GYNECOLOGY

In gynecological practice, hormonal treatment represents the most common prolonged treatment, with controversy regarding the risk-benefit ratio. Further details regarding these drugs are presented in Chapter 10.

Oral Contraceptives include estrogen and a progestin derivative. The estrogen component is ethynyl estradiol, but many progestin derivatives are available, involving several side effects, especially virilization. The side effects of contraceptive pills especially relate to their procoagulant properties. Thromboembolic complications are caused by the estrogenic component and emerge in 80/100,000 females taking a daily dose of ethynyl estradiol below five micrograms. At higher doses, this risk increases to about 112/100,000. The risk of myocardial or brain infarction is twice as high as that of nonusers, and even higher again in smokers. Considering these risks, there is a constant struggle to reduce the hormonal doses in contraceptive pills, the monthly dose being today lower than the daily dose used at the beginning of the 1960s [9, 10].

Hormone Replacement Therapy in Menopausal Females aims to abolish estrogen deficiency and prevent osteoporosis. However, this replacement is controversial. Monotherapy with estrogens proved to have a carcinogenic effect on the endometrium and breast. As a result, progestin components (with supposed protective effect on breast cancer) were added to these medications for some time. Nevertheless, some patients later developed breast cancer and the idea was abandoned. Moreover, synthetic progestins seem to stimulate secretions activity in rat endometrium and increase estrogens synthesis in the breast. In large multicentric trials, it has been shown that 41 of 10,000 women who used combined hormone replacement therapy in menopause presented noticeable time-dependent complications (eight with invasive breast cancer, seven with myocardial infarction, eight with pulmonary embolism, eight with brain infarction and 10 with peripheral vascular thrombosis). Considering the above-mentioned risks, initiation of hormone replacement therapy should be subject to a risk-benefit analys is [11, 12].

CONFLICT OF INTEREST

The authors confirm that this chapter content has no conflict of interest.

ACKNOWLEDGEMENTS

Declared none.

REFERENCES

[1] Vakili B, Chesson RR, Kyle BL, *et al.* The incidence of urinary tract injury during hysterectomy: a prospective analysis based on universal cystoscopy. Am J Obstet Gynecol 2005; 192: 1599-604. [http://dx.doi.org/10.1016/j.ajog.2004.11.016]

[2] Neuman M, Eidelman M, Eidelman A, *et al.* Iatrogenic injuries to the ureter during gynecological and obstetric operations. Surg Gynecol Obstet 1991; 173: 268-71.

[3] Higgins CC. Ureteral injuries during surgery a rewiew of 87 cases. JAMA 1967; 199: 82-8. [http://dx.doi.org/10.1001/jama.1967.03120020076013]

[4] Selzman AA, Spirnak JP. Iatrogenic ureteral injuries: A 20-year experience in treating 165 injuries. J Urol 1996; 155: 878-81. [http://dx.doi.org/10.1016/S0022-5347(01)66332-8]

[5] Sabharwal M. Large bowel injury during total laparoscopic hysterectomy. J Gynecol Endosc Surg 2009; 1: 57-8. [http://dx.doi.org/10.4103/0974-1216.51911]

[6] Vergers-Spooren HC, de Leeuw JW. A rare complication of a vaginal breech delivery. Case Rep Obstet Gynecol 2011; 2011: 306124. [http://dx.doi.org/10.1155/2011/306124]

[7] Bohrer JC, Walters MD, Park A, Polston D, Barber MD. Pelvic nerve injury following gynecologic surgery: a prospective cohort study. Am J Obstet Gynecol 2009; 201: 531.e1-7. [http://dx.doi.org/10.1016/j.ajog.2009.07.023]

[8] Kuponiyi O, Alleemudder DI, Latunde-Dada A, Eedarapalli P. Nerve injuries associated with gynaecological surgery. TOG 2014; 16: 29-36. [http://dx.doi.org/10.1111/tog.12064]

[9] Hormonal contraception: recent advances and controversies. Fertil Steril 2008; 90: S103-13. [http://dx.doi.org/10.1016/j.fertnstert.2008.08.093]

[10] Gerstman BB, Piper JM, Tomita DK, Ferguson WJ, Stadel BV, Lundin FE. Oral contraceptive estrogen dose and the risk of deep venous thromboembolic disease. Am J Epidemiol 1991; 133: 32-7. [http://dx.doi.org/10.1093/oxfordjournals.aje.a115799]

[11] Rossouw JE, Anderson GL, Prentice RL, *et al.* Risks and benefits of estrogen plus progestin in healthy postmenopausal womenprincipal results from the women's health initiative randomized controlled trial. JAMA 2002; 288: 321-33. [http://dx.doi.org/10.1001/jama.288.3.321]

[12] Beral V. Breast cancer and hormone replacement therapy in the Million Women Study. Lancet 2003; 362: 419-27. [http://dx.doi.org/10.1016/S0140-6736(03)14596-5]

CHAPTER 19

Iatrogenic Lesions in Neurosurgery

Alexandru Madaras and **Nicolae Dorin Gherasim***

Department of Neurosurgery, Clinical County Emergency Hospital, Tirgu-Mures, Romania

Abstract: Complications in neurosurgery can occur during diagnostic procedures, such as lumbar puncture, lumbar drainage, suboccipital cisternal tap or cerebral/spinal angiography, or during neurosurgical procedures. Severe complications during or subsequent to lumbar puncture are extremely rare and include brainstem herniation, infection, subdural hematoma and subarachnoid hemorrhage. Insertion of a catheter into the lumbar subarachnoid space to drain the cerebrospinal fluid (CSF) can also be followed by infection or overdrainage. The complications of cisternal tap include hemorrhage in the cisterna magna and piercing of the medulla oblongata that can cause cardiac or respiratory arrest. The iodine-based contrast agents used for cerebral angiography can cause allergic reactions and epileptic seizures. Iatrogenic complications during surgical procedures can occur at any stage pre-, intra- or immediately postoperative. Complications occur during patient positioning, rendering this step of paramount importance to the success of surgery. Infectious and cosmetic complications can occur during skin disinfection, incision of the skin of the scalp and surgical incision of the skull. Dural lesions can lead to cerebrospinal fluid leak or fistulae. Corticotomy or corticectomy should be realized cautiously and external to functional areas. Ligation or coagulation of brain vessels can lead to cerebral infarction (arterial or venous) with loss of cerebral function. Iatrogenic lesions in different regions of the brain lead to specific neurological manifestations. Lesions in the anterior fossa can lead to anosmia, abulia or behavioral alterations. Lesions in the middle fossa can lead to aphasia and motor deficits, while lesion in the posterior fossa can lead to cranial nerve deficits or coma.

Keywords: Anosmia, Aphasia, Brachial Paresis, Brain swelling, Brainstem herniation, Cerebrospinal fluid fistula, Chemical external otitis, Corticotomy, Duraplasty, Hearing loss, Ischemic stroke, Lumbar puncture, Meningitis, Osteonecrosis, Skull deformities, Thalamic infarction, Tonsillar herniation, Venous air embolism, Venous infarction, Ventriculitis.

* **Corresponding author Nicolae Dorin Gherasim:** Department of Neurosurgery, Clinical County Emergency Hospital, Tirgu-Mures, Romania; Tel/Fax: 0040-726-292627; E-mail: dorin.gherasim@gmail.com

Simona Gurzu & Ioan Jung (Eds.)

IATROGENIC LESIONS DURING DIAGNOSTIC PROCEDURES

Lumbar Puncture

In adults, the conus medullaris is located rostral to the termination of the thecal sac, being situated at the level of the L1-L2 vertebral bodies in the majority of cases. High (T12-L1) or low (L2-L3) variants of the conus medullaris are also encountered. A safe lumbar puncture should be realized at the level of the intercristal line (L4-L5). Following puncture, the overall risk of disabling or persistent symptoms is 0.1-0.5% only [1]. Severe complications are extremely rare and include brainstem herniation, infection, subdural hematoma and subarachnoid hemorrhage [2]. Tonsillar herniation can be acute, as in the case of an intracranial mass or a chronic lesion. Chronic herniation, also called acquired Chiari I malformation, is especially commonly reported following multiple traumatic lumbar punctures. Other possible complications are the following: infection (*e.g.*, spinal meningitis), spinal headache (usually positional), spinal epidural hematoma (usually associated with coagulopathy), spinal epidural collection of the cerebrospinal fluid (CSF), transplantation of the epidermal tissue *via* the needle with further development of a tumor, nerve root lesion by the needle (which can cause transient radicular pain), intracranial subdural hematoma or hygroma and sudden hearing loss. The latter may occur due to the drop in perilymph pressure through the cochlear aqueduct [1 - 3].

Lumbar Drainage

Insertion of a catheter into the lumbar subarachnoid space for the purpose of draining the CSF can be followed by: infection, overdrainage (if the drainage bag is situated too low), disconnection of the catheter and pneumocephalus. The latter can occur if the drainage occurs below the site of the CSF fistula and the air can be drawn through the fistula tract.

Cisternal Tap

This is an invasive procedure performed to achieve suboccipital access to the cisterna magna. It is usually realized with the patient in a sitting position with their neck flexed. The distance from the skin surface to the cisterna magna is about 4-6 cm, and from the dura to the medulla is 2.5 cm. Due to the tenting of the dura, the needle may infrequently touch the medulla. Peri-invasive complications include hemorrhage in the cisterna magna (due to perforation of a large vessel) and piercing of the medulla oblongata, which can cause cardiac or respiratory arrest [4].

Cerebral Angiography

This represents the gold standard in the diagnosis of cerebral vascular malformations (brain aneurysms, arteriovenous malformations, dural fistulae, *etc.*). Before Seldinger's technique was developed, cerebral angiography was realized through a direct carotid tap, meaning that bleeding to the puncture site could lead to a local compressive hematoma and respiratory distress. With Seldinger's technique, the usual puncture site is the femoral artery. Traumatic tap at this site can cause local hematoma that can extend into the retroperitoneal space. Transient femoral nerve injuries may also occur. The iodine-based contrast agents used for cerebral angiography can cause allergic reactions and epileptic seizures [5].

IATROGENIC COMPLICATIONS DURING SURGICAL PROCEDURES

Patient Position-Related Complications

Patient positioning is a key step during any surgical procedure and significant time must be spent to ensure that the position is as comfortable as possible for the patient, while offering, at the same time, the best approach for the surgeon. The sitting position for posterior fossa approaches can lead to venous air embolism, the mechanism of which involves perioperative negative pressure in the venous system of the head. Meticulous hemostasis, even for small bleedings, is mandatory [6]. The park bench position for cerebellopontine angle tumors can lead to brachial plexus elongation, while the lateral position can lead to contralateral axillary compression and brachial paresis. Head positioning is also of paramount importance. Forced rotation and flexion of the head can lead to impaired venous drainage, brain swelling and, in extreme situations, cervical luxation.

Lesions of the Skin and Scalp

During *skin disinfection*, surgical antiseptics can induce chemical conjunctivitis (if they reach the eye) or chemical external otitis (if they reach the ear). In cases of contact of the tympanum with iodine-based antiseptics, hearing impairment can arise.

Incision of the skin of the scalp should be performed behind the hairline in order to prevent unaesthetic scaring. Arcuate incisions of the scalp should have a fairly large pedicle in order to prevent scalp necrosis. In scalp lacerations, excision of the skin should be realized in a controlled manner in order to prevent skin defects. Tight suture of the skin can lead to scalp necrosis.

Surgical incision of the skull can also be followed by specific consequences. Craniotomy represents an important step of the surgical approach and should be carefully performed. If the bone is thin or infiltrated by tumor, the drill could pierce inside the skull and produce dural or brain injury. In depressed skull fractures, removal of bone fragments embedded in the dural sinuses can lead to life-threatening hemorrhage [7]. After surgery, improper bone repositioning can induce bone defects and unaesthetic skull deformities. Devascularized bone leads to osteonecrosis.

Dural Lesions

Before cutting the dura, the surgeon should always perform dural suspension on the overlying bone in order to prevent extradural hematoma formation. During dural suspension, special attention should be paid to the underlying subarachnoid vessels. Dural incision should be as thin and delicate as possible, using 11 or 15 blade scalpels and microscissors.

Duraplasty with bovine dura mater can lead to Creutzfeldt-Jakob disease. Inadequate dural manipulation or coagulation during tumor removal along the skull base can lead to CSF leakage. Tight dural closure is necessary in order to prevent CSF fistulae. Superior sagittal sinus ligature can be followed by venous infarction, especially in patients with ligature realized in the middle or posterior third [8].

Cerebral Lesions

Incision of the cerebral cortex is an extremely delicate procedure and must be carefully weighted. The corticotomy/corticectomy must be realized in as minimally invasive a manner as possible and externally to functional areas.

Vascular Lesions

Open lesions of the large arteries, such as the internal carotid artery or venous sinuses (superior sagittal sinus, transverse sinus, sigmoid sinus), can lead to catastrophic/fatal bleeding. Ligation or coagulation of brain vessels can lead to cerebral infarction (arterial or venous) with loss of cerebral function.

Iatrogenic Lesions Depending on the Location of Surgery

Anterior cranial fossa – inadequate manipulation of the frontal lobe, during a subfrontal approach, can lead to olfactory nerve injuries and consecutive anosmia.

Sella turcica – this represents an important anatomical landmark, with vital nervous and vascular structures in and around the sella turcica. Manipulation and/or damage to the pituitary stalk can lead to diabetes insipidus [9]. Opening of the cavernous sinuses can lead to severe bleeding and paresis of the oculomotor nerves (III, IV and VI). Manipulation of the optic nerves and chiasm can lead to loss of vision. Any injury to the internal carotid artery can lead to catastrophic bleeding or extensive cerebral infarction.

Middle cranial fossa – inadequate manipulation of the frontal and temporal lobes on the dominant hemisphere can lead to aphasia. In subtemporal approaches, care should be taken regarding the vein of Labbe, as its perforation can lead to significant vein infarction and brain swelling. Occlusion of the posterior communicating artery or anterior choroidal artery during aneurysm surgery leads to thalamic infarction.

Posterior cranial fossa – when removing the vestibular schwannomas through a cerebellopontine angle approach, injury to the cranial nerves can lead to facial paresis, hearing loss or swallowing difficulties. When approaching vestibular schwannomas through a translabyrinthine approach, transotic CSF fistulae can occur [8]. Injury to the rhomboid fossa on the fourth ventricle floor can cause brainstem infarction or facial paresis. Opening of a posterior fossa with increased intracranial pressure can lead to cerebellum herniation and infarction.

CAUSES OF IATROGENIC LESIONS

These causes can be defined by three phrases: "iatrogenic lesions are always realized by others"; "a surgeon's imagination is too weak to explore the diversity of iatrogenic complications that might occur"; and "the majority of iatrogenic lesions can be avoided and, if promptly recognized, safely treated".

CONFLICT OF INTEREST

The authors confirm that this chapter content has no conflict of interest.

ACKNOWLEDGEMENTS

Declared none.

REFERENCES

[1] Wiesel J, Rose DN, Silver AL, *et al.* Lumbar puncture in asymptomatic late syphilis. An analysis of the benefits and risks. Arch Intern Med 1985; 145: 465-8. [http://dx.doi.org/10.1001/archinte.1985.00360030105020]

[2] Fishman RA. Cerebrospinal fluid in diseases of the nervous system. Philadelphia: W. B. Saunders 1992.

[3] Sathi S, Stieg PE. Acquired Chiari I malformation after multiple lumbar punctures: case report. Neurosurgery 1993; 32: 306-9. [http://dx.doi.org/10.1227/00006123-199302000-00023]

[4] Ward E, Orrison WW, Watridge CB. Anatomic evaluation of cisternal puncture. Neurosurgery 1989; 25: 412-5.
[http://dx.doi.org/10.1227/00006123-198909000-00015]

[5] Earnest F, Forbes G, Sandok BA, *et al.* Complications of cerebral angiography: prospective assessment of risk. AJR 1984; 142: 247-53.
[http://dx.doi.org/10.2214/ajr.142.2.247]

[6] Standefer MS, Bay JW, Trusso R. The sitting position in neurosurgery. Neurosurgery 1984; 14: 649-58.
[http://dx.doi.org/10.1227/00006123-198406000-00001]

[7] Quinones-Hinojosa A. Schmidek and Sweet: Operative neurosurgical techniques: indications, methods and results. 6th ed., Saunders 2012.

[8] Greenberg MS. Handbook of neurosurgery. 7th ed., Thieme 2010.

[9] Verbalis JG, Robinson AG, Moses AM. Postoperative and posttraumatic diabetes insipidus. Front Horm Res 1985; 13: 247-65.
[http://dx.doi.org/10.1159/000410111]

SUBJECT INDEX

A

D

E

F

G

H

I

N

O

P

Q

R

S

T

U

V

W

Y

Made in United States
North Haven, CT
04 November 2026

21727464R00197